Proceedings in Life Sciences

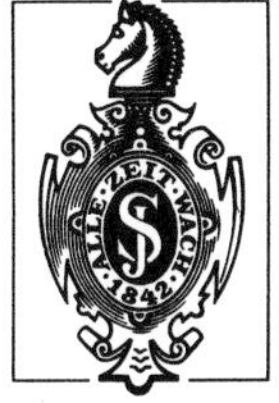

Environmental Endocrinology

Proceedings of an International Symposium
Held in Montpellier (France), 11-15 July 1977

Edited by
Ivan Assenmacher
Donald S. Farner

With 97 Figures

Springer-Verlag
Berlin Heidelberg New York 1978

IVAN ASSENMACHER, MD, DSc
Professor of Physiology, University of Montpellier, France

DONALD S. FARNER, PhD, DSc
Professor of Zoology, University of Washington, Seattle, USA

ISBN 3-540-08809-1 Springer-Verlag Berlin Heidelberg New York
ISBN 0-387-08809-1 Springer-Verlag Berlin Heidelberg New York

Library of Congress Cataloging in Publication Data. Main entry under title: Environmental endocrinology. (Proceedings in life sciences). "A satellite symposium of the 27th International Congress of Physiological Sciences, Paris, 18—23 July 1977." Bibliography: p. Includes index. Y. Endocrinology—Congresses. 2. Adaptation (Physiology)—Congresses. 3. Biological rhythms—Congresses I. Assenmacher, Ivan, 1927— II. Farner, Donald Sankey, 1915— QP187.E696 591.1'42 78-18840

Offset printing and bookbinding by Brühlsche Universitätsdruckerei, Lahn-Gießen

2131/3130-S43210

Preface

From 11 to 15 July 1977 about 60 physiologists, endocrinologists, ecologists and other biologists from 14 countries convened at the University Montpellier for a symposium on Environmental Endocrinology. This meeting was organized as a Satellite Symposium of the 27th International Congress of Physiological Sciences, Paris, 18-23 July 1977. This volume is a record of the communications presented at the symposium. The objectives of the program were to examine the role of the endocrine system in a wide spectrum of adjustments and adaptations to changes in environmental conditions by various species of animals, including man, and to promote an exchange of ideas among investigators who have approached these functions from diverse aspects. The diversity of the information and ideas communicated is great. Of necessity, they represent only an extremely modest selection of the many facets of endocrine function in the interaction of animals with their environments. Beyond the usefulness of the communications individually, we hope that they collectively demonstrate the substantial heuristic value of the concept of environmental endocrinology as it was perceived by the participants.

We acknowledge gratefully the kindness and sympathy of Professor Jaques ROUZAUD, President of the University of Montpellier II, for his generous extension of the hospitality of the University to the Symposium.

We are most grateful to Mrs. Monique VIEU who effected so well the secretarial organization of the Symposium, and to the staff members and technicians of the Department of Physiology who handled the diverse technical preparations so effectively.

We also acknowledge the support of the Division of Zoology of the International Union of Biological Sciences in the organization of the Symposium and in the preparation of the proceedings.

Montpellier and Seattle
October 1977

IVAN ASSENMACHER
DONALD S. FARNER

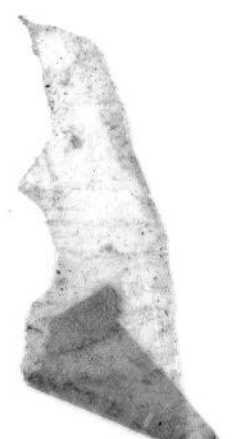

Contents

List of Participants and Contributors

ASCHOFF, J., Max Planck Institut für Verhaltensphysiologie, 8131 Erling Andechs / Fed. Rep. Germany

ASSENMACHER, I., Dept. Physiology, Univ. of Montpellier II, 34060 Montpellier /France

BERTHIER, J.L., Dept. Zoology, Museum National d'Histoire Naturelle, 75005 Paris / France

BOISSIN, J., Centre d'Etudes Biologiques des Animaux Sauvages, CNRS, Chizé, 79360 Beauvoir sur Niort / France

BRADSHAW, D., Dept. Zoology, Univ. of Western-Australia, Nedlands, Western Australia 6009 / Australia

BRANDENBERGER, G., Centre d'Etudes Bioclimatiques, CNRS, 67087 Strasbourg / France

BRIAUD, B., Dept. Physiology, Fac. of Sciences, Univ. of Strasbourg, 67000 Strasbourg / France

BROTMAN, J., Dept. Physiology-Anatomy, Univ. of California, Berkeley, California 94720 / USA

CAMPBELL, C.S., Dept. Biological Sciences, Northwestern Univ., Evanston, Illinois 60201 / USA

CAMPBELL, G.A., Dept. Physiology, Neuroendocrine Res. Lab., Michigan State Univ., East-Lansing, Michigan 48824 / USA

CHANDOLA, A., Dept. Zoology, Banaras Hindu Univ., Varanasi 221005 / India

CHENITI, T., Dept. Animal Physiology, Fac. of Sciences, Univ. of Tunis, Tunis / Tunisia

CIMINO, J., Dept. Physiology-Anatomy, Univ. of California, Berkeley, California 94720 / USA

CLEMENTI, G., Dept. Pharmacology, Univ. of Catania, Medical School, 95125 Catania / Italy

COLLINS, K.J., MRC Environmental Physiology Unit, London School of Hygiene & Tropical Medicine, London WC1 7HT / United Kingdom

DALLMAN, M.F., Dept. Physiology, School of Medicine, Univ. of California, San Francisco, California 94143 / USA

DE WILDE, J., Dept. Entomology, Agricultural Univ., 6700 EH-Wageningen / The Netherlands

EDHOLM, O.G., Chairman Commission Environmental Physiology IUPS, School of Environmental Studies, Wates House, Univ. College of London WC1H OQB / United Kingdom

EVANS, D.H., Dept. Biology, Univ. of Miami, Coral Gables, Florida 33124 / USA

FARNER, D.S., Dept. Zoology, Univ. of Washington, Seattle, Washington 98195 / USA

FAVINO, A., Istituto di Medicina del Lavoro, Univ. of Pavia, 27100 Pavia / Italy

FINKELSTEIN, J.S., Dept. Biological Sciences, Northwestern Univ., Evanston, Illinois 60201 / USA

FIORE, L., Dept. Pharmacology, Univ. of Catania, Medical School, 95125 Catania / Italy

FLETCHER, W.H., Dept. Anatomy, Duke Univ. Medical Center, Durham, North Carolina 27710 / USA

FOLLENIUS, M., Centre d'Etudes Bioclimatiques, CNRS, 67087 Strasbourg / France

GALLI-GALLARDO, S.M., Dept. Pharmacology, Columbia Univ. College of Physicians and Surgeons, New York, N. Y. 10032 / USA

GERENDAI, I., Dept. Pharmacology, Univ. of Catania, Medical School, 95125 Catania / Italy

GOGAN, F., Unité de Neurobiologie, U 109, Centre Paul-Broca INSERM, 75014 Paris / France

HEDE, K.E., Zoolophysiological Lab. A, August Krogh Institute, Univ. of Copenhagen, 2100 Copenhagen / Denmark

HERBERT, J., Dept. Anatomy, Univ. of Cambridge, Cambridge, CB2 3DY / United Kingdom

HERY, M., Unité de Neurobiologie, U 109, Centre Paul-Broca, INSERM, 75014 Paris / France

HOFFMANN, K., Max Planck Institut für Verhaltensphysiologie, 8131 Erling Andechs / Fed. Rep. Germany

HOLMES, W.N., Dept. Zoology, Univ. of California, Santa-Barbara, California 93106 / USA

HONTELA, A., Dept. Zoology, Univ. of Alberta, Edmonton T6G 2E9 / Canada

JALLAGEAS, M., Dept. Physiology, Univ. of Montpellier II, 34060 Montpellier / France

JOHANSSON, W., Heart Section, General Hospital, 21401 Malmö / Sweden

JØRGENSEN, C.B., Zoophysiological Lab. A, August Krogh Institute, Univ. of Copenhagen, 2100 Copenhagen / Denmark

KALRA, P.S., Dept. Obstetrics-Gynecology, Univ. of Florida, College of Medicine, Gainesville, Florida 32610 / USA

KALRA, S.P., Dept. Obstetrics-Gynecology, Univ. of Florida, College of Medicine, Gainesville, Florida 32610 / USA

KAWAKAMI, M.: Dept. Physiology, Yokohama City Univ., School of Medicine, Yokohama 232 / Japan

KLINOWSKA, M., Dept. Anatomy, Univ. of Cambridge, Cambridge CB2 3DY / United Kingdom

KOCH, B., Dept. Physiology, Fac. of Sciences, Univ. of Strasbourg, 67000 Strasbourg / France

KORDON, C., Unité de Neurobiologie, U 109, Centre Paul-Broca, INSERM, 75014 Paris / France

KUMAHARA, Y., Dept. Medicine-Geriatrics, Osaka Univ. School of Medicine, Osaka 553 / Japan

LACHIVER, F., Dept. General and Comparative Physiology, Museum National d'Histoire Naturelle, 75005 Paris / France

LAGOGUEY, M., Human Chronobiology Res. Unit, Dept. Physiology, Fondation A. de Rothschild, 75019 Paris / France

LARSEN, L.O., Zoophysiological Lab A, August Krogh Institute, Univ. of Copenhagen, 2100 Copenhagen / Denmark

LEATHEM, J.H., Dept. Zoology, Rutgers State Univ. of New Jersey, Nelson Biological Labs, Piscataway, New Jersey 08854 / USA

LOFTS, B., Dept. Zoology, Univ. of Hong Kong / Hong Kong

MACFARLANE, W.V., Dept. Animal Physiology, Univ. of Adelaide, Waite Agricultural Research Institute, Glen Osmond, South Australia 5064 / Australia

MARCHETTI, B., Dept. Pharmacology, Univ. of Catania, Medical School, 95125 Catania / Italy

MATSUSHIMA, M., 2nd Dept. Physiology, Yokohama City Univ., School of Medicine, Yokohama / Japan

MAUGET, R., Centre d'Etudes Biologiques des Animaux Sauvages CNRS, Chizé, 79360 Beauvoir sur Niort / France

MAUREL, D., Centre d'Etudes Biologiques des Animaux Sauvages CNRS, Chizé, 79360 Beauvoir sur Niort / France

METZ, B., Centre d'Etudes Bioclimatiques, CNRS, 67087 Strasbourg / France

MIALHE, C., Dept. Physiology, Fac. of Sciences, Univ. of Strasbourg, 67000 Strasbourg / France

NELSON, M., Dept. Anatomy and Reproductive Biology, Univ. of Hawaii, Honolulu, Hawaii 96822 / USA

NOUGUIER-SOULÉ, J., Dept. Physiology, Univ. of Montpellier II, 34060 Montpellier / France

OKADA, Y., Dept. Medicine-Geriatry, Osaka Univ. School of Medicine, Osaka 553 / Japan

ORTAVANT, R., Dept. Animal Physiology, INRA, Nouzilly, 37380 Monnaie / France

PANG, P.K.T., Dept. Pharmacology, Columbia Univ. College of Physicians and Surgeons, New York, N.Y. 10032 / USA

PELLETIER, J., Dept. Animal Physiology, INRA, Nouzilly, 37380 Monnaie / France

PETER, R., Dept. Zoology, Univ. of Alberta, Edmonton T6G 2E9 / Canada

PETTER, F., Dept. Zoology, Museum National d'Histoire Naturelle, 75005 Paris / France

PRATO, A., Dept. Pharmacology, Univ. of Catania Medical School, 95125 Catania / Italy

QUABBE, H.J., Dept. Endocrinology, Klinikum Steglitz, Free Univ. of Berlin, 1000 Berlin 45 / Fed. Rep. Germany

RAO, K.S.J., Division of Endocrinology, National Institute of Nutrition, Hyderabad 500007 / India

RAVAULT, J.P., Dept. Animal Physiology, INRA, Nouzilly, 37380 Monnaie / France

REINBERG, A., Human Chronobiology Res. Unit, Dept. Physiology, Fondation A. de Rothschild, 75019 Paris / France

ROTSZTEIJN, W.H., Unité de Neurobiologie, U 109, Centre Paul-Broca, INSERM, 75014 Paris / France

SAWYER, W.H., Dept. Pharmacology, Columbia Univ. College of Physicians and Surgeons, New York, N.Y. 10032 / USA

SABOUREAU, M., Centre d'Etudes Biologiques Animaux Sauvages CNRS, Chizé, 79360 Beauvoir sur Niort / France

SCAPAGNINI, U., Dept. Pharmacology, Univ. of Catania, Medical School, 95125 Catania / Italy

SEMPERE, A., Centre d'Etudes Biologiques Animaux Sauvages, CNRS, Chizé, 79360 Beauvoir sur Niort/ France

SKADHAUGE, E., Dept. Medical Physiology A, The Panum Institute, Univ. of Copenhagen, 2200 Copenhagen / Denmark

SKINNER, J.D., Dept. Zoology, Mammal Research Institute, Univ. of Pretoria, Pretoria 0002 / Rep. of South Africa

SREBNIK, H., Dept. Physiology-Anatomy, Univ. of California, Berkeley, California 94720 / USA

SUNDARARAJ, B.I., Dept. Zoology, Univ. of Delhi, New Delhi 110007 / India

SZAFARCZYK, A., Dept. Physiology, Univ. of Montpellier II, 34060 Montpellier / France

THAPLIYAL, J.P., Dept. Zoology, Banaras Hindu Univ., Varanasi 221005 / India

THIMONIER, J., Dept. Animal Physiology, INRA, Nouzilly, 37380 Monnaie / France

TIMIRAS, P.S., Dept. Physiology-Anatomy, Univ. of California, Berkeley, California 94720 / USA

TUREK, F., Dept. Biol. Sciences, Northwestern Univ., Evanston, Illinois 60201 / USA

VACCARI, A., Dept. Pharmacology, Univ. of Genova, 16146 Genova / Italy

WEIHL, A., Dept. Hyperbaric Medicine and Physiology Naval Medical Research Institute, Bethesda, Maryland 20014 / USA

WILKINSON, C.W., Dept. Physiology School of Medicine, Univ. of California, San Francisco, California 94143 / USA

WINGFIELD, J.C., Dept. Zoology, Univ. of Washington, Seattle, Washington 98195 / USA

YAMAOKA, S., Dept. Physiology, Saitama Medical School, Saitama 350-04 / Japan

Introduction: What is Environmental Endocrinology?

I. ASSENMACHER and D. S. FARNER

Most animals live in environments in which important physical and biologic factors vary both periodically and aperiodically. The maintenance of internal stability (homeostasis), and indeed the very survival of the individual, requires appropriately correcting physiologic and behavioral adjustments. These adjustments are based on information (signals) from external and/or internal sources detected (transduced) by adequate sensory receptors, and transmitted by nerve fibers to the central nervous system (integrating centers), where it is "processed" and transmitted to effectors, either as efferent nerve impulses, or as changes in the plasma levels of hormones. The maintenance of internal stability also requires feedback components between the effectors and various sites of the afferent communication system. Endocrine glands and hormones are essential components of both functions. It is now recognized that many nerve cells have typical endocrine functions (neurosecretion), while virtually all other nerve cells communicate with effectors by means of chemical transmitters. The distinctions long made among neurotransmitters, neurohormones, releasing factors, and hormones have become somewhat blurred. Thus, in a sense, the concept of environmental endocrinology, like those of many biologic "disciplines" in general, is an artificial consequence of reductionism. However, this in no way impedes its heuristic usefulness, as long as its artificiality is clearly recognized. Such recognition was abundantly clear in the formal communications and informal discussions in this symposium.

In the course of evolution the animal species have, by natural selection, acquired genotypes that permit nongenetic adaptations to differing ranges of variation of normally experienced environmental variables. Internal stability can be preserved by relatively rapid physiologic or behavioral adjustments. Examples are to be found in osmoregulation in many species of aquatic animals, in thermoregulation in homeotherms, including man, and in adjustments to changes in quantity and quality of food in the environment. Unusual environmental changes, including those imposed by man on himself, may lead to conditions that exceed the genetically established capability for maintenance of internal stability. Genuinely pathologic changes in the endocrine components of the system may then occur. It is often difficult to separate such states from extreme states of adjustment and, indeed, there is a range of states in which the distinction is semantic.

We have noted above that animals usually live in environments in which there are periodic changes in important variables. The daily photocycle and the annual cycle in day length, together with consequent cycles in environmental temperature, are the most striking examples. Most, if not all, animals have evolved endogenous circadian cycles as adaptations to the environmental 24-h photocycle that contribute towards maintenance of internal stability. There is evidence that some have evolved endogenous circennial (circannual) cycles with endocrine components.

Precise periodic environmental cycles can provide predictive information so that an animal can undergo the necessary physiologic development for performance of a vital function, such as reproduction or diapause at the appropriate season. For example, photoperiodic mechanisms, using day length as information, are widespread among species of mid and high latitudes. They have, of course, endocrine components.

Considering the field of environmental physiology in the broadest context as pertaining to the study of the system and physiologic regulations of organisms in relation with the various and varying factors of the environment, environmental endocrinology appears on the other hand to concern the highest level of regulations of the endocrine system and hormone-dependent functions that integrate reactions to changes in the environment.

Is environmental endocrinology then a new and discrete discipline? Since the so-called disciplines in biology are nondiscrete, this question has no rational answer. What has emerged clearly from the symposium is that the concept of environmental endocrinology is, indeed, a unifying and heuristic aspect from which a multitude of interesting and important functional adaptations and adjustments of animals to changes in their environments can be examined. We thus concur with the substantial number of participants who expressed the hope that further symposia on environmental endocrinology will be forthcoming.

Introductory Lecture—Emotion and Stress

O. G. EDHOLM

Many aspects of endocrinology are concerned, either directly or indirectly, with the concepts of emotion or stress. Both are themselves emotive words, and the purpose of this introductory paper is to examine these words and some of the physiologic ideas associated with them with the intention of seeking more objective criteria.

Emotion and stress are important concepts, particularly in connection with environmental physiology and, specifically, environmental endocrinology. From the general scientific point of view, it may be considered that biology is still dominated by Darwin's theory of evolution. The evolution of species depends on the interaction between inheritance or nature, and environment or nurture. The effects of environment on the living organism, whether it be insect, fish, bird, reptile, or mammal, must be regarded as central to the study of biology. The dominant theory in physiology is still that of CLAUDE BERNARD, who emphasized the constancy of the internal environment. He was followed by WALTER CANNON who developed the concept of homeostasis, and it is to WALTER CANNON also that we owe our principal ideas about the physiology of emotion.

In a recent review, MASON (1972) has written: "Physical stress may not be so involved in pituitary adrenal control. Emotional stimuli must be ruled out before concluding that a physical stress is capable by itself of eliciting adrenal cortical activity." MASON goes on to examine HANS SELYE'S concept of stress. SELYE claimed: "Effects of diverse nocuous (sic) agents, including severe muscular exercise, trauma, cold, fasting, spinal shock and acute infections, appeared similar." He concluded that the pituitary adrenal cortical system responds in a nonspecific manner to many different stimuli as part of a general adaptation syndrome. MASON comments: "Is it not disturbing to consider that most if not all of the situations described by SELYE involve some degree of emotional reaction, discomfort or pain?"

Returning to the physiologists, and the work that has been developing over a number of years on the physiology of emotion, HILTON (1965) discussed the role of the limbic system: "Certain specific regions of the brain become specialised early in vertebrate phylogeny for the mobilisation of all the resources of the organism in response to the signals of dangerous situations." It is obvious that survival would frequently depend on the ability to respond to and avoid dangerous situations, and hence in the evolution of species the mechanisms involved would persist and develop. This emphasis on the importance of having mechanisms to respond to the signals of dangerous situations helps one to understand its significance. It may be that one may think of "emotional" effects as perhaps rather trivial, that "emotion" in general is not to be taken seriously, and certainly not to be considered as a fundamental and widespread biologic characteristic. However, some 25 years ago, UVNAS in Sweden and SIDNEY HILTON in England described the existence of the emotional tract, and the effects of stimulating the various portions of the limbic system. Such stimulation in the brain evoked widespread muscle vasodilation, characteristic of what was beginning to be described as the defense reaction, and it appeared that this reaction was a fundamental physiologic mechanism. It was HESS and BURGER who termed the emotional response "defense reaction", and such a term is less evocative than "emotional response". The defense reaction can be shown to be a widespread, indeed all-embracing, physiologic response. In the earlier phase, often called the alerting stage, charaterized in the cat by the pricking of ears, pupillary dilation and increased respiratory rate, muscle vasodilation is already widespread. With more powerful signals, baroceptor reflexes are inhibited, and multitudinous visceral and hormonal changes develop. Both emotion and stress are of interest to psychologists as well as physiologists, but it is surprising how little contact there is between the two disciplines. Even within physiology, however, there are quite marked divisions, and endocrinology is, to a considerable extent, apart from the main field of physiology. To the physiologists emotion is largely a question of muscle dilation, and to the endocrinologist it is essentially catecholamines all the way, and nothing else in sight. To quote MASON again: "What really is needed is a closer two-way relationship between psycho-endocrinology and physiology." MASON elso emphasizes that "a survey must be made of the number of endocrine responses that actually occur during emotional disturbances; there is a multiple endocrine response."

It would be out of place, indeed presumptuous, to include a review in this paper of present knowledge concerning these multitudinous endocrine responses. However, hopefully, there will be more work devoted to the whole animal (including man), so that the effects predominantly due to the activity of the limbic system may be distinguished from and integrated with the endocrine responses. There can be little doubt that studying the defense reaction must be considered to be fundamental to our understanding both of animals and man. To quote CANNON: "Fear, rage and pain and the pangs of hunger are all primitive experiences which human beings share with the lower animals. These experiences are properly classed as among the most powerful that determine the action of men and beasts. A knowledge of the conditions which attend these experiences is of general and fundamental importance in the interpretation of behaviour." This statement by CANNON is still true and relevant to contemporary research.

The concept of "stress" current today owes much to SELYE'S ideas, but it has become much wider and less precise. There are many definitions of "stress"; most physiologists today would have difficulty in providing one that would command universal acceptance. We can describe how environmental stresses produce strains on the organism, but we should avoid the use of the word stress as a description of a bodily state. This linguistic point may not be any longer of much importance, and it would probably be difficult to eradicate the misuse of the word. So we have "the stress of modern life", "discussion of the causes of stress disease", "the stress of the urban environment", etc.

The physical effects of the environment, heat and cold, low and high almospheric pressure, of injury and hemorrhage, have been studied in great detail by physiologists and the physiologic aspects are by now well understood. However, the concept of stress which is so popular today has little or nothing to do with such crude or violent happenings. The contemporary idea is, as mentioned above, concerned with the effects of "stress of modern life, or the urban environment, or with the exhausting effects of constant decision-taking". The practical importance of this idea of stress is the associated concept of disease resulting from "stress", including coronary heart disease, peptic ulcers, and hypertension. Another major area of disease includes neurosis and possibly psychosis; it is widely considered that "stress" plays a dominating role in the etiology of such conditions.

At present, it is difficult to sort out the confusion due to the use of the word "stress". MASON has pointed out that many, if not all, of the situations described by SELYE as stressful and leading to the general adaptation syndrome, also must arouse emotional responses, i.e., evoke the defense reaction. This comment also applies to the contemporary ideas of "stress", that is, to situations what cause anger or fear or resentment or frustration, all of which can produce the defense reaction. Such a summary indicates that in many respects "stress" and "emotion" describe the same state. There can be little doubt that the two words are sometimes used interchangeably, as well as there being on occasions an emotional element in a conventionally stressful situation. The physiologist cannot evade his responsibility to clarify such a confusion. If he is interested in environmental physiology, he must be concerned to know what part "emotion" or the defense reaction may have played in the changes occurring in a subject exposed, e.g., to a heat stress. It is not possible in this paper to examine all the environmental conditions listed above as being stressful, so heat will be used as an example.

Although a number of studies have been done in the field, meaning outside the laboratory, most have been carried out in climatic chambers with precise control of environmental factors (temperature, humidity, radiation, and air movement). When subjects are exposed to particular conditions on successive days, the physiologic changes during exposure alter. On the first day, body temperature will rise to a high level, as will heart rate; but sweat rate may be only moderate, and the subjects will experience considerable discomfort, and even distress. On subsequent occasions, body temperature and heart rate at the end of exposure will diminish from day to day, whereas sweat rate will increase, and the discomfort is reduced. After 10 to 14 days of exposure, the subjects experience virtually no discomfort, and certainly no distress. It has been common experience amongst those making such observations that there is a considerable difference between day 1 and day 2; cases of collapse or distress are virtually confined to day 1, and there is a greater difference between body temperature and heart rate recorded on day 1 and day 2 than on any other day. The stress of the environment produces a physiologic strain, and it is the resulting strain in the form of a raised body temperature that initiates the process of acclimatization. The question that needs answering is whether there is an emotional element. It seems probable that there will be apprehension amongst some subjects when they first enter the climatic chamber, but any initial emotional reaction should manifest itself in the early period of exposure, during the first hour, if fear is the dominant emotion. During this initial period discomfort is slight, and the obvious signs of fear or apprehension should be noticeable. None of the published accounts of climatic chamber trials describes such signs. Negative evidence is not satisfactory, and certainly not conclusive. It seems possible that emotional factors may occur together with the physiologic strains induced by the environment, but the emotional factors are secondary.

There is a further question: do situations that evoke the defense reaction also call into play the physiologic responses due to strain? This question can be put in another form: are the various phenomena that are considered as stressful identical with those that bring on the defense reaction or, more succintly, are "emotion" and "stress" identical? Much published work does not appear to distinguish between emotion and stress. CARRUTHERS (1976), in an article entitled <u>Biochemical Response to Environmental Stress</u>, has a sub-heading <u>Anxiety</u>,

Aggression and Catecholamines. It is clear from the introductory paragraphs of his excellent paper that CARRUTHERS considers that environmental stress arouses emotion.

If we consider the list of environmental stresses that elicit physiologic strains as given above, i.e., heat, cold, trauma, severe infection, high and low atmospheric pressure, high levels of noise and vibration, then one may propose that emotional factors are either absent or secondary.

Emotions such as anger, fear, desire, and hunger elicit the defense reaction. There are the further and major problems of mental disturbance. MILLS and EDEN (1976), discussing the increasing number of admissions to hospital for attempted suicide, write: "The final incident which triggers off taking an overdose is frequently a relatively trivial event when looked at in isolation, but a more detailed study of the patient's preceding life frequently reveals a variety of stresses and strains that many of us would find difficult to cope with."

In this article MILLS describes the increasing incidence of other associated conditons; anorexia nervosa, drug-taking, consumption of alcohol, etc., and relates these to the changing conditions of modern life with the resulting strains, particularly in adolescents or the age group 15-24. It seems possible that in addition to those conditions summarized under the heading of environmental stress, and those described by "emotion", there may be a third group related both to environmental stress and to emotions, prolonged and frequent, that entails the CNS and perhaps endocrine mechanisms additional to those concerned with the defense reaction.

As far as environmental endocrinology is concerned, it should be relatively easy to distinguish these two or perhaps three sets of phenomena. Certainly there is here still a large and exciting field for further research.

References

CANNON, W.B.: Bodily Changes in Pain, Hunger, Fear and Rage. New York: Appleton, 1929

CARRUTHERS, M.: Biochemical responses to environmental stress. In: Man in Urban Environments. Harrison, G.A., Gibson, J.B. (eds.). Oxford: University Press, 1976, pp. 247-273

HILTON, S.M.: Emotion. In: The Physiology of Human Survival. Edholm, O.G., Bacharach, A.L. (eds.). London-New York: Academic Press, 1965, pp. 353-376

MASON, J.W.: Organisation of psycho-endocrine mechanisms: a review and reconsideration of research. In: Handbook of Psychophysiology. Greenfield, N.S., Sternbach, R.S. (eds.). New York: Holt, Rinehart & Winston Inc., 1972, pp. 3-124

MILLS, I.H., EDEN, MARY: Social disturbances affecting young people in modern society. In: Man in Urban Environments. Harrison, G.A., Gibson, J.B. (eds.). Oxford: University Press, 1976, pp. 217-246

Appendix

A recent obituary of Professor GRAHAM WILSON, a distinguished pharmacologist, had been published in The Times, and it had been suggested that his death could be attributed to overwork. His widow, Dr. ELIZABETH WILSON wrote:

"Sir, Today's edition (April 18) of The Times carries a thoughtful and detailed obituary of my husband, Professur GRAHAM WILSON. However, there is one important point with which I must take issue. He died of cancer of the stomach which had probably been present for a long time before it was discovered nine months ago. There is absolutely no scientific evidence that stress, hard work or travelling have any connexion whatever with this condition and very little that they are a relevant factor in cardiovascular or any other disease.

There has been a great deal of emphasis in the media recently about the hypothetically adverse effects of so-called "over" work. My husband, a medical scientist, felt strongly that this supposition had no basis in fact and would have been most indignant if he had known that the possibility had been raised in his own obituary.

Stress is the loosely applied term which is supposed to provide the causal relationship. However, there is far more stress in coming home at five o'clock to a nagging wife and rebellious children than in completing 14 hours of worthwhile and largely enjoyable work.........
People who work hard do so because they want to - some live long like CHURCHILL and some die before their time as did my husband, but to believe that one can be killed by overwork is an unscientific as to associate the common cold with wet feet."

Chapter I. Annual Endocrine Rhythms and Environment

1. Seasonal States and Endocrine Levels in Insects

J. DE WILDE

The Problem

Early in this century, biologists had already become aware that animals are involved in two, seemingly contradictory types of functional relationship. Internal relationships lead to stability, external relationships to adaptability with regard to the environment. This had already been conceptualized in 1900 by the French physiologist RICHET, but the contradiction emerges clearest in comparing respective statements of the physiologist and the ecologist who first formulated clearly these two types of relationships.

In 1878, CLAUDE BERNARD, the father of physiology made the famous statement: "La fixeté du milieu intérieur est la condition de la vie libre." JACOB VON UEXKÜLL, one of the forerunners of modern ecology and ethology, stated in 1909: "Die Umwelt ... ist immer ein Teil des Tieres selbst, durch seine Organisation aufgebaut und verarbeitet zu einem unauflöslichen Ganzen mit dem Tiere selbst."

Now there are environmental influences that have such far-reaching consequences for the physiologic condition of animals, that totally different levels of life result. One may wonder how, in such cases, the information that an animal receives from its environment is so transferred that the homeostatic processes are not disturbed. It is to the merit of E. and B. SCHARRER (1963) that they recognized in neuroendocrine integration a mechanism that guarantees the integrity of the organism, and at the same time enables a strong adaptability to environmental changes. "Channels must exist, through which these modifying influences enter the control system and become integrated with or supertede the feedback mechanism. This integration can only take place in the central nervous system" (E. and B. SCHARRER, 1963).

Now that ecophysiological research has confirmed the supposition of the SCHARRERs, the question is raised: how is environmental information channeled through the neuroendocrine pathway in different animal species?

I attempt here to answer this question for the case of the Colorado beetle (*Leptinotarsa decemlineata* Say) emphasizing especially the extrinsic control of the functional state of adults.

Environmental Effects, State Levels, Tokens

Two Categories of Environmental Impact. In Figure 1 a distinction is made between two types of environmental effects.

1. Direct effects on the peripheral processes, of a more quantitative nature. This category comprises, among others, the effect of temperature on metabolism, the effect of light gradients on phototaxis, the

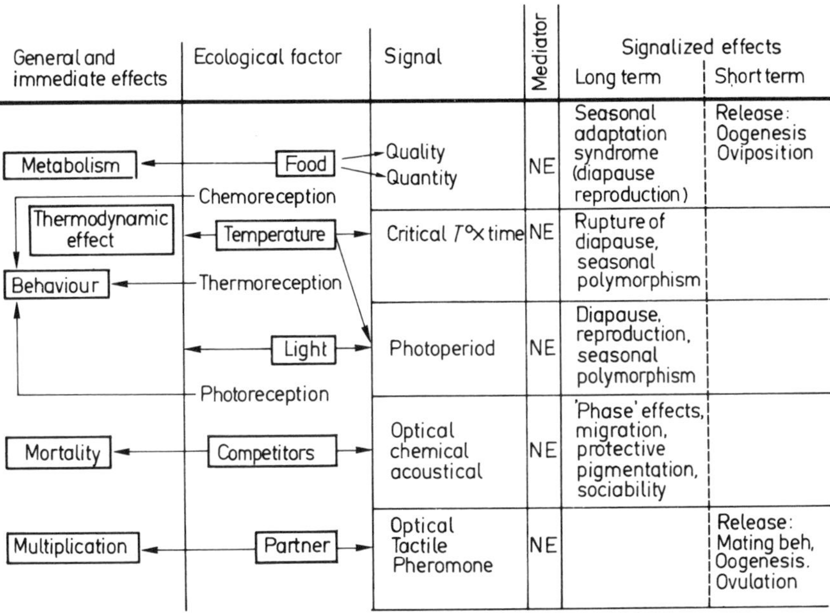

General and immediate effects
Ecological factor
Signal
Mediator
Signalized effects
Long term
Short term
Metabolism
Food
Quality
Quantity
NE
Seasonal adaptation syndrome (diapause reproduction)
Release: Oogenesis Oviposition
Chemoreception
Thermodynamic effect
Temperature
Critical T°x time
NE
Rupture of diapause, seasonal polymorphism
Behaviour
Thermoreception
Light
Photoperiod
NE
Diapause, reproduction, seasonal polymorphism
Photoreception
Mortality
Competitors
Optical chemical acoustical
NE
'Phase' effects, migration, protective pigmentation, sociability
Multiplication
Partner
Optical Tactile Pheromone
NE
Release: Mating beh, Oogenesis. Ovulation

Fig. 1. Two types of environmental effects. Left, Effects that do not determine states but concern more direct and peripheral responses, which last as long as the factor concerned. Right, Signalized effects which determine homeostatic states and syndromes, mediated by the neuroendocrine system

effect of nutrition on growth, the effect of competitors on available requisites.

2. Signalized effects, whose point of attack is more central, and whose effect involves the release of new processes, and the induction of adaptation syndromes of a varied nature. In this case it is not so much the quantitative, but more the configurative element that is important: it concerns the effect of specific molecules such as pheromones, certain patterns of light and darkness, certain temperatures acting during a certain time, specific optical configurations, etc. These factors have a token value. It is this second category of factors that will occupy us further in this chapter. The syndromes that they cause are physiologic and morphogenetic states: reproductive state, migration, diapause, ecomorphs such as phases, castes, aphid morphs, etc. The effect on the central nervous system is in many cases direct, that is, without the interference of the sensory system.

Homeostasis in Different State Levels. The conflict of relations cited above may be avoided if the environment induces different physiologic states characterized by their own homeostatic levels.

In the Colorado beetle two adaptive states can be distinguished:

1. The reproductive state, characterized by oviposition, sexual behavior, feeding, and simetimes flight behavior. This condition usually persists for about six weeks, after which senescence occurs; 75-100 eggs are produced each day or every other day.

2. The state of diapause, characterized by absence of reproduction and feeding, by rest or burrowing behavior, and by a very low metabolic rate. This condition lasts under natural circumstances 7-8 months, and takes place in the soil.

The reproductive condition is preceded by a maturation period, the diapause condition by a pre-diapause period, during which the above-mentioned levels are installed.

Reproduction may occur either directly after emergence, or after the elapse of diapause, which, under natural circumstances, occurs in the following spring. Diapause can begin already in late summer, but usually coincides with the winter season.

On one hand it was found that a number of processes that characterize both conditions are under endocrine influence. On the other hand, ecologic investigation have shown that diapause and reproduction are determined by specific environmental conditions. The Colorado beetle is a very suitable experimental object for the study of the relationships between the environment and the inner world of an insect in the above sense.

Signals Determining Diapause and Reproduction. The primary signal, daylength, which in the temperate and subtropical regions determines reproduction and diapause, has a cosmic origin. The photoperiodic response curve of the Colorado beetle shows a steep decline at 15 h. It is a long-day animal in which day lengths greater than 15 h induce reproduction in 70% to 80% of the beetles. On the contrary, day lengths shorter than 14 h induce diapause in 100% of the individuals. Thus day length synchronizes the life cycle with the astronomic season.

A third factor is the physiologic condition of the potato plant. When physiologically old potato foliage is given as food, oviposition ceases and diapause ensues even under long-day conditions. We have here a veto factor that synchronizes the life-cycle of the beetle with the host plant season.

Comparable relations have also been found in other insects. The sensitive stage (in the Colorado beetle, mainly the adult) and the reacting stage may be identical, but they may also be widely separated. Temperature above 25° inhibits the short-day effect in most insects of the temperate zone. In the commercial silkworm (*Bombyx mori* L.), which is a short-day species, and in which diapause occurs under long-day conditions, there is the paradoxical situation in which high temperatures promote (egg) diapause! There are, however, also insects that are insensitive to day length. In the mealworm, *Tenebrio molitor*, neither short nor long days influence reproduction; diapause does not occur in this insect.

In considering the question of the perception or measurement of day length, it must be emphasized that photoperiodic mechanisms contain cyclic components (LEES, 1971), and that several vital functions, such as feeding and oviposition, also have typical diurnal rhythms. A discussion of the actual mechanisms of time measurement in photoperiodic responses is beyond the scope of this presentation. However, the measurement of day length must involve photoreception, the sites for which can be identified by topographic exclusion experiments. The Colorado beetle lacks occeli. Its compound eyes are not involved, since removal or covering with nontransparent lacquer leaves the effect of day length unimpaired.

The brain is the most probable site of perception. Above the midbrain, the cuticle of the head capsule is transparent. In the diapause pupa of the silkworm, *Anthereya pernyi*, which is much more suitable for this type of experiment than the adult Colorado beetle, this perception has been investigated in more detail. This pupa, which is very heavily pigmented and thus essentially nontransparent, has a transparent cuticular window just above the brain. In this pupa, long day is a condition for adult development in spring. Differential illumination of the rostral and caudal part of the pupa with long and short days, respectively, reveals that development ensues after long-day illumination of the rostral end. When the brain is transplanted to the tip of the abdomen, and an artificial window is fixed in the cuticle at that site, development, on the contrary, is activated by long-day illumination of the caudal end. The initiation of development is due to an effect of the pars intercerebralis.

Returning to the Colorado beetle, we may question whether, in the neuroendocrine hierarchy, the medial neurosecretory cells are the highest center governing reproduction and diapause. It appears that diathermic cauterization of these cells may bring several complications. In cases in which this operation has been performed "cleanly", reproduction does not occur even under long-day conditions, while after some time diapause behavior develops. The probability that the "primum movens" is in the MNSC, is increased by the observation that after feeding with physiologically old potato foliage, the neurosecretory cells, according to their histologic appearance, retain their product. When subsequently young foliage is given, the transport of the neurosecretory substance is resumed. Parallel with this, in the first-mentioned case, egg production is inhibited and subsequently accelerated. SCHOONEVELD (1970, 1974) who was able to distinguish no less than seven types of cerebral NSC in the Colorado beetle, was able to show that in four of these, the histologic activity pattern runs parallel with reproduction and diapause.

However, neurosecretory substance accumulates conspicuously only in the second half of prediapause, and only after several weeks has the secretory transport ceased completely. That the activity of the cerebral neurosecretory cells is nevertheless the "pacemaker" of the activity of the corpora allata is supported further by experiments, in which the postcerebral complexes in females were inactivated by short-day treatment and subsequently reactivated by long days. This was done in animals in which the corpora allata had been transplanted into the abdominal cavity, so that the brain could only have an effect on the corpora allata via the hemolymph.

Clearly, the corpora allata are under the continuing dominance of the neurosecretory system of the brain. This system can, under the circumstances described, release its neurosecretory product via the regenerated complex of corpora cardiaca (DE WILDE and DE BOER, 1969).

Adult Diapause as Pseudo-Allatectomy

Extirpation of the corpora allata in the Colorado potato beetle is followed by a number of events that are similar to those observed under short-day treatment. The beetle feeds abundantly, but oviposition does not occur, or is arrested after a very short time. The ovaries are or will be in regression. An extensive fat body is formed which, being filled with protein granules, has a pale color.

The beetle subsequently burrows into the soil and enters into a state of rest. The basic rate of oxygen consumption decreases to less than 20% of the former intensity.

STEGWEE (1964) and DE KORT (1969) have investigated more closely the cause of this strong decline in respiratory activity. The basic metabolism of winged insects is accounted for preponderantly by the flight muscles and their giant mitochondira, the sarcosomes. Now it was shown that under short-day treatment or after allatectomy the flight muscles atrophy. As a consequence, when diapause has started, the sarcosomes have mainly disappeared or are strongly reduced. DE KORT has determined the activity of a number of enzymes of energy metabolism in the flight muscles, parallel with the ultrastructure of these muscles, during pre-diapause, when the flight muscles initially develop, but later regress. He came to the conclusion that the activities of mitochondrial enzymes such as SDH and αGPox show a sharp decline during the degeneration of the sarcosomes, while plasmatic extramitochondrial enzymes, such as GAPDH and GDH, change their activities much more gradually.

At the end of diapause, the flight muscles again develop and, as a consequence, when the beetle emerges, their structure has been restored.

It is remarkable that allectomy in an insect such as the mealworm, *Tenebrio molitor*, is followed only by a cessation of reproduction; motility and respiratory intensity remain unchanged. The flight muscles are less developed in *Tenebrio* than in *Leptinotarsa*, but the ultrastructure remains intact after allatectomy.

It is tempting to seek differences between the diapause condition in allatectomized and short-day beetles, respectively. A marked difference is that allatectomy diapause is never broken either spontaneously nor by external factors. We have kept such beetles for more than $1^1/_2$ years in a state of diapause; they remained in the substrate until they died. This difference is by itself not astounding. What was, however, remarkable was the difference in the effect of implantation of active corpora allata. Whereas in beetles that have entered diapause after allatectomy, implantation of two pairs of corpora allata from reproductive animals were sufficient to break the resting condition, this was much more difficult in short-day diapause. Some 10 active corpora allata were necessary to obtain a brief re-activation. The cause of this difference is discussed below. Implantation of corpora allata can be replaced by treatment with juvenile hormone, which has given some remarkable results. As was expected, diapause could be broken by external application of rather high doses of juvenile hormone. According to results of SCHOONEVELD et al. (1977), this re-activation is only of a short duration if the beetles are kept under short day. If, after such application, long day is given, a normal oviposition period of 6 weeks results.

Histologic investigations have shown that cerebral neurosecretory activity in diapause beetles begins one day after treatment with fuvenile hormone (JH). This shows that there is a positive feedback of the hormone titer on neurosecretory activity. In addition, it was shown that the corpora allata of the treated beetles do not increase in size but remain at the level of diapause, which suggests inactivity. Moreover, they are not essential for the above-mentioned activation process since treatment with juvenile hormone is as effective after the glands have been exstirpated. This suggests that, next to the increase in the JH titer, the activity of the MNSC is essential for breaking diapause.

The situation in male animals should be mentioned. Diapause behavior and lowering of the metabolic rate ensue also in male beetles after either short-day treatment or allatectomy, but, after allatectomy under long-day conditions, the males copulate before entering diapause, while this is not the case after short-day treatment.

With regard to reactivation by implantation of active corpora allata, the same differences occur between allatectomized and short-day males as are observed in the female. With regard to reproduction, the activity of the accessory glands first requires attention. Length and diameter of these very elongated glands decrease considerably after either short-day treatment or allatectomy, and also their ultrastructure suggests inversion. Such effects are not observed in the testes (DE LOOF and LAGASSE, 1972). Short-day diapause in both sexes is, therefore, nearly identical with the allatectomy syndrome but not completely, the term pseudo-allatectomy being thereby justified.

From the above data, it follows that the problem posed in the introduction can partly be retraced to the environmental effect on the homeostatic regulation of the juvenile hormone titer in the hemolymph.

The Juvenile Hormone Titer and Its Regulation

We now come to the essential question: is the titer of the juvenile hormone regulated at distinctly different levels in reproduction and diapause? and when this is so, what mechanism sets the "hormostat"? This is related to the question of whether the titer that we determine has a physiologic meaning, and to the mechanism that brings the regulation into effect.

By means of the *Galleria* test we have followed the titer of the juvenile hormone (mainly JH-III) in the course of adult life in short-day as well as long-day beetles; the volume of the corpora allata was also measured (Fig. 2). After the adult moult there is, in both cases, an initial increase of the titer, after which it may occur at one of two different levels, both clearly distinguishable, and correlated with processes that characterize two different physiologic states, reproduction and diapause. This correlation suggests that these titers are indeed of physiologic significance (DE WILDE et al., 1968; SCHOONEVELD et al., 1977).

What rates of secretion and decomposition of the hormone are involved in the regulation of its titer? To study the rate of incretion we had initially at our disposal only an indirect parameter, i.e., indications that the size of the corpus allatum increases with its activity. We now know that the rate of juvenile hormone synthesis is the best parameter for the rate of incretion, as the gland apparently has very little storage capacity for JH. Methods developed by TOBE and PRATT (1975) to measure the rate of JH synthesis in isolated corpora allata in vitro should soon provide more direct data. Measurements of CA volume made by SCHOONEVELD et al. (1977), by which it was shown that application of JH causes the gland to regress, give us some indication of the feed-back relations involved in regulation of its titer.

The rate of inactivation of JH in the hemolymph has been found to be considerable, with "half-life" values of 25 min having been observed at room temperature. However, regulation can occur only if there is a feed-back relation between the hormone titer and the rate of incretion and/or inactivation. Among the several possible mechanisms for inactiva-

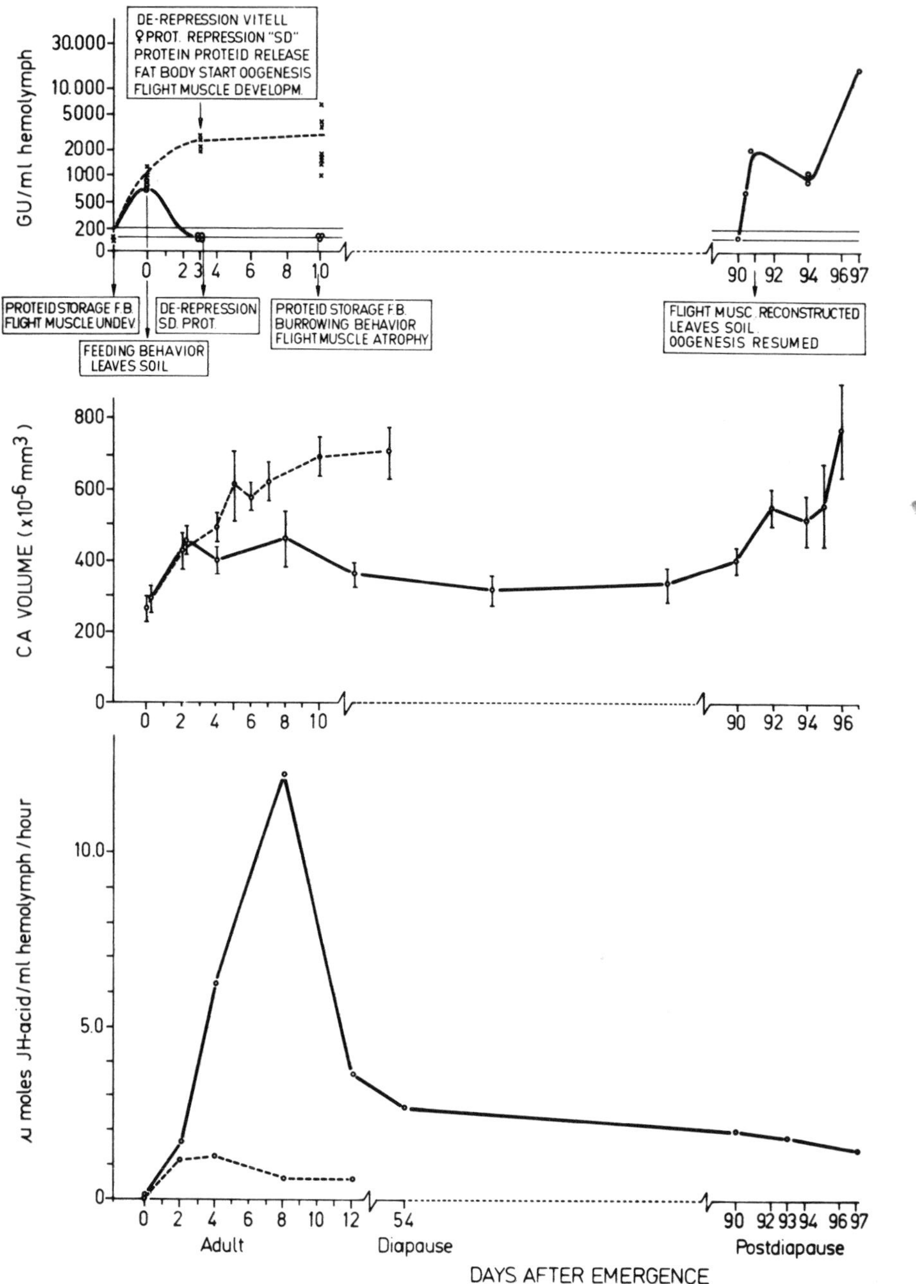

Fig. 2. Juvenile hormone titer in the adult Colorado beetle in two state levels. From above downwards: JH titer in the hemolymph; Volume of corpus allatum; Activity of JH-specific esterase; ----, long-day treatment; ——, short-day treatment

tion of JH, that involving JH-specific esterase (JH esterase) is most important in the Colorado beetle, since it has been shown that the activity of JH esterase is most clearly related to the physiologic condition of the animal and its JH titer. A K_m value of 5.10^{-7} M has been determined (KRAMER and DE KORT, 1976a, b). Figure 2 shows activity of this esterase in adults subjected to long and short days. It is important to note here that JH application during short-day diapause immediate causes an increase of JH esterase activity.

The role of the brain in the induction of the JH esterase activity is suggested by experiments performed by RETNAKARAN and JOLY (1976), who after cauterization of the neurosecretory A and B cells observed a strong decrease of esterase activity. It had already been found earlier by GIRARDIE that this operation in some cases seems to support the effect of the corpus allatum. The fact that the persistence of JH in the Colorado beetle is much increased after ligature of the head, and that after this operation in diapausing beetles, JH esterase activity no longer reacts to application of JH is a further indication in this direction. The localization of the "hormostat" now seems to be within reach.

JH esterase is synthesized in the fat body. Here also other blood proteins are formed, including a lipo-protein of MW > 100,000, which can bind the C_{18} juvenile hormone and is to be considered a "carrier protein." This then provides for transport of JH in the hemolymph, and also protects it to a certain degree against JH esterase. The affinity to JH is low in the Colorado beetle, but the binding capacity is high. One must imagine that the "carrier protein" molecules capture the JH molecules as they are released at the surface of the corpus allatum. They, however, do not offer much protection against JH esterase, as witnessed by the short "half-life" of JH in the hemolymph (KRAMER and DE KORT, 1977).

From Cosmic Signal to Subcellular Response

From the outer world to the inner world of the insect, a long chain of processes now becomes apparent. Day length is registered in the brain of the Colorado beetle by a mechanism with a certain degree of freedom. An insect such as the mealworm lacks this mechanism, and in the Colorado beetle it disappears in some phases of the life cycle, e.g., immediately after breaking of diapause. The response to day length is such that a narrow critical region separates two types of induction. Long days mainly induce reproduction whereas short days induce diapause. The critical region is so narrow that it is almost an all-or-none effect. Long days activate the cerebral neurosecretory cells and at the same time set the "hormostat" of the JH titer at a high level. As a consequence, the corpora allata are activated and their product, JH, is broken down only slowly. The resulting high JH titer, together with one or more neurosecretory hormones from the brain, initiates vitellogenesis, which is supported simultaneously by feeding. JH activity maintains cerebral neurosecretion that results in a buffering effect upon transition from long day to short day.

Under the influence of short days, the "hormostat" for JH is set at a low level; a relatively low JH titer already induces a high catabolic rate. It would seem that the low initial JH titer that always occurs after emergence induces a cerebral neurosecretory activity of a type that activates the synthesis of JH esterase in the fatbody. The JH titer is subsequently lowered to very low values, well below the minimum perceptibile of the regulatory system. As a consequence there is no vitellogenesis; instead of this a "short-day protein" is formed. At the same time, the synthesis of JH esterase decreases to very low values. The vitellaria of the ovarioles regress, the behavior of the beetle changes from feeding to burrowing, and subsequently to complete rest.

These physiologic changes imply several subcellular components of the two state levels induced by day length. We have already noted the regression in the synthesis of mitochondrial enzymes (DE KORT, 1969) during the atrophy of the flight muscles in short-day beetles. BARTELINK and DE KORT (1975), who continued these investigations, have found that application of JH in pre-diapause beetles results in an increased rate of ^{14}C-leucine incorporation in the isolated sarcosomes of these beetles. Protein synthesis in the sarcosomes is therefore influenced significantly by the JH titer in the blood. The above changes take place in the Colorado beetle; however, in the mealworm, behavior and the structure of flight muscles are not controlled by the juvenile hormone. In bark beetles, a high JH titer even induces the flight muscles to atrophy. It is therefore obvious that the "message" which is transferred by a hormone is a function of the receptive tissues.

Between the astronomic signal and the subcellular response lies the homeostatically regulated JH titer. That temperature and food quality have effects perfectly analogous to day length proves that information of a varied nature, fed into the system of neuroendocrine integration, influences the same homeostatic center. The freedom in the correlations observed in the environmental endocrinology of different insect species proves that the ecologic niche has its profound physiologic consequences.

References

BARTELINK, A.K.M., DE KORT, C.A.D.: Effects of diapause induction and juvenile hormone administration on mitochondrial formation in the flight muscles of the Colorado beetle. Proc. Roy. Neth. Acad. Sci. Ser. C 78, 1-11 (1975)

BERNARD, CL.: Leçons sur les phénomènes de la vie communs aux animaux et aux végêtaux. Paris: Baillière, 1978-1979, 2 vols.

KORT, C.A.D. DE: Hormones and the strucutral and biochemical properties of the flight muscles in the Colorado beetle. Med. Landb. Hogesch. Wageningen 69-2, 1-63 (1969)

KRAMER, S.J., DE KORT, C.A.D.: Age-dependent changes in juvenile hormone esterase and general carboxyesterase activity in the hemolymph of the Colorado potato beetle, *Leptinotarsa decemlineata*. Mol. Cell. Endocrinol. 4, 43-53 (1976a)

KRAMER, S.J., DE KORT, C.A.D.: Some properties of hemolymph esterases from *Leptinotarsa decemlineata* Say. Life Sci. 19, 211-218 (1976b)

KRAMER, S.J., DE KORT, C.A.D.: Juveline hormone carrier lipoprotein in the hemolumph of the Colorado potato beetle, *Leptinotarsa decemlineata*. Insect Biochem. (1977) in press

LEES, A.D.: The role of circadian rhythmicity in photoperiodic induction in animals. Proc. Int. Symo. Circadian Rhathm. Pudoc Wageningen 1971, pp. 87-110

LOOF, A. DE, LAGASSE, A.: The ultrastructure of the male acessory reproductive glands of the Colorado beetle. Z. Zellforsch. Mikrosk. Anat. 130, 545-552 (1972)

RETNAKARAN, A., JOLY, P.: Neurosecretory control of juvenile hormone inactivation in *Locusta migratoria* L. Colloque Int. C.N.R.S. 251, 317-324 (1976)

SCHARRER, E., SCHARRER, B.: Neuroendocrinology. New York-London: Columbia University Press, 1963, 289 pp.

SCHOONEVELD, H.: Structural aspects of neurosecretory and corpus allatum activity in the adult Colorado beetle, *Leptinotarsa decemlineata* Say. Neth. J. Zool. 20, 151-237 (1970)

SCHOONEVELD, H.: Ultrastructure of the neurosecretory system of the Colorado beetle, *Leptinotarsa decemlineata* Say. I. Characterization of the protocerebral neurosevretory cells. Cell Tissue Res. 154, 275-288 (1974)

SCHOONEVELD, H., OTAZO SANCHEZ, A., DE WILDE, J.: Juvenile hormone-induced break and termination of diapause in the Colorado potato beetle. J. Insect Physiol. 23, 689-696 (1977)

STEGWEE, D.: Respiratory chain metabolism in the Colorado beetle. II. Respiration and oxygative phosphorylation in "sarcosomes" from diapausing beetles. J. Insect Physiol. 97-102 (1964)

TOBE, S.S., PRATT, E.: Corpus allatum activity in vitro during ovarian maturation in the Desert Locust, *Schistocarca gregaria*. J. Exp. Biol. 62, 611-627 (1975)

TRAUTMANN, K.H., MASNER, P., SCHULER, A., SUCKÝ, M., WIPA, H.K.: Evidence of the juvenile hormone methyl (2E,6E)-1',11-epoxy-3,7,11-trimethyl-2,6-dodecadienoata (JH-3) in insects of four orders. Z. Naturforsch. 29C, 757-759 (1974)

UEXKÜLL, J.: Umwelt und Innenwelt der Tiere. Berlin: Julius Springer, 1909

WILDE, J. DE: Diapause and seasonal synchronization in the adult Colorado beetle (*Leptinotarsa decemlineata* Say). Symp. Soc. Exp. Biol. 33, Dormancy and Survival, pp. 263-284, Campbridge: University Press, 1969

WILDE, J. DE: Hormones and insect diapause. Mem. Soc. Endocrinol. 18, 487-514 (1971)

WILDE, J. DE, DE BOER, J.A.: Humoral and nervous pathways in photoperiodic induction of diapause in *Leptinotarsa decemlineata* Say. J. Insect Physiol. 15, 661-675 (1969)

WILDE, J. DE, DE LOOF, A.: Reproduction-endocrine control. In: Physiology of Insecta, Vol. 1, M. Rockstein (ed.). New York: Academic Press, 1973, pp. 97-157

WILDE, J. DE, STAAL, G.B., DE KORT, C.A.D., BAARD, G.: Juvenile hormone titer in the hemolymph as a function of photoperiodic treatment in the adult Colorado beetle (*Leptinotarsa decemlineata* Say). Proc. Roy. Neth. Acad. Sci. C71, 321-326 (1968)

WILLIAMS, C.M., ADKISSON, P.L.: Physiology of diapause. XIV. An endocrine mechanism for the photoperiodic control of pupal diapause in the oak silkworm, *Anthereya pernyi*. Biol. Bull. Wood's Hole 127, 511-525 (1964)

2. Annual Gonadal Cycles in Teleosts: Environmental Factors and Gonadotropin Levels in Blood

R. E. PETER and A. HONTELA

The seasonal reproductive cycle, involving recrudescence of the gonad, ovulation or spermiation, and spawning, is the most frequently cited example of an annual endocrine cycle in teleost fishes. Since this cycle is supposedly timed to be adaptive for survival of the species, in more constant climates, such as in the tropics or deep ocean, an annual reproductive cycle could not be predicted. Indeed, in a number of species of Caribbean reef fishes, a portion of the individuals were found to be in reproductive condition throughout the year (MUNRO et al., 1973). However, even in these species a peak of reproductive activity occurs in one period of the year, and in the majority there is a seasonal cycle in which reproductive activity is confined to one period of the year, generally when water temperatures are minimal. When the climatic conditions have greater extremes, as in temperate zones, the conditions appropriate for reproduction are obviously more restricted in time than in tropical climates. The reproductive cycle in this case may then be even more evident, in that spawning in many species occurs only once in a given year and individual populations may spawn en masse.

In order to be able to spawn at a certain time of year, fishes must use various environmental cues to initiate gonadal recrudescence so that the gametes are matured in time for spawning. In turn, there must be a set of environmental conditions to cue spawning. The environmental factors involved in cuing reproductive activity will be only briefly reviewed here, and will also be discussed in Chapter I.3 of this volume. Another approach to the endocrinology of annual reproductive cycles is to examine the cycles of secretion of gonadotropin (GtH) that might underlie or relate to the more obvious cycle of maturation of the gametes and spawning. This will be the main emphasis of this paper.

Annual Gonadal Cycles and Environmental Cues

The annual cycle of activity of the testes and ovary can be divided in a number of semiarbitrary phases. For example, the annual ovarian cycle of the Indian catfish, *Heteropneustes fossilis*, has been divided into preparatory, prespawning, spawning, and postspawning phases by SUNDARARAJ and VASAL (1976). The recrudescence of the ovary of the goldfish, *Carassius auratus*, has been described as occurring in nine stages (YAMAZAKI, 1965), and atretic oocytes and postovulatory follicles in five and three stages, respectively (KHOO, 1975). Similar categorizations have been made for the ovarian cycles of a variety of other species: e.g., Longjaw Goby, *Gillichthys mirabilis* (DE VLAMING, 1972c); and Shiner Seaperch, *Cymatogaster aggregata* (WIEBE, 1968). Six stages of the testicular cycle of *G. mirabilis* has been described by DE VLAMING (1972c): quiescent, mitotic, meiotic, prespawning, postspawning, and regressing. Similarly, the testicular cycles of a number of other species have also been categorized semiarbitrarily: e.g., Brook Trout, *Salvelinus fontinalis* (HENDERSON, 1963); *C. aggregata* (WIEBE, 1968); and Golden Shiner, *Notemigonus crysoleucas* (DE VLAMING, 1975).

Of the various possible environmental factors that may be used to cue gonadal cycles, duration of the daily photophase (photoperiod) and temperature have been assumed to be of prime importance in most of the species investigated (for reviews: SUNDARARAJ and VASAL, 1976; DE VALMING, 1972a, 1974). Depending on the environmental conditions of adaptation by the species, one factor or the other may be of more importance. For example, BAGGERMAN (1972), has shown that the Threespine Stickleback, *Gasterosteus aculeatus*, undergoes gonadal recrudescence during the winter following exposure to artificial long days and warm (16L 8D/20°C) conditions, but responds poorly or not at all when exposed to a short days and warm (8L16D/20°C) conditions. In spring long days induce more rapid gonadal maturation than short days in both warm and cold (9°C), although significantly the fish undergo gonadal maturation even under short days in the spring. During the summer, after termination of the normal spawning season, long days and warm conditions do not induce another cycle of gonadal recrudescence. This suggests that, although the animals are most responsive to a long days and warm conditions in the winter and spring, there is some refractoriness that occurs following spawning that prevents another cycle of gonadal maturation in the summer, in spite of the presence of supposedly favorable conditions. Furthermore, there seems to be a change in threshold, since in the winter short photophases are not stimulatory, whereas during the spring gonadal maturation can occur even under a short photophase continuous with the short photophase of winter. BAGGERMAN (1972) has demonstrated that there is a daily rhythm in responsiveness to light in the stickleback, the sensitive period for inducing gonadal maturation being about 12-18 h after the onset of the daily photophase. A similar cycle has also been shown to occur in *H. fossilis* (SUNDARARAJ and VASAL, 1976). On this basis, perhaps the response of the sticklebacks to short photophase in the spring may involve a shift of the photosensitive phase to closer to the onset of the daily photophase.

In a number of species, in addition to the Threespine Stickleback, the combination of long days and warm temperature is highly favorable for gonadal recrudescence: e.g., *C. aggregata* (WIEBE, 1968); Golden Shiner (DE VLAMING, 1975); Green Sunfish, *Lepomis cyanellus* (KAYA and HASLER, 1972); and *H. fossilis* (SUNDARARAJ and VASAL, 1976). On the other hand, Brook Trout, a fall-spawning species, has been shown by HENDERSON (1963) to respond primarily to photophase. Acceleration of the spring-through-fall photophase cycle caused earlier gonadal maturation in both male and female adult trout, but not in fish undergoing gonadal maturation for the first time.

Temperature may be the main factor cuing the gonadal cycle of a number of cyprinids (see DE VLAMING, 1972a), but there is good evidence for this only for the Lake Chub, *Couesius plumbeus* (AHSAN, 1966). However, the Longjaw Goby, *G. mirabilis*, is highly dependent on temperature (DE VLAMING, 1972b, c). In this species high temperatures (22°C in females, 24°C in males) block gonadal recrudescence, regardless of day length. At low temperatures (10°-20°C) gonadal recrudescence occurs. This effect of low temperature on gonadal recrudescence is accelerated by short daily photophases whereas long photophases are somewhat favorable to maintenance of the gonad in a mature state.

A wide variety of environmental factors, in addition to temperature and day length, impinge on fishes, and could also be adopted as cues for timing gonadal cycles. For example, flooding has been suggested as an important cue for some Australia fishes (LAKE, 1967). Some other more obvious cues may be various social interactions, food, vegetation, running or static water, and water quality. In designing experiments to investigate environmental cues for gonadal recrudescence, investigators must be cautious not to introduce unwittingly or fail to introduce some important factor, leading to misinterpretation of results regarding the factors controlled. From what is known about environmental factors used to cue gonadal cycles, it would be premature at this point to speculate about generalizations for phylogenetic groups.

Gonadatropin

Hypophysectomy blocks the occurrence of ovarian or testicular cycles in teleosts (for review: FONTAINE, 1976), which demonstrates the necessity of a pituitary factor (or factors), presumably GtH. Annual cycles of activity of GtH cells in the pituitary, correlated with gonadal cycles, have been described for a number of species (for review: FONTAINE, 1976) and therefore will not be presented here again. The implication from these observations is that the pituitary must be releasing GtH to cause gonadal recrudescence, and spermiation or ovulation. Presumably this would be reflected by changes in the concentrations of GtH in blood.

CRIM et al. (1973) found that the plasma levels of GtH during gonadal recrudescence in male and female Pink Salmon, *Oncorhynchus gorbuscha*, were nondetectable (< 6.0 ng/ml) in the majority (61%) of the fish. In some fish "low" levels (6.0-17.5 ng/ml) were detectable and in a number of cases (16%) inexplicably high levels (22-760 ng/ml) were found. Plasma GtH levels were detectable in all fish captured on spawning beds, with the females, most of which had ovulated, having average GtH levels of 74.9 ± 1.9 ng/ml.

Using a radioimmunoassay of improved sensitivity for salmon and trout GtH (minimum detectable level 2 ng/ml), CRIM et al. (1975) still could not detect GtH in plasma from male or female Brook Trout that were immature or in early stages of gonadal recrudescence. However, plasma GtH was measurable in Brook Trout and land-locked Atlantic Salmon (*Salmo salar*) that had spermatozoa present in the testis or mature oocytes in the ovary. Ovulated fish of both species consistently had significantly higher plasma GtH levels than preovulatory fish. Spermiation in Atlantic Salmon, but not in Brook Trout, was also associated with significantly higher plasma GtH levels.

Clearer evidence for increasing levels of plasma GtH in correlation with ovarian development was found by CRIM et al. (1975) in female Sockeye Salmon, *O. nerka* (3.3 ng/ml in preliminary vitellogenesis to 9.4 ng/ml during advanced vitellogenesis). Very high levels of plasma GtH were again found in ovulated fish (ca. 300 ng/ml). Parallel studies on male Sockeye Salmon did not show as clear a correlation between testicular development and plasma GtH levels, because up to final stages of spermatogenesis relatively few males had detectable plasma GtH. However, as the males progressed through recrudescence, more and more had detectable plasma GtH levels, until the testes contained spermatozoa, when all had measurable levels. Spermiating Sockeye had significantly higher plasma GtH than fish in earlier stages. BRETON et al. (1975) have made similar observations on Rainbow Trout.

Thus, for salmonids there is good evidence for an increase in blood concentrations of GtH in correlation with gonadal development. Females have a much more pronounced cycle due to the very high GtH levels that occur in association with ovulation. This generalization may also extend to cyprinids, as similar changes in plasma GtH have been found in the tench during gonadal recrudescence and ovulation or spermiation (BRETON et al., 1975), and significantly higher plasma GtH levels have been found in goldfish on the day of ovulation (BRETON et al., 1972).

Environmental factors that influence gonadal cycles, such as day length and temperature (see previous section), will presumably do so partially through influences on the secretion of gonadotropin. Unfortunately there is little information available on this topic. However, GILLET et al. (1977) have studied the effects of temperature on plasma GtH levels in male goldfish. The study commenced in January by placing fish under certain temperature regimes or natural conditions, and continued through to July, encompassing the normal period of testicular recrudescence and spawning for goldfish. The photoperiodic regime at the beginning the experiment was 8L 16D; it was lengthened at intervals to 16L 8D by the end of the experiment. Blood samples were taken monthly. The fish held continuously at 10°C, the lowest of the experimental temperatures, had a slight but nonsignificant increase in plasma GtH through June. The fish held at 17°, 24° or 30°C had plasma GtH levels that were basically similar to each other, but the 30°C fish were higher in March and all three groups were higher than the 10°C fish from February through May. In May the fish held at 17°, 24° and 30°C began to have a decline in plasma GtH levels and in June they were similar to the 10°C fish. Fish that were subjected to a gradual increase in temperature from 10°C to 22°C from February to June had plasma GtH levels similar to the fish at 10°C in February and March, and then had increasing levels with the highest levels in May; following the high in May, plasma GtH declined to a level similar to all the other groups. Fish under normal conditions were most similar to the fish held at 10°C, but, except for July, consistently had somewhat higher plasma GtH levels. Together with information on the state of the testes, the data indicate that temperatures of 17° and 24°C can accelerate the cycle of testicular maturation and regression in goldfish, and this acceleration is associated with higher plasma GtH levels during recrudescence. At 30°C spermatogenesis does not occur in spite of high plasma GtH levels. At 10°C GtH levels change very little, but resticular recrudescence still occurs, albeit more slowly. Regression of the testes is associated with a decrease in plasma GtH at all temperatures. From these results it is obvious that plasma GtH levels need not change greatly in order to accomplish gonadal recrudescence. Also, temperature conditions obviously influence GtH secretion in goldfish.

A significant daily cycle in plasma GtH levels was found in female goldfish with mature ovaries by BRETON et al. (1972). No cycle in secretion of GtH was found in males. For this experiment the fish were exposed to the natural day length of about 15-16 h and the water temperature changed about 10°C during the 24-h period of sampling. It is difficult from these results to assess the effects of temperature and day length on GtH secretion.

We (A. HONTELA and R.E. PETER, unpublished results) have studied the effects of temperature (11°-13°C vs 20°-22°C) and day length (16L 8D vs 8L 16D) on the daily variations in serum GtH in female goldfish at three different stages of ovarian development. For the experiments the fish were acclimated in groups of about 40 to the environmental conditions in 293-l flow-through aquaria. Sampling from each group was spread out over a 3-day period to avoid the possible stress of repeated disturbance during a single 24-h period. To avoid stress influences during sampling, the fish were netted in groups of about six, anesthetized, and blood samples were taken, following which the fish were killed. Fish with mature and maturing oocytes had daily variations in the levels of serum GtH that were statistically significant or near significance under each of the four temperature-photophase combinations. Fish with regressed or immature ovaries in general had less variation in the levels of serum GtH, although there were significant differences in the two groups at the high temperature. It is interesting to note that at any stage of ovarian development the fish adapted to the higher temperatures had higher serum GtH levels at certain times of the day than the fish at the cold temperatures. Some differences in the cycles could also be attributed to differences in day length. Finally, under any one set of environmental conditions, similar serum GtH levels were found in the three different groups of fish at certain times of day, generally the basal level being the most common. The significant difference between the fish with immature ovaries and the other two groups, therefore, is that the latter tend to have more marked daily variations in serum GtH levels from the basal level. Thus, these data indicate that the concept of progressive increase in GtH secretion as the female goldfish proceeds through ovarian recrudescence does not hold as a generality. Instead this concept must be modified to include the idea that there can be a daily cycle in secretion of GtH, the presence or absence of which is somewhat dependent on the state of ovarian development, and modified by the temperature-photoperiodic conditions. Also, because of the similarity of the basal levels of GtH in immature, maturing and mature females under any one set of environmental conditions, it is likely that surges in secretion of GtH have more significance for producing effects in the gonad than do the basal levels of GtH.

Acknowledgements. We wish to thank M.D. WIEGAND and L.W. CRIM for critical comments on this manuscript. Unpublished work reported herein was supported by a grant from the National Research Council of Canada.

References

AHSAN, S.N.: Effects of temperature and light on the cylcical changes in the spermatogenetic activity of the lake chub, *Couesius plumbeus*. Can. J. Zool. 44, 161-171 (1966)

BAGGERMAN, B.: Photoperiodic responses in the stickleback and their control by a daily rhythm of photosensitivity. Gen. Comp. Endocrinol. Suppl. 3, 466-476 (1972)

BRETON, B., BILLARD, R., JALABERT, B.: Specificité d'action et relations immunologiques des hormones gonadotropes de quelques téléostéens. Ann. Biol. Anim. Bioch. Biophys. 13, 347-362 (1973)

BRETON, B., BILLARD, R., JALABERT, B., KANN, G.: Dosage radioimmunologique des gonadotropines plasmatiques chez *Carassius auratus*, au cours du nycthémère et pendant l'ovulation. Gen. Comp. Endocrinol. 18, 463-468 (1972)

BRETON, B., JALABERT, B., FOSTIER, A., BILLARD, R.: Étude sur le cycle reproducteur de la Truite arc-en-ciel et de la Tanche. Effect de variations experimentales de la température. J. Physiol. (Paris) 30, 561-564 (1975)

CRIM, L.W., MEYER, R.K., DONALDSON, E.M.: Radioimmunoassay estimates of plasma gonadotropin levels in spawning pink salmon. Gen. Comp. Endocrinol. 21, 69-76 (1973)

CRIM, L.W., WATTS, E.G., EVANS, D.M.: The plasma gonadotropin profile during sexual maturation in a variety of salmonid fishes. Gen. Comp. Endocrinol. 27, 62-70 (1975)

FONTAINE, M.: Hormones and the control of reproduction in aquaculture. J. Fish. Res. Bd. Can. 33, 922-939 (1976)

GILLET, C., BILLARD, R., BRETON, B.: Effets de la température sur le taux de gonadotropine plasmatique et la spermatogenèse du poisson rouge *Carassius auratus*. Can. J. Zool. 55, 242-245 (1977)

HENDERSON, N.E.: Influence of light and temperature on the reproductive cycle of the eastern brook trout, *Salvelinus fontinalis* (Mitchill). J. Fish. Res. Bd. Can. 20, 859-897 (1963)

KAYA, C.M., HASLER, A.D.: Photoperiod and temperature effects on the gonads of green sunfish, *Lepomis cyanellus* (Rafinesque), during the quiescent, winter phase of its annual cycle. Trans. Am. Fish. Soc. 101, 270-275 (1972)

KHOO, K.H.: The corpus luteum of goldfish (*Carassius auratus* L.) and its functions. Can. J. Zool. 53, 1306-1323 (1975)

LAKE, J.S.: Rearing experiments with five species of Australian freshwater fishes. I. Inducement to spawning. Aust. J. Man. Freshwater Res. 18, 137-153 (1967)

SUNDARARAJ, B.I., VASAL, S.: Photoperiod and temperature control in the regulation of reproduction in the female catfish *Heteropneustes fossilis*. J. Fish. Res. Bd. Can. 33, 959-973 (1976)

VLAMING, V.L. DE: Effects of photoperiod and temperature on gonadal activity in the cyprinid teleost, *Notemigonus crysoleucas*. Biol. Bull. 148, 402-415 (1975)

VLAMING, V.L. DE: Environmental and endocrine control of teleost reproduction. In: Control of Sex in Fishes. Schreck, C.B. (ed.). Blacksburg: Virginia Polytechnic Institute and State University, 1974, pp. 13-83

VLAMING, V.L. DE: Environmental control of teleost reproductive cycles: a brief review. J. Fish. Biol. 4, 131-140 (1972a)

VLAMING, V.L. DE: The effects of diurnal thermoperiod treatments on reproductive function in the estuarine gobiid fish, *Gillichys mirabilis* Cooper. J. Exp. Mar. Biol. Ecol. 9, 155-163 (1972b)

VLAMING, V.L. DE: The effects of temperature and photoperiod on reproductive cycling in the estuarine gobiid fish *Gillichthys mirabilis*. Fish. Bull. 70, 1137-1152 (1972c)

WIEBE, J.P.: The reproductive cycle of the viviparous seaperch, *Cymatogaster aggregata* Gibbons. Can. J. Zool. 46, 1221-1234 (1968)

YAMAZAKI, F.: Endocrinological studies on the reproduction of the female goldfish, *Carassius auratus* L., with special reference to the function of the pituitary gland. Mem. Fac. Fish., Hokkaido Univ. 13, 1-64 (1965)

3. Environmental Regulation of Annual Reproductive Cycles in the Catfish *Heteropneustes fossilis*

B. I. SUNDARARAJ

Teleost fishes, which occupy a wide variety of ecologic niches, generally exhibit an annual reproductive rhythm (see DE VLAMING, 1972, 1974; SUNDARARAJ and VASAL, 1976). Many species breed in spring and early summer, while others do so either in monsoon or in autumn. The time of breeding of each species is so precisely regulated that fry are produced in a favorable environment when the chances of survival and growth are optimal. Fishes must anticipate the favorable period by using the various environmental cues to initiate gonadal recrudescence to accomplish spawning at a particular time of year. PETER and HONTELA have briefly reviewed the environmental factors involved in cuing of reproductive activity of teleost fishes in the preceding paper (Ch. I.2, this vol.). In this discussion paper, the investigations performed in my laboratory on environmental regulation of ovarian cycling in the catfish, *Heteropneustes fossilis*, will be briefly summarized.

The catfish is a seasonal breeder and its annual ovarian cycle in the vicinity of Delhi (lat. 28° 35'N; long. 77° 12'E) is divisible into four periods: the preparatory period (February to April), the prespawning period (May to June), the spawning period (July to August), and the postspawning period (September to January). Two consecutive sets of physiologic events intimately interwoven with environmental changes are involved in the completion of the circannual reproductive cycle in the catfish. The first set of phenomena leads to the gradual enlargement of the ovary, with concomitant formation of yolky oocytes during the prespawning period when in nature both the daily photofraction and mean environmental temperature increase progressively (SUNDARARAJ and VASAL, 1976; VASAL and SUNDARARAJ, 1976). The second set of physiologic events, involving ovulation and spawning of the oocytes, seems to be triggered by a host of environmental factors prevailing during the monsoon season (July to August), the prime time for breeding in the environmental niche.

Exposure of catfish in the preparatory period (February) to 12- or 14-h daily photophases at ambient water temperature (15.5° to 17°C), 25°, 30° or 34°C for 36 days results in a significant increase in ovarian weights associated with the formation of yolky oocytes only in those exposed to 25°C and above, regardless of day length, whereas during the postspawning period (November) a significant increase in ovarian weight with concomitant formation of yolky oocytes in observed only in catfish exposed to 30°C for 60 days, irrespective of day length. However, early vitellogenic oocytes are formed, albeit in very low proportions, even when the temperature is below 25°C. Thus, the threshold temperature for the formation of yolky oocytes appears to be 25°C, and above it the rate of vitellogenesis is proportional to increasing temperature. This catfish is capable of regulating its body temperature by behavioral means; the preferred temperature is 28.6° to 32°C. Thus, it is not surprising that the rate of ovarian recrudescence is rapid around 30°C (VASAL and SUNDARARAJ, 1976).

During the postspawning period, ovarian regression is retarded more effectively by a temperature of 30°C than by cooler temperatures (25°C), regardless of photoperiodic manipulations. Even so, ovaries eventually regress in the first week of October (VASAL and SUNDARARAJ, 1976).

Mature female catfish exposed from November 1969 to August 1972 to continuous light (LL) or continuous darkness (DD) at 25°C clearly show an ovarian rhythm comparable to that seen in fish collected from nature (NL). For animals in LL and DD, a circannual rhythm was demonstrated by fitting a 1-year cosine curve with the single cosinor technique. Evidence for a change in period length, at least in LL, is clearly apparent from the fact that the acrophase in LL occurs earlier than in DD or NL, and what is more important, the interval estimate of the circannual acrophase in LL does not overlap the corresponding interval estimate for the data from NL. With 150 fishes contributing the data in NL and 56 fishes contributing those in LL, it can be safely concluded that the computed acrophase differences establish, at least indirectly, a circannual rhythm desynchronization (SUNDARARAJ, VASAL and HALBERG, unpublished results). Thus it is apparent that in this species the termination of the reproductive phase is endogenously timed, and the postspawning ovarian regression under constant laboratory conditions is obligatory.

The annual ovarian cycle of the catfish is primarily influenced by seasonal temperature variations. A circannual ovarian rhythm expresses itself, albeit slightly out of phase in LL, even when catfish are placed under constant environmental conditions. Day length and temperature may act as synchronizers to bring the ovarian rhythm into phase.

Acknowledgments. Supported in part by research grants GF-34379 and OIP72-02845 AOI from the National Science Foundation, Washington, D.C., U.S.A.

References

SUNDARARAJ, B.I., VASAL, S.: Photoperiod and temperature control in the regulation of reproduction in the female catfish *Heteropneustes fossilis*. J. Fish. Res. Bd. Can. 33, 959-973 (1976)

VASAL, S., SUNDARARAJ, B.I.: Response of the ovary in the catfish, *Heteropneustes fossilis* (Bloch), to various combinations of photoperiod and temperature. J. Exp. Zool. 197, 247-264 (1976)

VLAMING, V.L. DE: Environmental control of teleost reproductive cycles: a brief review. J. Fish Biol. 4, 131-140 (1972)

VLAMING, V.L. DE: Environmental and endocrine control of teleost reproduction. In: Control of Sex in Fishes. Schreck, C.B. (ed.). Blacksburg: Virginia Polytechnic Institute and State University, 1974, pp. 13-83

4. Environmental Control of Annual Ovarian Cycle in the Toad *Bufo bufo bufo* L.: Role of Temperature

C. B. JØRGENSEN, K.-E. HEDE, and L. O. LARSEN

The annual ovarian cycle in the toad *Bufo bufo bufo* (L.) represents a functional pattern that has been observed in many anuran amphibians of temperate zones. In the mesic climates that predominate in the temperate zones of the higher latitudes, temperature and day length are the most obvious factors to consider in environmental control of reproductive, as well as of other annual cycles. In the common toad we have found that the annual temperature cycle is the main environmental factor in securing the normal annual ovarian cycle, whereas the annual cycle in day length appeared less important (K. POULSEN, personal communication).

Natural Annual Ovarian Cycle in Adult Female Toads

In order to evaluate possible effects on ovarian function of exposing toads to artificial environments, we must know the natural ovarian cycle, which we have followed in wild toads throughout the year by analysis of ovarian biopsies. In recaptured animals it has been possible to describe ovarian cycles of individual toads in nature.

In Denmark, populations of *Bufo bufo bufo* exhibit a short breeding period, usually in April, when the mature eggs are ovulated. After the breeding season, the ovaries enter a resting phase in which only smaller oocytes are present (Fig. 1). Eventually, some of these oocytes will begin rapid growth by depositing yolk. The period of recruitment to this final growth stage lasts about a month, whereas growth continues until the oocytes have reached full size within about three months. In wild toads in Denmark, an ovarian cycle is initiated only in late spring or summer (Fig. 2).

Oocytes in the final growth stage tend to grow synchronously. This tendency can be seen in the size-frequency distribution of the growing oocytes. Figure 3 shows frequency distribution curves of growing oocytes, measured in ovarian biopsies from recaptured wild toads. The curves exhibit pronounced peaks. From the change in location of the peaks between first and second capture of the toads, it is possible to estimate the mean growth rate of the oocytes in the time interval between captures, that is, the growth rate of oocytes in nature.

The height of the peak of the curves of size frequency distribution of oocytes during final growth can be used as an indicator of the synchrony of oocyte growth. The degree of synchrony may be expressed as the percentage of oocytes falling within a certain size range under the peak. The higher this percentage, the narrower the peak, and the more synchronous the growth of oocytes. The size range adopted was such that if the number of growing oocytes within the range amounted to about 30%, growth was asynchronous, all oocyte sizes being about equally represented within the growth phase. Percentages of 31%-50% would suggest moderate synchrony of growth, 51%-70% pronounced synchrony, and

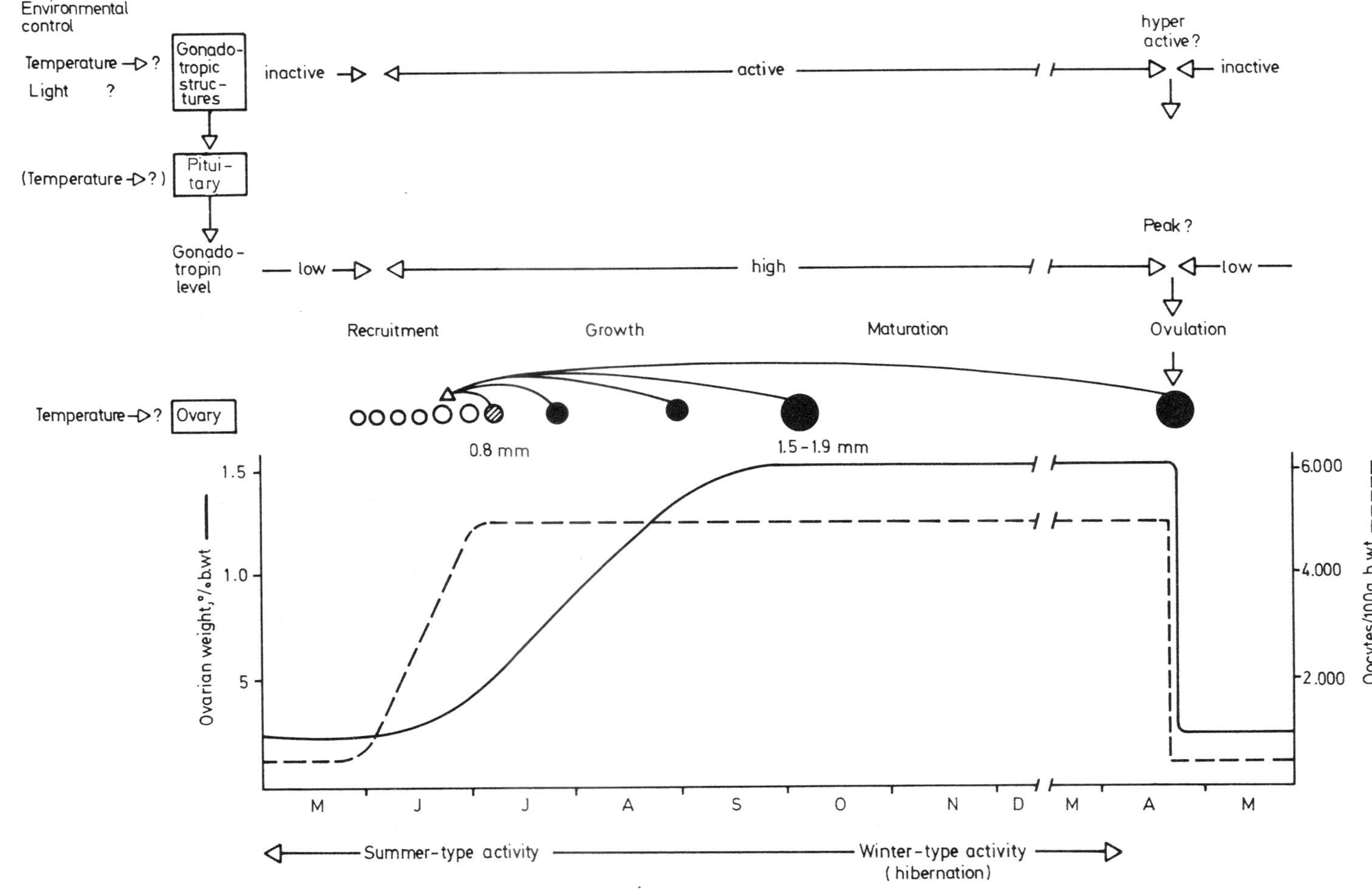

Fig. 1. Diagram of annual ovarian cycle in the toad *Bufo bufo bufo* in Denmark, its neuroendocrine regulation and control by external factors, especially temperature. Arrow pointing towards the small oocytes indicates inhibitory effect of large oocytes on further recruitment of oocytes to the final growth stage

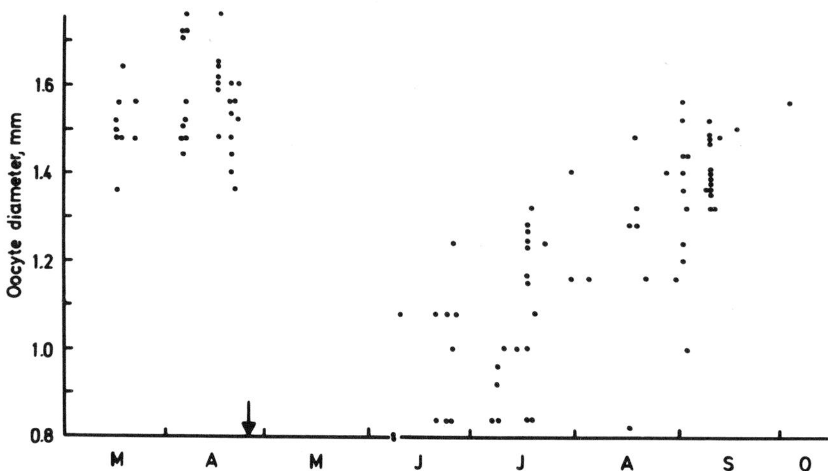

Fig. 2. Pattern of annual ovarian cycle, as observed in a population of toads, near Copenhagen. Abscissa, months; ordinate, dominant oocyte sizes, determined from size frequency distribution curves (see Fig. 3). Values from second half of July to early October are from 1976; values from March to early July are from 1977. Arrow indicates time of spawning

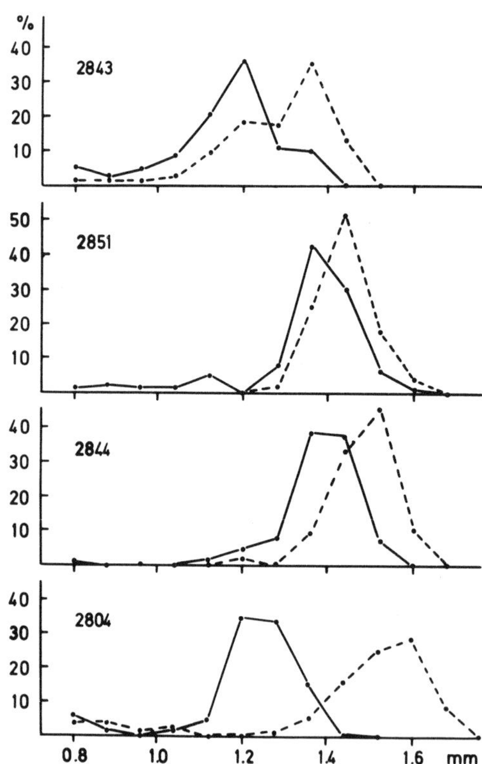

Fig. 3. Size-frequency distribution curves of final growth stage oocytes in ovaries of recaptured wild toads. Full lines indicate frequency distribution in ovarian biopsies taken at first capture, broken lines at subsequent capture. # 2804, biopsies taken 17 July and 2 September; # 2844, 30 July and 18 August; # 2851, 6 August and 27 August; # 2843, 30 July and 18 August

more than 70%, a high degree of synchronous growth of the oocytes. Table 1 shows that in the wild population, most of the toads exhibited an oocyte growth pattern characterized by pronounced synchronous growth.

Table 1. Degree of synchronous growth of oocytes in final growth phase

Environment and experimental conditions	Percentage of oocytes of peak size			
	≤ 30	31-50	51-70	> 70
Wild controls, biopsies	0	9	19	4
Intact toads, in laboratory at 20°C	7	25	18	2
Hypophysectomized toads, in laboratory at 20°C, treated with hCG	0	9	15	11

Ovarian Function in Adult Female Toads Maintained at a Constant High Temperature (20°C)

In order to study the importance of the annual temperature cycle for the ovarian cycle, we followed the functional state of the ovaries in toads brought into the laboratory after breeding, and kept at 20°C. Ovarian biopsies obtained in the middle of July all contained large numbers of oocytes in the final growth stage. The peak sizes of the oocytes varied greatly (Fig. 4). Peak values of oocyte diameters ranged from about 0.8 mm to 1.6 mm. Oocytes of 0.8 mm in diameter are in the early part of the final growth stage, whereas diameters around 1.6 mm are within the range of full-grown oocytes, as measured in wild toads. The size frequency distribution of the oocytes tended to be less regular than in the wild toads (Table 1).

Growth patterns of the ovarian cycles in the laboratory-acclimated toads were also compared with the growth pattern in ovaries of hypophysectomized toads exposed to the same laboratory environment, but treated with constant daily doses of gonadotropin (human chorionic gonadotropin, hCG). The ovaries of such toads all exhibited synchronous growth of oocytes in the final growth stage. The synchrony even tended to be higher than in the ovaries of wild toads (Table 1).

Subsequent biopsies of the intact toads kept at 20°C showed that the oocytes continued to grow, and by November final peak sizes of 1.8 to 2.0 mm oocyte diameter were attained, that is, larger than usually seen in nature (Fig. 2). Oocytes also continued to grow in toads that were hypophysectomized early October and treated with hCG (JØRGENSEN, 1975).

In November, the ovaries contained large oocytes and oocytes smaller than about 0.6 mm in diameter, whereas oocytes of intermediate sizes were absent or few in number. This agrees with previous findings that the presence of a pool of oocytes in the final growth stage prevents further oocytes from entering this stage, as indicated by the arrow in Figure 1 (JØRGENSEN, 1975). When the large oocytes became atretic, they were replenished by small oocytes that started to grow in numbers, approximating the pool of oocytes lost by atresia. Early in March this second generation of large oocytes had reached sizes that varied from about 1.0 to 1.4 mm in diameter (Fig. 4). Presumably, therefore, the original generations of large oocytes had become atretic shortly after

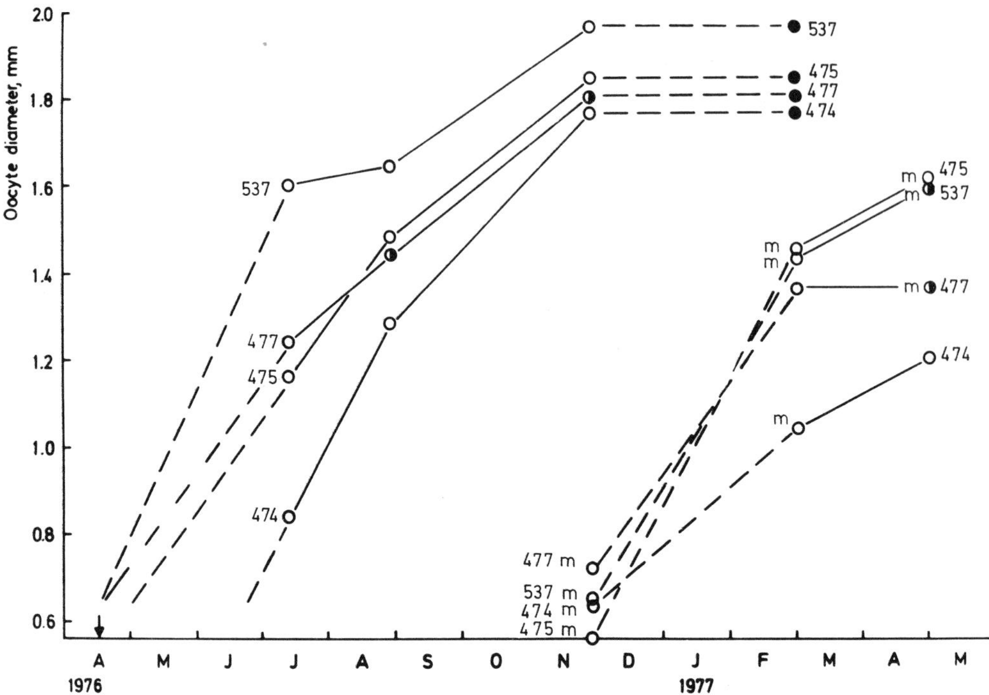

Fig. 4. Examples on pattern of growth of oocytes in toads maintained at 20°C. Abscissa, months; ordinate, dominant oocyte size. m, Maximum oocyte size when oocyte growth was asynchronous (see text). Open circles indicate no or slight atresia among oocytes; half filled circles, moderate to extensive atresia; filled circles, complete atresia. Arrow indicates time of spawning and subsequent transfer into the laboratory

the end of November. This agrees with previous findings that when toads with full-grown eggs in the ovaries are brought into the laboratory in the fall and maintained at room temperature, atresia starts to progress rapidly by December (JØRGENSEN, 1970).

The full-grown oocytes were never observed to be ovulated.

The second generation of large oocytes observed in the toads exhibited abnormal growth patterns, and mostly oocytes did not show well-defined peaks in the size-frequency distribution curves. This increasingly abnormal growth pattern of oocytes could not be correlated with obvious nutritional deficiencies. Toads killed after one year, in early May, had normal livers and mostly moderate to large fat bodies.

Lack of Vitellogenetic Growth at Low (Hibernation) Temperatures

Presumably ovarian cycles are not initiated in toad ovaries so late in the summer that the oocytes cannot complete their growth before hibernation (JØRGENSEN, 1975). It was, therefore, of interest to see whether low (hibernation) temperatures are incompatible with oocyte growth.

Twelve toads with ovaries containing oocytes in their final growth stage were cooled to 4°C, and after two and a half months returned to 20°C. Ovarian biopsies showed no growth in any of the toads during the stay at low temperature, whereas normal growth rates were resumed when the toads regained the high body temperature.

Ovarian growth has been stated to continue during hibernation in other anurans, e.g., *Bufo fowleri* (BUSH, 1963) and *Rana pipiens* (MIZELL, 1964; BRENNER and BRENNER, 1969).

Effect of Low Temperature on Sensitivity of Fullgrown Oocytes to Gonadotropin

It has been stated that exposure to low temperature during hibernation is necessary for the full-grown oocytes to mature and ovulate (BARTHÉLEMY, 1926; HOLZAPFEL, 1937, p. 70; SU and YU-LAN, 1963a, b). In order to study the effect of low body temperature on the maturation of full-grown follicles, we exposed sexually mature female toads caught in the fall to low temperature for varying lengths of time, and tested the sensitivity of the ovaries toward single injections of ovulation-inducing hormone, hCG. Table 2 shows that the sensitivity of the follicles increased with duration of exposure to hibernation temperatures.

Table 2. Sensitivity of full-grown follicles toward ovulation hormone (hCG): effects of exposure to low (hibernation) temperature in fall

Duration of exposure to low temperature, months	Dosage of hCG, i.u. 100 +	100 -	500 +	500 -	1,000-1,500 +	1,000-1,500 -
0					0	21
2-3			11	21	6	4
4-6	6	22	64	7		

Symbols: +, profuse ovulation; -, no or slight ovulation.

Breeding in Non-Hibernators in Winter at Intermediate Temperatures

As mentioned, a constant high environmental temperature was compatible with growth of oocytes in their final growth stage, but the follicles did not mature and ovulate. Low environmental temperature was incompatible with oocyte growth, but enhanced maturation of full-grown follicles. It remains to be seen how ovaries function at intermediate environmental temperatures.

In the month of September, mixed groups of male and female toads were placed in two large containers in an unheated basement room where the mean monthly temperatures varied from 18°C in September and October, 15°C in November, 14°C in December and January, 13°C in February, to 14.5°C in March. One group of toads was force-fed on heart meat, the other group fed spontaneously on living food, flies (*Musca domestica*), and *Tenebrio* larvae.

In early March, the first couples were observed in amplexus. At the end of March all the toads were transferred to concrete basins situated in the room and supplied with water and twigs for support of egg strings. Spawning commenced immediately. The toads were not followed individually, but a minimum of 9 out of about 15 sexually mature females were in amplexus, and most of them spawned profusely. The eggs developed into tadpoles. There was no obvious difference in the breeding performance of the toads that had been force-fed on meat and those that had eaten living food.

It can thus be concluded that maturation of full-grown follicles, normal sexual behavior, and normal breeding can take place in Danish toads that remain feeding and nonhibernating throughout the winter. In nature, toads do not feed from shortly before hibernation until after breeding the following spring (HEUSSER, 1968a; KNUD-ERIK HEDE, unpublished observations).

Conclusions and Interpretations

The annual ovarian cycle in the toad, and presumably in many other annually breeding anurans, depends upon the proper timing of activation and inactivation of gonadotropic structures within the central nervous system, especially the hypothalamus, as indicated in Figure 1 (VIJAYAKUMAR et al., 1971; JØRGENSEN, 1975). In the activated state the gonadotropic structures serve to stimulate the high rate of gonadotropin secretion from the pituitary gland that is needed to maintain normal growth of oocytes (JØRGENSEN, 1973).

The mechanisms responsible for initiating a new ovarian cycle after spawning are not well understood. As mentioned, day length is not of decisive importance. Temperature is of importance, but presumably mainly indirectly. The environmental temperature must be high enough for the toads to feed. Resumed feeding after spawning will restore energy reserves in the body. It may primarily be the nutritional state that determines when gonadotropic structures are activated after spawning and initiate an ovarian cycle.

In nature, if the gonadotropic central nervous structures have not become activated before late summer, some mechanism seems to build up, preventing the activation of the structures during that season. The nature of the mechanisms is not known, but it may involve an endogenous rhythm (JØRGENSEN, 1975).

The completion of the ovarian cycle depends upon the maintenance of the active state of the gonadotropic central nervous structures. This active state appears to be labile and sensitive to adverse environmental factors, including lack of food (JØRGENSEN, 1970).

Toads exposed to the artificial environment of the laboratory tended to exhibit irregular ovarian cycles, often associated with atresia of large oocytes. Such abnormalities in ovarian function in the laboratory are presumably secondary to deficiencies in gonadotropin secretion, which again reflects deficient function of the gonadotropic central nervous structures. This interpretation is supported by the finding that the adverse effects of the laboratory environment on the ovarian cycle may be totally compensated if the toads are hypophysectomized and the ovarian cycles are initiated and maintained by administration of exogenous gonadotropin (JØRGENSEN, 1973).

Temperature again becomes an important environmental factor in controlling the ovarian cycle during the fall, when decreasing temperature protects the large follicles from degenerating and enhances their maturation. If the toads are kept at abnormally high temperatures during the fall and winter, the follicles degenerate. This does not necessarily mean that the gonadotropic structures have become inactivated, because the large atretic oocytes are immediately replaced by new oocytes entering the final growth stage. The high temperature may, therefore, act at the peripheral level, the ovary, rather than at the central level, the gonadotropic central nervous structures.

The exposure to low temperature during hibernation presumably determines the normal time course of the ovarian cycle in toad populations in nature. The finding that toads may breed when kept during winter at temperatures of 13°C or more shows, however, that hibernation, or exposure to low temperatures are not indispensable environmental factors for oocyte maturation and ovulation in *Bufo bufo bufo* populations in Denmark. It remains to be seen whether populations of *Bufo bufo bufo* in Denmark and *Bufo bufo asiaticus* in the Shanghai region (SU and YU-LAN, 1963a, b) differ in the role low temperature during winter and/or hibernation plays in follicle maturation.

The timing of breeding is presumably controlled by environmental factors, of which temperature is one, as well as an endogenous rhythm (HEUSSER, 1968b, c). By analogy with observations made in other vertebrates, it may be assumed that ovulation results from passing high rates of gonadotropin secretion (Fig. 1). This assumption agrees with the finding that the dose of hCG needed to induce ovulation in sexually mature female toads in the spring is about 10 times higher than the dosage level needed to produce normal growth of oocytes in the final growth stage in the ovaries of hypophysectomized toads (JØRGENSEN, 1973).

References

BARTHÉLÉMY, H.: Recherches biométriques et expérimentales sur l'hibernation, la maturation et la surmaturation de la Grenouille rousse ♀ (*Rana fusca*). C.R. Acad. Sci. (Paris) 182, 1653-1654 (1926)

BRENNER, F.J., BRENNER, P.E.: The influence of light and temperature on body fat and reproductive conditions of *Rana pipiens*. Ohio J. Sci. 69, 305-312 (1969)

BUSH, F.M.: Effects of light and temperature on the gross composition of the toad, *Bufo fowleri*. J. Exp. Zool. 153, 1-13 (1963)

HEUSSER, H.: Die Lebensweise der Erdkröte, *Bufo bufo* (L.). Der Magenfüllungsgrad in Abhängigkeit von Jagdstimmung und Wetter. Sitzungsber. Ges. Naturf. Freunde Berlin 8, 148-156 (1968a)

HEUSSER, H.: Die Lebensweise der Erdkröte *Bufo bufo* (L.); Wanderungen und Sommerquartiere. Rev. Suisse Zool. 75, 927-982 (1968b)

HEUSSER, H.: Die Lebensweise der Erdkröte, *Bufo bufo* (L.); Laichzeit: Umstimmung, Ovulation, Verhalten. Vierteljahrsschr. Naturforsch. Ges. Zürich 113, 257-289 (1968c)

HOLZAPFEL, R.A.: The cyclic character of hibernation in frogs. Quart. Rev. Biol. 12, 65-84 (1937)

JØRGENSEN, C.B.: Hypothalamic control of hypophysial function in anurans. In: The Hypothalamus. Martini, L., Motta, M., Fraschini, F. (eds.). New York: Academic Press, 1970, pp. 649-661

JØRGENSEN, C.B.: Pattern of recruitment of oocytes to second growth phase in normal toads, and in hypophysectomized toads, *Bufo bufo bufo* (L.), treated with gonadotropin (HCG). Gen. Comp. Endocrinol. 21, 152-159 (1973)

JØRGENSEN, C.B.: Factors controlling the annual ovarian cycle in the toad *Bufo bufo bufo* (L.). Gen. Comp. Endocrinol. 25, 264-273 (1975)

MIZELL, S.: Seasonal differences in spermatogenesis and oogenesis in *Rana pipiens*. Nature (London) 202, 875-876 (1964)

SU, T., YU-LAN, W.: L'hibernation, facteur detèrminant de la maturation ovulaire chez le crapaud (*Bufo bufo asiaticus*). Sci. Sinica 12, 1161-1164 (1963a)

SU, T., YU-LAN, W.: La succession d'ovogenèse et l'impossibilité de maturation ovulaire chez le crapaud femelle élevée dans le milieu à haute température pendant toute une année. Sci. Sinica 12, 1165-1168 (1963b)

VIJAYAKUMAR, S., JØRGENSEN, C.B., KJAER, K.: Regulation of ovarian cycle in the toad *Bufo bufo bufo* (L.): Effects of autografting pars distalis of the hypophysis, of extirpating gonadotropic hypothalamic region, and of partial ovariectomy. Gen. Comp. Endocrinol. 17, 432-443 (1971)

5. Reptilian Reproductive Cycles and Environmental Regulators

B. LOFTS

Introduction

Reptiles generally have precise seasonal reproductive patterns. Only for some tropical species is there occasional reference to continuous breeding throughout the year. Thus, CHURCH (1962) has observed continuous breeding in several species of geckos in Java; and in Malaysia, BERRY and LIM (1967) have noted females of the aquatic, ovoviviparous snake, *Hopolopsis buccatta*, with large ovarian follicles and oviducal eggs during every month. Even in the tropics, however, many reptiles have seasonal reproductive patterns. The female equatorial lizard, *Agama agama lionotus*, for example, produces eggs only in July and August in Kenya, even though males have testes with bunched spermatozoa throughout the year (MARSHALL and HOOK, 1960). Sperm production throughout the year has also been reported in other tropical and semitropical lizards (e.g., LICHT and GORMAN, 1970). In Hong Kong waters, a well-marked seasonal pattern in testis weight occurs in the sea snake *Hydrophis cyanocinctus*, even though spermatozoa are present in the seminiferous tubules in every month. The peak occurs in December, followed by a decline to a minimum level in March. Presumably this decline in testis weight is due to a reduction in the rate of germ-cell propagation, but whether this also reduces fertility is not known.

The extensive literature on the reproductive patterns in reptiles has been excellently reviewed by SAINT GIRONS (1963) and FITCH (1970). Temperate-zone species copulate shortly after the emergence from hibernation in the spring, and in females, this is followed by a fairly rapid vitellogenic growth of the follicles with ovulation and egg laying in May or June. Young are usually born in late summer. Some of the ovoviviparous *Sceloporus* lizards are a notable exception in that follicular development and ovulation occur later in the year, before hibernation, and the young are born in the following spring or early summer. In males, following the copulatory phase, the testes regress and seminiferous tubules become spermatogenetically inactive. The duration of this sexual quiescence varies from species to species. In some it is comparatively brief, and a recrudescence of spermatogenetic activity occurs in late summer. The degree of spermatogenetic advancement reached before winter differs among species. In others, the gonads remain quiescent throughout the winter, and spermatogenesis resumes in early spring.

Some colubrid snakes and turtles breed at the time at which the testes are sexually regressed. Spermatozoa come from an epididymal reservoir in which they have remained over winter.

Endogenous Reproductive Cycles

It has frequently been claimed that some reptiles possess an endogenous reproductive rhythm that is largely independent of external environmental influence. That some reptiles breed in captivity at the same time of year as in their natural environment, though experiencing different changes in day length and ambient temperature at different latitudes, has sometimes been put forward as evidence that such an endogenous rhythm exists. Experimentally, FISCHER (1968) has demonstrated that male *Lacerta sicula campestris* kept in continuous darkness at 5°C from late summer onwards, show some testicular recrudescence in the following March at about the same time as the naturally occurring event. Specimens kept under constant 14-h daily photophases at 28°-30°C also recovered spontaneously in March. The desert iguana, *Dipsosaurus dorsalis*, also has been shown to recover spermatogenetic activity at the normal time of year when maintained under constant conditions of temperature and day length beginning from the time of estival regression of the testes (LICHT, 1971a).

It is perhaps premature to conclude from such data that an endogenous circannual reproductive rhythm exists in reptiles; since in many cases in which such claims have been made, information of other environmental parameters, such as rainfall or seasonal availability of food, is lacking. In *Agama agama*, for example, seasonal breeding in females is timed by the appearance of insects used as food. The duration of investigations have generally been insufficient to determine whether further cycles would occur in succeeding years. In the case of *Dipsosaurus*, for example, only one single specimen out of fifteen apparently showed some signs of a second cycle in the following year (LICHT, 1971a). More research needs to be done to demonstrate unequivocally the presence of a circannual rhythm.

Day Length and Ambient Temperature

The evidence in support of exogenous influences on reptilian breeding cycles by day length and temperature, is much stronger, although in many cases, the relative roles played by these two factors is still contentious. Day length has been claimed to be the most important environmental regulator in several species of lizards (review by LICHT, 1971a) and in the turtle *Pseudemys elegans*. However, in many of these early investigations, adequate controls of ambient temperature were lacking and there has often been a failure to recognize that manipulation of the day length may cause changes in ambient temperature that, in turn, influence testicular response. Elevated temperatures alone have been shown to stimulate gonadal development in male *Lacerta sicula* and *L. muralis* (LICHT et al., 1969), and in female *Sceloporus undulatus* (MARION, 1970).

We have been investigating the effects of temperature and day length on the reproductive cycle of the male Chinese cobra, *Naja naja*. Breeding is towards the end of April, after which the testes regress rapidly, and remain spermatogenetically inactive until late August. In January seminiferous tubules are well stocked with spermatocytes and occasional spermatids. At this time of year, specimens kept at a January day length (11.25 h), but subjected to April temperatures (22°C) for four weeks, show a significant increase in testicular weight (Fig. 1) compared with controls kept under similar day length, but maintained at a January temperature (15°C). In a second experiment, two groups kept at

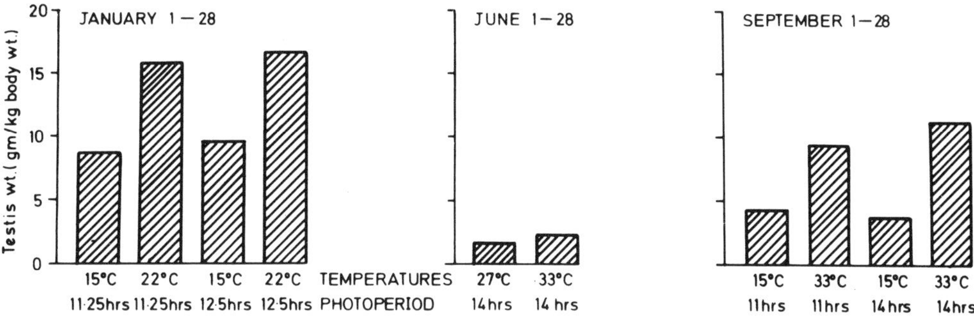

Fig. 1. The effects of ambient temperature and day length on the testicular cycle of the cobra. High temperatures in the spring accelerate testicular development, but different photophases have no effect. During the period of testicular regression higher temperatures and longer daily photophases have no effect, but during the autumn recovery phase, higher ambient temperature stimulates testicular recrudescence

15°C and 22°C, respectively, but maintained under an April day length (12.5 h), again showed an acceleration of testicular development at the higher temperature only. There appeared to be no significant difference in the mean testis size of the two high-temperature groups. When the effects of temperature and day length were investigated on sexually regressed snakes in June, specimens exposed to a high summer temperature of 33°C (6°C above the mean monthly temperature) and a maximum Hong Kong day length of 14 h, remained unstimulated. However, in September an acceleration of testicular development was achieved with 33°C even in a group kept under a mid-December day length of 11 h. A contralateral group kept at 15°C (mid-December mean) and under 14-h daily photophase, however, failed to show significant testicular development.

Thus, it would appear that in *Naja*, environmental temperature may be the major exogenous regulatory factor in the testicular cycle. Thus, increasing ambient temperature in the spring, therefore, may stimulate the hypothalamo-hypophysial-gonad axis into full sexual activity. A spontaneous thermorefractory period, analogous to the photorefractory phase of many avian species may be responsible for the sudden regression in May, and persists until approximately the end of August. In Hong Kong, environmental temperature remains high until well into November. Because of a recovery of thermal sensitivity in September, these high temperatures possibly stimulate a recrudescence of spermatogenetic activity which then declined during the colder winter months. Evidence of gonadal refractoriness has also been found in lizards (*Xantusia vigilis*, BARTHOLOMEW, 1953; *Uta stansburiana*, TINKLE and IRWIN, 1965).

The cobra cycle is very similar to that of two European lizards *Lacerta sicula* and *L. muralis* (LICHT et al., 1969). In these species, changes in experimental day length had no effect on the annual testicular cycle, whereas temperature fluctuations greatly affected them. In these two species, however, testicular activity developed later in the year than in *Naja*, and regression did not occur until July. LICHT and colleagues calculated that the thermorefractory period lasts until the end of December. The data differ from those for the cobra in one respect. In *Lacerta* the testes regressed on transferral to high temperatures in autumn, whereas lower temperatures had a stimulatory effect. This difference between the lizards and cobra may be due to the earlier termination of the thermorefractory phase in the latter. The lizards remained refractory until January; when exposed to high temperatures in this month, resticular development was stimulated in just the same way as in the cobra at the termination of its refractory phase.

Although the results of LICHT et al. (1969) indicate that day length is unlikely to be an important timing cue in *Lacerta*, some more recent data of FISCHER and EWALD (1972) suggest that day length may have a modifying effect on the duration of the refractory phase. At constant high temperatures (28°-30°C) refractory male *L. sicula* kept under different daily photophases (14, 16 and 18 h) regained their spermatogenetic activity at different times; and the longer the daily photophase the greater the delay. With an 18-h daily photophase, gonadal recrudescence was delayed for two months after the natural event.

Whereas the data on *Naja* and *Lacerta* suggest that fluctuations on ambient temperature are probably the major proximate timing cues in these species, the extensive investigations carried out by LICHT (1971a, b) on *Anolis carolinensis* have demonstrated a complex, seasonally changing interaction between day length and ambient temperature. There is a clear photoperiodic response to decreasing day lengths between July and October. This is the time of year in which testicular regression occurs in this species, and although exposure to high summer temperatures of 32°C does not prevent it, artificially increased day length will restimulate testicular development. Apparently, photosensitivity is then lost, and the regenerative phase of spermatogenesis between late autumn and spring is controlled primarily by ambient temperature (LICHT, 1971b).

Rainfall

Rainfall does not appear to act as a major timing cue in temperate-zone species; also in tropical reptiles, testicular cycles appear to be independent of seasonal rainfall. However, rainfall seems to be important for the female cycle, and appears to act as a timing cue for the regulation of egg production in some tropical species. LICHT and GORMAN (1970) have demonstrated a strong correlation between egg production and rainfall in several tropical species of *Anolis* on the Caribbean Islands, particularly in *A. grahami*, *A. lineatopus* and *A. sagrei*, and we have found a similar correlation in the cobra (LANCE and LOFTS, unpublished results). The cobras of the Kwantung Province of Southern China and Hong Kong have a conspicuous maximal ovarian weight during March to April. Vitellogenesis begins about mid-April and ovulation occurs in late May or early June, with oviposition occurring some two weeks later. By the end of July the ovaries and oviducts regress to a nonbreeding condition, and remain quiescent until the following March. The young are born in late August or September. The deposition of eggs in May to June in Hong Kong coincides with the beginning of the summer monsoon rains; a similar coincidence also occurs in India (May-June), Java (September-October) and Ceylon (January-February). Whether rainfall per se is the proximate factor, or whether the accompanying increase in humidity is the cue, is not known. Recently BROWN and SEXTON (1973) have demonstrated that humidity can be a controlling factor in reproduction in *Anolis sagrei*. In Costa Rica this lizard has an annual breeding cycle that coincides with the annual rainy season. These investigators have shown that experimental manipulation of ambient temperature and day length fails to stimulate reproduction; but with ambient temperature and daily photophase constant, egg laying can be induced when the humidity is held above 75%. Egg laying is greatly reduced at a humidity of approximately 25%.

Endocrine Cycles

Based on data obtained from a series of investigations involving bioassays and the observed effects of exogenous mammalian and avian FSH and LH on lizards and turtles (summarized by LICHT, 1972), LICHT and colleagues have proposed that the functions of both interstitial tissue and seminiferous tubules in reptiles is under the control of a single gonadotropic hormone of an FSH-like nature, and that the secretion of this single hormone is modified by the seasonal temperature cycle. They suggest that ambient temperature affects the sensitivity of the target tissues so that they may respond, at different times in temporal sequence, to this single gonadotropic hormone. Thus, it is suggested that in the natural cycle low ambient temperature suppresses circulating gonadotropins, so that only the early stages of spermatogenesis occur in response, and so that development of the accessory structures is prevented. Increasing ambient temperature in spring stimulates increased gonadotropin release, leading to a rapid completion of spermatogenesis and a restimulation of the interstitial cells with a consequent hypertrophy of the epididymis and sex segment of the kidney.

In this context, it is worth drawing attention to earlier investigations on frogs, where maintenance of *Rana temporaria* (VAN OORDT and LOFTS, 1963) and *R. esculenta* (DE KORT and VAN OORDT, 1965) at high temperatures in winter induced stimulation of spermatogenetic activity with a concomitant suppression of activity of the interstitial cells. Furthermore, DE KORT (1971) demonstrated in addition that injections of mammalian LH into *R. esculenta* had a much greater effect at lower than at higher ambient temperature.

Confirmation that lower ambient temperatures stimulate secretion of gonadotropic hormone during the winter regenerative phase of *Anolis carolinensis* has recently been produced by investigations on the pituitary-gonad axis, involving observations at both the light and electron microscopy level of pituitary, testes, accessory sexual organs, together with radioimmunoassay measurements on plasma testosterone levels (PEARSON et al., 1976). The results demonstrated that production of gonadotropins in *Anolis* was stimulated at 20°C in late winter. Plasma testosterone levels in this group were higher than in a second group kept at 31°C, but evoked only a limited response in the epididymis and renal sex tubules. Testicular enlargement occurred at both temperatures, but whereas 31°C stimulated full spermatogenetic activity, spermatogenesis was blocked at the spermatocyte level at lower temperature. At the higher temperature plasma testosterone levels were lower, but accessory sexual structures were more sensitive to androgen and showed better development.

In the case of the cobra, it is unnecessary to speculate that differential sensitivities of the two testicular tissues to a single gonadotropin, since the functional activity of both follow a parallel seasonal cycle. The seasonal pattern of testicular androgen synthesis, based on in vitro estimations using labeled precursors and chromatographic analysis, indicate a close correlation between testosterone synthesis and spermatogenesis. Such a pattern would suggest an increasing output of gonadotropic hormone(s) with increasing temperatures in spring, an abrupt cessation as animals become thermorefractory, and a resumption of secretion following the termination of refractoriness. Increasing levels of secretion occur during the warm autumn months of Southern China and Hong Kong (mean September temperature is 27.1°C, then decline during the colder months of the December-February period (17°-15°C).

The Male Soft-Shelled Turtle, *Trionyx sinensis*

This animal has a spermatogenetic cycle that recrudesces immediately after the copulatory period in April and is completed by early autumn. The spermatozoa are evacuated from the seminiferous tubules and are stored in the epididymal canals over winter. In spring, at the time of breeding, the seminiferous tubules are completely regressed and spermatogenetically inactive, but the adjacent interstitium is highly active. About a month after breeding, the situation is completely reversed, and spermatogenetic activity builds up parallel to the decline of interstitial cell activity (LOFTS and TSUI, 1977). In this species, therefore, the cycle does not fit the concept of differing target tissue sensitivities suggested by LICHT and colleagues. The increasing temperatures from April onwards stimulate spermatogenetic activity while, at the same time, interstitial tissue activity is inhibited. This is therefore, the reverse of that proposed for *Anolis*, and is more analogous to the observed experimental effects in amphibians. However, it is unclear as to how such a differing sensitivity to temperature could be applied to the August-October part of the *Trionyx* cycle. The mean monthly temperatures over these three months vary by only about 3°C (27.7°-24.6°C) and are higher than the mean temperature in May (25.2°C), yet this is the time of year when the active propagation of new germinal cells has more or less ceased and rehabilitation of interstitial cells and synthesis of testosterone are increasing (LOFTS, 1977). In other words, the reverse of the May events.

In attempting to evaluate the relevance of thermal effects on the cycles of the snake and turtle, I am conscious of the fact that I have not taken into account any behavioral patterns. It is well established that reptiles exercise considerable control over their body temperatures by utilizing behavioral means, and it is conceivable that a change in behavior could have altered the internal body temperatures, and thus affect physiologic mechanisms, even when environmental temperatures remain high. Evidently, there is a need for further research along these lines before any firm conclusions can be reached. There is also a need for the application of immunoreactive techniques for establishing in vivo hormone levels and determining the effects that changes in day length and ambient temperature changes have on them.

References

BARTHOLOMEW, G.A.: The modification by temperature of the photoperiodic control of gonadal development in the lizard *Xantusia vigilis*. Copeia 1953, 45-50 (1953)

BERRY, P.Y., LIM, G.S.: The breeding pattern of the puff-faced water snake *Homalopsis buccata* Boulenger. Copeia 2, 307-313 (1967)

BROWN, K.M., SEXTON, O.J.: Stimulation of reproductive activity of female *Anolis sagrei* by moisture. Physiol. Zool 46, 168-172 (1973)

BURGER, J.W.: Experimental sexual photoperiodicity in the male turtle *Pseudemys elegans* (Wied). Am. Nat. 71, 481-487 (1937)

CHURCH, G.: The reproductive cycles of the Javanese house geckos, *Cosymbotus platyurus*, *Hemidactylus frenatus* and *Peropus mutilatus*. Copeia 2, 262-269 (1962)

FISCHER, K.: Untersuchungen zur Jahresperiodik der Fortpflanzung bei männlichen Ruineneidechsen (*Lacerta sicula campestris* Betta). I. Die Refraktärperiode. Z. Vergl. Physiol. 60, 244-268 (1968a)

FISCHER, K.: Untersuchungen zur Jahresperiodik der Fortpflanzung bei männlichen Ruineneidechsen (*Lacerta sicula campestris* Betta). II. Einflüsse verschiedener Photoperioden und Temperaturen auf die Progressions- und die Regressionsphase. Z. Vergl. Physiol. 61, 394-419 (1968b)

FISCHER, K., EWALD, R.: Untersuchungen zur Jahresperiodik der Fortpflanzung bei männlichen Ruineneidechsen (*Lacerta sicula campestris* Betta). IV. Langzeiteinwirkung verschiedener, langer Photoperioden bei 28-30°C von der Refraktärperiode an. J. Comp. Physiol. 77, 190-207 (1972)

FITCH, H.S.: Reproductive cycles in lizards and snakes. Univ. Kansas Mus. Nat. Hist. Misc. Publ. 52, 1-247 (1970)

KORT, E.J.M. DE: Het interstitium testis bij de groene kikker, *Rana esculenta*. Een histometrisch en histochemisch onderzoek. Terborg, the Netherlands: Thesis Utrecht Publ. Lammers and Zn., 1971

KORT, E.J.M. DE, OORDT, P.G.W.J. VAN: The effects of high temperature upon the testes and thumb pads in the green frog, *Rana esculenta*. Gen. Comp. Endocrin. 9, 692-693 (1965)

LICHT, P.: Problems in experimentation on timing mechanisms for annual physiological cycles in reptiles. In: Hibernation and Hypothermia. South, F. (ed.). Amsterdam: Elsevier, 1971a, pp. 681-711

LICHT, P.: Regulation of the annual testis cycle by photoperiod and temperature in the lizard *Anolis carolinensis*. Ecology 52, 240-252 (1971b)

LICHT, P.: Environmental physiology of reptilian breeding cycles: Role of temperature. Gen. Comp. Endocrin. Suppl. 3, 477-488 (1972)

LICHT, P., GORMAN, G.C.: Reproductive and fat cycles in Caribbean *Anolis* lizards. Univ. Calif. Publ. Zool. 95, 1-52 (1970)

LICHT, P., HOYER, H.E., OORDT, P.G.W.J. VAN: Influence of photoperiod and temperature on testicular recrudescence and body growth in the lizards, *Lacerta sicula* and *Lacerta muralis*. J. Zool. 157, 467-501 (1969)

LOFTS, B.: Patterns of spermatogenesis and steroidogenesis in male reptiles. In: Reproduction and Evolution. Calaby, J.H., Tyndale-Biscoe, C.H. (eds.). Canberra: Australian Acad. Sci., 1977, pp. 127-136

LOFTS, B., TSUI, H.W.: Histological and histochemical changes in the gonads and epididymides of the male soft-shelled turtle, *Trionyx sinensis*. J. Zool. 181, 57-68 (1977)

MARION, K.R.: Temperature as the reproductive cue for the female fence lizard *Sceloporus undulatus*. Copeia 1970, 562-564 (1970)

MARSHALL, A.J., HOOK, R.: The breeding biology of equatorial vertebrates: Reproduction of the lizard *Agama agama lionotus* Boulenger at lat. 0° 01'N. Proc. Zool. Lond. 134, 197-205 (1960)

OORDT, P.G.W.J. VAN, LOFTS, B.: The effects of high temperature on gonadotropin secretion in the male common frog (*Rana temporaria*) during autumn. J. Endocrinol. 27, 137-146 (1963)

PEARSON, A.K., TSUI, H.W., LICHT, P.: Effect of temperature on spermatogenesis, on the production and action of androgens and on the ultrastructure of gonadotropic cells in the lizard *Anolis carolinensis*. J. Exp. Zool. 195, 291-304 (1976)

SAINT GIRONS, H.: Spermatogènese et evolution cyclique des caractères sexuels secondaires chez les squamata. Ann. Sci. Nat. Zool. 5, 461-478 (1963)

TINKLE, D.W., IRWIN, L.N.: Lizard reproduction: refractory period and response to warmth in *Uta stansburiana* females. Science 148, 1613-1614 (1965)

6. Environmental Endocrinology and the Control of Annual Reproductive Cycles in Passerine Birds

D. S. FARNER and J. C. WINGFIELD

The endocrine glands and the hormones secreted by them are components of a communication system that, among other functions, is involved in adjustment to changes in the external environment. The spectrum of such adjustments in endocrine functions induced by changes in the environment ranges from rather direct adjustments such as those involved in osmoregulation or thermoregulation to those involved in periodic reproductive function. The latter are the subject of this communication.

A substantial fraction of the more than 8600 contemporary species of birds live in annually periodic environments. Natural selection has favored the survival of populations and species in which individual reproductive effort is timed so that young are produced at the time of the year in which the probability of survival is optimized. Despite the gross simplification involved, there is perhaps some heuristic merit in the designation of two very different possible bases for the attainment of reproductive function at the optimal time:

Near-Tonic Control Systems

Maintenance of the reproductive system in a near-functional state permits the direct and rapid induction of reproductive function by those environmental conditions that enhance survival of the young. Natural selection would operate against such systems in areas of reasonably precise annual environmental periodicities because they are energetically wasteful, and would not be consistent with the evolution of migration and the enhancement of reproductive potential that it confers. Nevertheless, although experimental evidence is sparse, it appears that systems that approach this type must occur in at least some species of the Australian deserts in which seasons are aperiodic (FARNER, 1967; IMMELMANN, 1963; SERVENTY, 1971).

Annually Periodic Control Systems

These systems permit the gonads and accessory reproductive organs to remain in a relatively quiescent state for most of the year, and to become functional only briefly at the time that maximizes the probability of survival of the young. A common characteristic of these systems is their dependence on periodic environmental information. The time that must elapse between the onset of development of the quiescent reproductive system and the hatching or onset of independence of the young is usually a matter of at least several weeks. It therefore follows that the environmental information that induces the onset of reproductive function must have a precise temporal relationship with the time of optimal conditions for the survival of the young, i.e., it must have a predictive quality (FARNER, 1970a). As first stated clearly by BAKER (1938), it is necessary to distinguish two important sets of environmental factors with respect to annually periodic reproductive cycles. The ultimate environmental factors are those that select those individuals that produce young at the optimal time for survival. The proximate factors are those that constitute the information that causes gonadal development that results in the production of young at the time at which the probability of survival is maximal. Proximal factors have been discussed usefully and in some detail by IMMELMANN (1963, 1973).

Among the proximal factors our knowledge is almost overwhelmingly limited to day length. Indeed it is the single known proximal factor that has been subjected to extensive experimental investigation (DOLNIK, 1976; FARNER and LEWIS, 1971; LOFTS and MURTON, 1968). This great bias on the investigation of the role of day length is doubtless due to the ease with which it can be manipulated experimentally and the residence of most avian endocrinologists and their experimental facilities in mid-latitudes where, for most species of birds, day length is the primary source of environmental information in the control of annual cycles.

As early as the 17th century, Dutch bird netters had learned that song associated with reproductive activity could be induced in autumn in the males of several passerine species by holding them in darkness from May until August and then returning them to natural day length (HOOS, 1937). These singing males were used to decoy southward migrants into nets. However, the first scientific demonstration of the role of day length in the control of gonadotropic function was that of ROWAN (1925) in experiments on *Junco hyemalis*. Much of the extensive literature on photoperiodic control systems in passerine birds has been reviewed by DOLNIK (1975a, 1976), FARNER and LEWIS (1971) and LOFTS and MURTON (1968).

In this communication we illustrate the role of day length as a proximate environmental factor that provides predictive information for the gonadotropic function of the hypothalamo-hypophysial system. We draw heavily on our own investigations on the White-Crowned Sparrow, *Zonotrichia leucophrys*. In making this choice we must, for at least two reasons, urge caution with respect to generalization concerning the passeriform species as a group. First, annual reproductive cycles occur in many species of the tropics and subtropics in which the small or negligible changes in day length can scarcely serve as a source of information. Second, it is highly probable that photoperiodic control systems within the order Passeriformes are of multiple evolutionary origin (FARNER, 1964). Indeed the differences among those of *Passer domesticus*, *Zonotrichia leucophrys* and *Sturnus vulgaris* are sufficiently great to make it very probable that they were independently evolved (FARNER et al., 1977).

As in the other photoperiodic species that have been adequately investigated (e.g., BENOIT, 1970; MENAKER and KEATTS, 1971; McMILLAN et al., 1975; HOMMA and SAKAKIBARA, 1971), photoreceptors of the photoperiodic control system of *Zonotrichia leucophrys* are primarily, if not exclusively, hypothalamic (YOKOYAMA and FARNER, 1976; YOKOYAMA et al., 1978) rather than retinal. Indeed, in female *Z. leucophrys* the retina may transmit information that inhibits the secretion of luteinizing hormone and the final development of the ovary (YOKOYAMA and FARNER, 1976).

When male *Zonotrichia leucophrys* are subjected experimentally to constant daily, 9-h or longer, photophases at intensities of 200 lux or greater, the testes increase in weight from the resting state of 2 mg to the fully developed and functional state with a weight of 400-500 mg. Until a weight of 250 mg is attained, growth is a logarithmic function of time. The logarithmic growth-rate constant is a positive function of the duration of the daily photophase over the range of 9-20 h (FARNER, 1975). These laboratory-established testicular growth rates predict well the development of the testes under natural conditions for *Zonotrichia leucophrys*, *Fringilla chloris* and *Fringilla coelebs* (DOLNIK, 1963), and other species (FARNER and LEWIS, 1971). Although we do not have direct evidence, because of the lack of an adequate assay, it is reasonable to assume that the testicular growth induced by long days is caused by an increase in the plasma level of FSH (FOLLETT, 1976). We have established in *Zonotrichia leucophrys* that long days cause an increase in the plasma level of LH (FOLLETT et al., 1975), that the level is a direct function of the length of the daily photophase (MATTOCKS and FARNER, unpublished), and that the level of testosterone is a direct but complex function of the level of LH.

Because the logarithmic rate of testicular growth and the plasma level of LH are both positive functions of the duration of the daily photophase, it follows that the system must have a component that measures the duration of the daily photophase. It appears (FOLLETT et al., 1974; FARNER, 1965, 1975) in *Zonotrichia leucophrys* that this is effected by an external coincidence system involving an entrained circadian cycle in photosensitivity, consistent with the hypothesis originally proposed by BÜNNING (1936) and formulated more precisely by PITTENDRIGH and MINIS (1964). Similar conclusions have been reached for other photoperiodic passerine species (FARNER, 1975). DOLNIK (1976), however, has proposed that day length is measured in *Fringilla coelebs* and *Passer domesticus* by a two-oscillator internal-coincidence system, similar in principle to that proposed by TYSHCHENKO (1966) to explain the photoperiodic control of diapause in some species of insects. The available information suggests, however, that a hypothesis of this complexity may be unnecessary for the photoperiodic species of birds thus far investigated.

There is now substantial literature (e.g., BERTHOLD, 1974, 1977; DOLNIK, 1974, 1975a, b, 1976; GWINNER, 1968, 1973, 1975, 1977) on certain species of passerine birds that appears to support the concept (ASCHOFF, 1955; IMMELMANN, 1963) that annual cycles in birds are entrained endogenous circennial cycles, and that in the photoperiodic species the role of day length as a source of information is that of a Zeitgeber, which entrains the circennial cycle to a period of one year, rather than a more direct role of generating or driving the annual cycle. There are difficulties in a general application of this hypothesis. Basically the occurrence of an endogenous cycle can be established only by its persistence through several periods in constant conditions. However, a very large fraction of the data that appear to support the concept of endogenous circennial cycles comes from experiments in which birds have been held on 24-h light-dark cycles with photophases of constant duration. Does this constitute the constant conditions necessary for demonstration of an endogenous periodicity? If birds, like some species of insects, can "count" daily light-dark cycles, then day length of constant duration certainly cannot be regarded as a constant condition for testing the hypothesis. Furthermore, general application of the hypothesis includes in a single scheme systems of diverse evolutionary origins, some of which, such as in *Zonotrichia leucophrys*, are clearly driven basically by an environmental cycle such as that of day length. Semantic difficulties arise because, in many species, such as *Fringilla coelebs* and *Z. leucophrys*, the cyclic events of late summer are indirect sequelae of the long days of spring (DOLNIK, 1976; FARNER, 1964). It is perhaps heuristically useful to consider, without evolutionary implications, a spectrum that ranges from truly endogenous cycles that are merely entrained by annually periodic environmental cycles to those largely or entirely dependent on environmental cycles recognizing that there may be very different "damping" constants among them when they are subjected to constant conditions (FARNER and LEWIS, 1973; KING and FARNER, 1974).

In the control of annual reproductive cycles mechanisms that terminate reproductive function are second in importance only to the mechanisms that initiate gonadotropic function. In *Zonotrichia leucophrys* (FARNER, 1964), as in at least some of the other passerine species (e.g., LOFTS and MURTON, 1968; FARNER and LEWIS, 1971; DOLNIK, 1974, 1975a), this is effected by the development of photorefractoriness, a state in which no known pattern of illumination induces gonadotropic function and whose etiology is unknown. Since castrated birds become photorefractory (MATTOCKS et al., 1976) it is necessary to conclude tentatively that photorefractoriness is induced somehow by long days (FARNER, 1964; DOLNIK and GAVRILOV, 1972) but without the involvement of a negative feedback from the gonads. The site of photorefractoriness is either at hypothalamic or higher level in the brain (ERICKSON, 1975; FARNER, 1970b). Whatever its etiology may be, the onset of photorefractoriness in *Zonotrichia leucophrys* is followed by a regression in the gonads because of reduced secretion of FSH, and a marked reduction in the plasma levels of LH and sex hormones (LAM and FARNER, 1975; MATTOCKS et al., 1976; WINGFIELD and FARNER, 1977). MEIER and his colleagues (e.g., MEIER, 1976) have accumulated considerable evidence, primarily from experiments with *Zonotrichia albicollis*, from which they propose that the phases of the annual cycle, including photorefractory and photoinducible phases, are controlled by the changing phase angle between daily cycles in the circulating levels of corticosterone and prolactin. This hypothesis has not been tested on other species or in other laboratories.

The recent development of microradioimmunoassays and appropriate field techniques (WINGFIELD and FARNER, 1976) has permitted an expanded basis for examination of the applicability in nature of conclusions drawn from laboratory experiments. In our combined laboratory and field investigations we have accumulated information on the annual cycle in gonadal development and the levels of LH, sex hormones and corticosterone in the plasma in the northwestern race of the White-crowned Sparrow, *Zonotrichia leucophrys gambelii*, which breeds principally in Alaska and the Yukon, and winters principally in southern California, Arizona and New Mexico.

In the males of *Z. l. gambelii* the plasma concentration of immunoreactive luteinizing hormone (irLH) begins to increase in March and April from a winter level of no greater than approximately 1 ng/ml and continues to increase through migration to reach a maximum of about 5 ng/ml on the breeding grounds in the Fairbanks area in Alaska (64°N) in late May and early June. This maximum level of plasma LH is coincident with the maximum weight and development of the testes, with the maximum plasma levels of testosterone (4-5 ng/ml), and with courtship behavior and defense of territory. During the incubation period there is a precipitous decline in plasma concentration of testosterone to ca. 1 ng/ml although the male does not participate in the incubation of the clutch. This decrease in testosterone is accompanied by a marked reduction in frequency of song and by a sharp decrease in territorial encounters. There is also a less precipitous decline in the concentration of irLH to ca. 3 ng/ml. By the time of the post-nuptial molt in July plasma irLH and testosterone reach basal levels of ca. 1 ng/ and ca. 0.1 ng/ml, respectively.

Females arrive in the breeding territories with plasma levels of irLH (ca. 3 ng/ml), estradiol (ca. 250 pg/ml), and estrone (ca. 250 pg/ml) that are substantially higher than in winter (less than 1 ng/ml of irLH, and undetectable levels, i.e., less than 50 pg/ml, of estrone and estradiol). They attain maximum concentrations (ca. 5 ng/ml irLH, ca. 800 pg/ml estradiol, and estrone combined) during courtship and egg-laying. The plasma level of testosterone also becomes maximal (ca. 0.4 ng/ml) at this time in a temporal pattern similar to that of males but at a lower level. Females participate in territorial defense. During incubation and feeding of the young the plasma levels of irLH, estrone, and estradiol decline, reaching basal levels during the post-nuptial molt.

In both sexes the decrease in plasma concentration of irLH coincides with the onset of photorefractoriness. The levels of all hormones studied are generally low throughout autumn and winter.

It is not possible in this brief communication to present an adequate integration of the results of our investigations in laboratory and field on the control of the reproductive cycle of *Z. l. gambelii*. Since we lack quantitative data on FSH and prolactin and because we still do not know the etiology of photorefractoriness, our model is incomplete. Nevertheless, it rationalizes sufficiently well the existing quantitative information to be of genuinely heuristic value. It is clear in this species (FARNER, 1964, 1970a, 1975), as in several other photoperiodic passerine species (FARNER and LEWIS, 1971; DOLNIK, 1976), that the development of the testes is almost completely under the control of day length through a photoperiodically induced increase in secretion of FSH. Its endocrine function is regulated, at least in part, through the photoperiodically controlled secretion of LH (LAM and FARNER, 1976; FOLLETT et al., 1975). Although the control system is slightly sensitive to ambient temperature (FARNER and LEWIS, 1973) and to the level of caloric intake (FARNER, LEWIS and MATTOCKS, unpublished), it is unlikely that the natural variation in these factors can effect changes of more than a few days in the temporal course of the annual testicular cycle. Because the testes are maintained in a fully functional state for about a month (KING et al., 1966), the control system is adequately adapted to the range of onset-times of breeding imposed by temporal variations in the annual phenologic cycle of the breeding area.

The situation is different in the female in that the control system has so evolved that the extensive energy involved in the production of the clutch is not committed until the phenologic development of the breeding area has reached the stage that optimizes the chances of success of the reproductive effort. When female *Z. l. gambelii* are subjected to daily photophases of constant stimulatory duration there is logarithmic, apparently FSH-induced, initial slow growth phase of the follicles, the largest attaining a diameter of about 2.5 mm. During this phase the ovary increases in weight from about 5 to about 70 mg (FARNER et al., 1966). This is the maximum development attained by photoperiodic stimulation of intact females in the laboratory and is the phase in which females in nature arrive in the breeding territories. The failure of the ovaries of females held under long-day conditions in the laboratory to continue into the second phase of development during which the follicles grow rapidly with deposition of yolk is associated with an inadequate level of plasma LH, apparently because the control system receives inhibitory information from the retina (YOKOYAMA and FARNER, 1976). Although completely sufficient evidence is lacking, it is now a good hypothesis that the final rapid growth of follicles to ovulatory size, which requires about 5 or 6 days, is brought about by increased secretion of LH induced by such environmental information as a singing male, cortship, availability of nesting material, and other properties of the phenologically appropriate territory (FARNER and LEWIS, 1971).

Thus the female effects the fine temporal adjustment of the onset of reproduction within a temporal frame of two or three weeks although basic timing is controlled overwhelmingly by the continuous use of day length as predictive information beginning in February in the wintering area 4800 km southward!

Acknowledgment. Some of the information presented herein is from a series of investigations supported by grants from the National Science Foundation to the senior author.

References

ASCHOFF, J.: Jahresperiodik der Fortpflanzung beim Warmblütern. Stud. Gen. 8, 742-776 (1955)

BAKER, J.R.: The evolution of the breeding seasons. In: Evolution: Essays on Aspects of Evolutionary Biology. De Beer, G.R. (ed.). London: Oxford University Press, 1938, pp. 161-177

BENOIT, J.: Étude de l'action des radiations visibles sur la gonadostimulation et de leur pénétration intra-crânienne chez le oiseaux et les mammifères. In: La photorégulation de la reproduction chez les oiseaux et les mammifères. Benoît, J., Assenmacher, I. (eds.). Paris: CNRS, 1970, pp. 121-149

BERTHOLD, P.: Endogene Jahresperiodik. Innere Jahreskalender als Grundlage der jahreszeitlichen Orientierung bei Tieren und Pflanzen. Konstanzer Universitätsreden, 1974, 46 pp.

BERTHOLD, P.: Endogene Steuerung des Vogelzugs. In: Ökophysiologische Probleme in der Ornithologie. Berthold, P., Gwinner, E. (eds.). Vogelwarte, 30 (Sonderheft), 4-15 (1977)

BÜNNING, E.: Die endogene Tagesrhythmik als Grundlage der photoperiodischen Reaktion. Ber. Deut. Bot. Ges. 54, 590-607 (1936)

DOLNIK, V.R.: Kolichestvennoe issledovanie zakonomernostei vesennovo rosta semenikov u neskolkikh vidov vyukovykh ptits (Fringillidae). Dokl. Acad. Nauk SSSR 149, 191-193 (1963)

DOLNIK, V.R.: Okologodovaya tsiklichnost migratsionnovo otlozheniya zhira, polovoi aktivnosti i linki pri postoyannykh photoperiodakh u zyablika (*Fringilla coelebs*). Zh. Obshch. Biol. 34, 543-555 (1974)

DOLNIK, V.R.: Fotoperiodicheskii kontrol sezonnykh tsiklov vesa tela, linki i polovoi aktivnosti u zyablikov (*Fringilla coelebs*). Zool. Zhur. 54, 1048-1056 (1975a)

DOLNIK, V.R.: Migratsionnoe Sostoyaniye Ptits. Moscow: Academiya Nauk SSSR, 1975b

DOLNIK, V.R.: Fotoperiodizm u ptits. In: Fotoperiodizm Zhivotnykh i Rastenii. Zaslevsky, V.A. (ed.). Akademiya Nauk SSSR, Leningrad, 1976, pp. 47-81

DOLNIK, V.R., GAVRILOV, V.M.: Fotoperiodicheskie kontrol godovykh tsiklov u zyablika-migranta v predelakh umerennoi zony. Zool. Zhur. 51, 1685-1696 (1972)

ERICKSON, J.E.: Hypothalamic gonadotropin-releasing hormone and the photoperiodic control of the testes of the White-crowned Sparrow, *Zonotrichia leucophrys gambelii*. Doctoral Dissertation, University of Washington, Seattle, 1975

FARNER, D.S.: The photoperiodic control of reproductive cycles in birds. Am. Sci. 52, 137-156 (1964)

FARNER, D.S.: Circadian systems in the photoperiodic responses of vertebrates. In: Circadian Clocks. Aschoff, J. (ed.). Amsterdam: North Holland, 1965, pp. 357-369

FARNER, D.S.: The control of avian reproductive cycles. In: Proc. 14th Int. Ornithol. Cong. Snow, E.S. (ed.). Oxford: Blackwell, 1967, pp. 107-133

FARNER, D.S.: Predictive functions in the control of annual cycles. Environm. Res. 3, 119-131 (1970a)

FARNER, D.S.: Day length as environmental information in the control of reproduction of birds. In: La photorégulation de la reproduction chez les oiseaux et les mammifères. Benoit, J., Assenmacher, I. (eds.). Paris: CNRS, 1970b, pp. 71-91

FARNER, D.S.: Photoperiodic controls in the secretion of gonadotropins in birds. Am. Zool. 15 (Supplement), 117-135 (1975)

FARNER, D.S., DONHAM, R.S., LEWIS, R.A., MATTOCKS, P.W., DARDEN, T.R., SMITH, J.P.: The circadian component in the photoperiodic mechanism of the House Sparrow, *Passer domesticus*. Physiol. Zool. 50, 247-268 (1977)

FARNER, D.S., FOLLETT, B.K., KING, J.R., MORTON, M.L.: A quantitative examination of ovarian growth in the White-crowned Sparrow. Biol. Bull. 130, 67-75 (1966)

FARNER, D.S., LEWIS, R.A.: Photoperiodism and reproductive cycles in birds. Photophysiology 6, 325-370 (1971)

FARNER, D.S., LEWIS, R.A.: Field and experimental studies of the annual cycles of White-crowned Sparrows. In: The Environment and Reproduction in Mammals and Birds. Perry, J.S., Rolands, I.W. (eds.). J. Repr. Fert., Suppl. 19, 1973, pp. 35-50

FOLLETT, B.K.: Plasma follicle-stimulating hormone during photoperiodically induced sexual maturation in male Japanese quail. J. Endocrinol. 69, 117-126 (1976)

FOLLETT, B.K., FARNER, D.S., MATTOCKS, P.W.: Luteinizing hormone in the plasma of White-crowned Sparrows, *Zonotrichia leucophrys gambelii*, during artificial photostimulation. Gen. Comp. Endocrinol. 26, 126-134 (1975)

FOLLETT, B.K., MATTOCKS, P.W., FARNER, D.S.: Circadian function in the photoperiodic induction of gonadotropin secretion in the White-crowned Sparrow, *Zonotrichia leucophrys gambelii*. Proc. Nat. Acad. Sci. USA 71, 1666-1669 (1974)

GWINNER, E.: Circannuale Periodik als Grundlage des jahreszeitlichen Funktionswandels bei Zugvögeln. J. Ornithol. 109, 71-95 (1968)

GWINNER, E.: Circannual rhythms in birds: Their interaction with circadian rhythms and environmental photoperiod. In: The Environment and Reproduction in Mammals and Birds. Perry, J.S., Rolands, I.W. (eds.). J. Repr. Fert. Suppl. 19, 1973, pp. 51-65

GWINNER, E.: Circadian and circannual rhythms in birds. In: Avian Biology, Vol. V. Farner, D.S., King, J.R. (eds.). New York: Academic Press, 1975, pp. 221-288

GWINNER, E.: Circannuale Rhythmen bei Vögeln und ihre photoperiodische Synchronisation. In: Ökophysiologische Probleme in der Ornithologie. Berthold, P., Gwinner, E. (eds.). Vogelwarte 30 (Sonderheft), 16-25 (1977)

HOMMA, K., SAKAKIBARA, Y.: Encephalic photoreceptors and their significance in photoperiodic control of sexual activity in Japanese quail. In: Biochronometry. Menaker, M. (ed.). Washington: Nat. Acad. Sci. 1971, pp. 333-341

HOOS, D.: De vinkenbaan. Hoe het er toeging en wat er mee in verband stond door. Ardea 26, 173-203 (1937)

IMMELMANN, K.: Tierische Jahresperiodik in ökologischer Sicht. Zool. Jahrb. Abt. 1 Systematik Oekol. 91, 91-200 (1963)

IMMELMANN, K.: Role of the environment in reproduction as source of "predictive" information. In: Breeding Biology of Birds. Farner, D.S. (ed.). Washington: Nat. Acad. Sci. 1973, pp. 121-147

KING, J.R., FARNER, D.S.: Biochronometry and bird migration. In: Chronobiology. Scheving, L.E., Halberg, F., Pauly, J.E. (eds.). Tokyo: Igaku Shoin, 1974, pp. 625-630

KING, J.R., FOLLETT, B.K., FARNER, D.S., MORTON, M.L.: Annual gonadal cycles and pituitary gonadotropins in *Zonotrichia leucophrys gambelii*. Condor 68, 476-487 (1966)

LAM, F., FARNER, D.S.: The ultrastructure of the cells of Leydig in the White-crowned Sparrow, *Zonotrichia leucophrys gambelii*, in relation to plasma levels of luteinizing hormone and testosterone. C. Tiss. Res. 169, 93-100 (1976)

LEWIS, R.A., FARNER, D.S.: Temperature modulation of photoperiodically induced vernal phenomena in White-crowned Sparrows, *Zonotrichia leucophrys*. Condor 75, 279-286 (1973)

LOFTS, B., MURTON, R.K.: Photoperiodic and physiological adaptations regulating avian breeding cycles and their ecological significance. J. Zool. 155, 327-394 (1968)

MATTOCKS, P.W., FARNER, D.S., FOLLETT, B.K.: The annual cycle in luteinizing hormone in the plasma of intact and castrated White-crowned Sparrows, *Zonotrichia leucophrys gambelii*. Gen. Comp. Endocrinol. 30, 156-161 (1976)

McMILLAN, J.P., UNDERWOOD, H.A., ELLIOTT, J.A., STETSON, M.H., MENAKER, M.: Extraretinal light perception in the Sparrow. IV. Further evidence that the eyes do not participate in photoperiodic photoreception. J. Comp. Physiol. A. 97, 205-213 (1975)

MEIER, A.H.: Chronoendocrinology of the White-throated Sparrow. In: Proc. 16th Int. Ornithol. Cong. Frith, H.J., Calaby, H.J. (eds.). Canberra: Aust. Acad. Sci., 1976, pp. 369-382

MENAKER, M., KEATTS, H.: Extraretinal light perception in the sparrow. II. Photoperiodic stimulation of testis growth. Proc. Nat. Acad. Sci. USA 60, 146-151 (1968)

PITTENDRIGH, C.S., MINIS, D.H.: The entrainment of circadian oscillations by light and their role as photoperiodic clocks. Am. Nat. 98, 261-294 (1964)
ROWAN, W.: Relation of light to bird migration and developmental changes. Nature (London) 115, 494-495 (1925)
SERVENTY, D.L.: Biology of desert birds. In: Avian Biology, Vol. 1. Farner, D.S., King, J.R. (eds.). New York: Academic Press, 1971, pp. 287-341
TYSHCHENKO, B.P.: Dvukhostsillyaornaya model fisiologicheskovo mekhanizma fotoperiodicheskoi reaktsii nasekomykh. Zh. Obshch. Biol. 27, 209-222 (1966)
WINGFIELD, J.C., FARNER, D.S.: Avian endocrinology - field investigations and methods. Condor 78, 570-572 (1976)
WINGFIELD, J.C., Farner, D.S.: Zur Endokrinologie des Fortpflanzungszyklus von *Zonotrichia leucophrys pugetensis*. In: Ökophysiologische Probleme in der Ornithologie. Berthold, P., Gwinner, E. (eds.). Vogelwarte 30 (Sonderheft), 25-32 (1977)
YOKOYAMA, K., FARNER, D.S.: Photoperiodic responses in bilaterally enucleated female White-crowned Sparrows, *Zonotrichia leucophrys gambelii*. Gen. Comp. Endocrinol. 30, 528-533 (1976)
YOKOYAMA, K., OKSCHE, A., FARNER, D.S., DARDEN, T.R.: The sites of encephalic photoreception in the photoperiodic induction of the growth of the testes in the White-crowned Sparrow, *Zonotrichia leucophrys gambelii*. Cell Tiss. Res. (1978) in press

7. Annual Endocrine Cycles and Environment in Birds with Special Reference to Male Ducks

I. ASSENMACHER and M. JALLAGEAS

Man has presumably discovered long ago that "spring bade the sparrows pair" (Browning), and it is more than likely that annual cycles in the behavior of birds are among the most familiar environmental cues in human perception of the recurring seasons. As a matter of fact, the obvious dependence on cycling environmental factors of the major biological events of annual cycles, such as sexual display and song, nuptial molts, nesting and migration, has led through recent decades to an increasing amount of experimental investigation of environmental physiology in birds. Since most annual physiologic rhythms are closely related to the reproductive cycle or to hormone-dependent metabolic cycles, it is understandable that birds have been used as very useful tools for the study of the general mechanisms and concepts of annual endocrine cycles.

Among the common laboratory birds, Pekin Ducks (*Anas platyrhynchos*) are distinctive in that they have retained through centuries of domestication a very prominent annual pattern in reproduction. Therefore they serve as classical experimental "models" along with other domestic species such as the domestic fowl, the pigeon (*Columbia livia*), and the Japanese Quail (*Coturnix coturnix*).

Experimental data on domestic ducks compared with investigations on a related wild species, the teal (*Anas crecca*), and with complementary studies on other domestic species, will be reviewed in this section.

Hormones were measured by radioimmunoassay (LH, testosterone, aldosterone), or by the protein-binding method (thyroxine, corticosterone), whereas a 2-h perfusion method of labeled hormones was used for the evaluation of metabolic clearance rates (MCR) of several steroid hormones.

Annual Endocrine Cycles in Ducks and in Teal

Pekin Ducks were studied in 400-m^2 enclosures at Montpellier (43° 50' N) whereas a population of teal, captured in their winter quarters in the Rhone delta area, were held in 2400 m^2 of "natural" environment with a large pond and located in immediate proximity to the seashore.

Sexual Cycle. The sexual cycle of the Pekin Duck exhibits a clear biphasic pattern (GARNIER, 1971; JALLAGEAS et al., 1974). In a typical annual cycle (Fig. 1.1) the plasma concentrations of LH and testosterone begin to increase in January to culminate during the reproductive phase (March-April), after 3- and 9-fold augmentations in LH and testosterone, respectively. The testis weight, on the other hand, has increased 30-fold by that time. The reproductive phase comes to a sudden termination by late May or early June, with an acute decrease in testosterone, usually but not always (JALLAGEAS et al., 1974) associated with a correlated decrease in LH, whereas testis weight has decreased by only

50%. Even by taking into consideration a temporary increase of MCR of testosterone (from 106 ± 3 to 189 ± 19 ml/min/kg), the secretion rate of the hormone appears to decrease by at least half in June (ASSENMACHER et al., 1975). This blockade of sexual function is followed by a transient rebound of all measured sexual parameters in August to September before the final onset of the autumnal phase of sexual quiescence.

Although a few individuals may lack the temporary hormonal rebound in late summer, a rather similar profile of the annual plasma LH cycle has been observed in Khaki Campbell Ducks at Kiel (lat 54° N; HAASE et al., 1975). In this experiment, a further small transient increase in LH was noticed for several birds in November to December, when BALTHAZART and HENDRICK (1976) also measured a significant increase in plasma testosterone in another bread (Rouen) of domestic ducks. Using a heterologous radioimmunoassay system for the measurement of plasma FSH in these ducks, the latter authors claimed that FSH increased progressively from September through February, but began to decline already in March to April, i.e., by the height of the breeding season, which would indicate a lack of clear correlation with either testosterone levels or testis enlargement.

Finally the pituitary concentrations of prolactin display in Pekin Ducks an annual cycle that parallels the testis cycle (GOURDJI and TIXIER-VIDAL, 1966), a fact that argues against an "anti-gonadal" effect of this hormone at least in this species.

The sex-hormone levels in teal (Fig. 1.2) also revealed a very comparable annual excursion (JALLAGEAS et al., 1976b). The maximum concentrations were found from April to June for LH, (a four-fold increase over January) and in June for testosterone (a 30-fold increase over January). By July the hormone levels fell by two thirds for LH, and by seven times for testosterone, prior to a short rebound in August.

The testis weight followed a comparable pattern with a maximum in June (30-fold increase over January), but failed to undergo a partial recovery in September. Rather close correlations were observed between the annual cycle in sex hormones and sexual behavior. The classical pattern of sexual behavior (song and nuptial display) increased progressively from February to June, and then disappeared completely by mid-June. During the hormonal rebound in September, a slight resumption of song was noticed, together with isolated components of sexual displays which never reached full nuptial sequences.

Among the very few nonpasserine birds in which cycles of sexual hormones have been measured, the Red Grouse (*Lagopus scoticus*) seems to display a less complex cycle, with a sharp increase in both LH and testosterone from February to April (reproductive phase), followed by a gradual decrease through June until August, and a moderate resumption from September to January, associated with a slight increase in territorial behavior (SHARP et al., 1975).

Thyroid Cycle. The annual excursion of the plasma thyroxine levels in ducks exhibits a very sharp increase in June (almost two-fold increase over April) preceding a progressive decline through July and August, and a slight rebound in September (Fig. 1.1; ASSENMACHER et al., 1975). Thus the cycle of thyroxine clearly followed an inverse phase relationship to the testosterone cycle.

Quite similarly, the salient feature of the thyroxine cycle in teal is an acute increment (65%) in July, culminating at + 140% in August, before decreasing in September (Fig. 1.2). In this case, also the annual

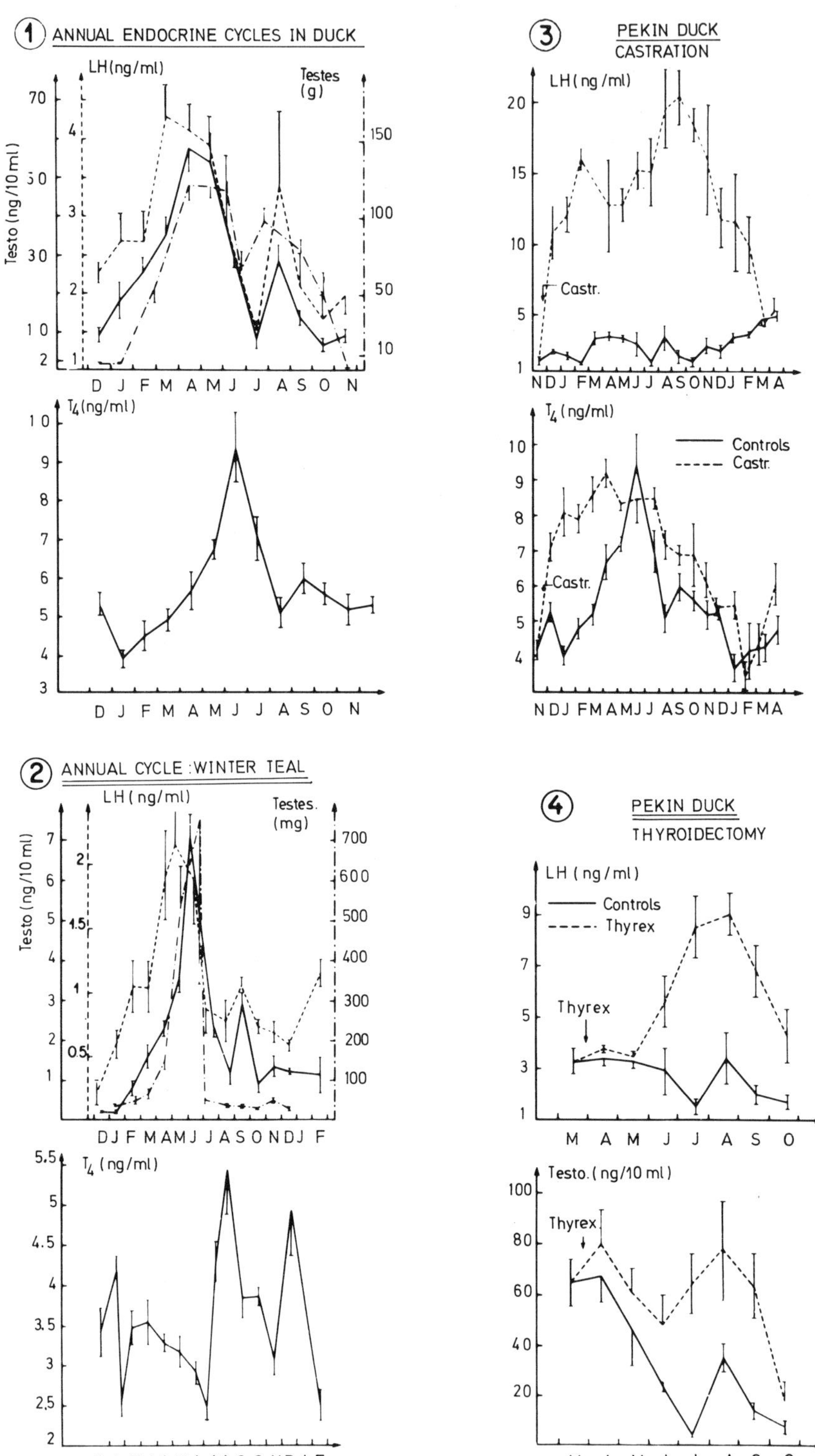
1 ANNUAL ENDOCRINE CYCLES IN DUCK
LH(ng/ml)
Testes (g)
Testo (ng/10 ml)
70
50
30
10
2
4
3
2
1
150
100
50
10
D J F M A M J J A S O N
T4(ng/ml)
10
9
8
7
6
5
4
3
D J F M A M J J A S O N
3 PEKIN DUCK
CASTRATION
LH (ng/ml)
20
15
10
5
1
Castr.
N D J F M A M J J A S O N D J F M A
T4 (ng/ml)
Controls
Castr.
10
9
8
7
6
5
4
Castr.
N D J F M A M J J A S O N D J F M A
2 ANNUAL CYCLE: WINTER TEAL
LH (ng/ml)
Testes. (mg)
Testo (ng/10 ml)
7
6
5
4
3
2
1
2
1.5
1
0.5
700
600
500
400
300
200
100
D J F M A M J J A S O N D J F
5.5
T4 (ng/ml)
5
4.5
4
3.5
3
2.5
2
D J F M A M J J A S O N D J F
4 PEKIN DUCK
THYROIDECTOMY
LH (ng/ml)
Controls
Thyrex
9
7
5
3
1
Thyrex
M A M J J A S O
Testo. (ng/10 ml)
100
80
60
40
20
Thyrex.
M A M J J A S O

maximum in plasma thyroxine coincided with the severe decline in plasma testosterone. However unlike Pekin Ducks, the teal displayed a second maximum in December. This peak was of varying amplitude and could be related to no precise meteorologic event.

Although the literature is rather poor in biochemical investigations of annual thyroid cycles in related bird species, earlier histologic studies in the mallard had evidenced a phase of increased thyroid activity at the end of the reproductive phase (HÖHN, 1949).

Annual Molt Cycle. Pekin Ducks, as well as teal, undergo the postnuptial molt in June or July. This major metabolic event always occurs in close correlation with a marked hormonal imbalance characterized by a sharp augmentation of the ratio between plasma thyroxin and testosterone which is 3.5 times higher than during the reproductive phase.

On the other hand, the molt of body feathers that leads the teal from the eclipse to the breeding plumage occurred in November to December. Whether this second molt may be correlated with the second annual peak in plasma thyroxin in December, awaits further clarification.

Adrenal Cycle. In ducks, plasma concentration of corticosterone is augmented by 50% during the reproductive phase (ASSENMACHER et al., 1975). As a matter of fact, this increment reflects essentially a 60% increase of the binding capacity of the plasma transcortine, which has been shown itself to be the result of a stimulatory effect of testosterone (DANIEL and ASSENMACHER, 1974). On the other hand plasma aldosterone remains close to 11 ng/100 ml throughout the year. Considering that the MCR of corticosterone is elevated by 25%, and the MCR of aldosterone by 100% in June, as a result of a stimulatory effect of high thyroxine levels, the secretion rate is increased by 30 to 40% during the reproductive phase through June for corticosterone and two-fold in June for aldosterone (ASSENMACHER et al., 1975).

The annual cyclic variations in secretion and metabolism of both major metabolic corticosteroids appear therefore essentially as secondary to the sexual cycle.

Experimental Studies on the Mechanism Controlling Annual Endocrine Cycles

Initiation of the Sexual Cycle

Environmental Factors. During the past four decades, the stimulatory role of long days on the sexual function of a great variety of temperate-zone and tropical bird species has been well demonstrated. However, recent studies have established that the seasonal fluctuations of the day length may act as a primary synchronizer for the so-called "endogenous" sexual rhythms, which have been demonstrated in

Fig. 1. Annual endocrine cycles; *1*, annual cycles in male ducks; *2*, annual cycles in male teal; *3*, annual cycles in gonadectomized ducks; *4*, annual cycles in thyroidectomized ducks

some species of birds held for several years in a nonfluctuating environmént (ASSENMACHER, 1974).

Table 1. Environmental factors and sexual function in ducks (December)

Treatment	Testis weight (g)	Plasma concentrations Testosterone (ng/10 ml)	LH (ng/ml)
Controls	3.2 ± 1.3 (15)	3.2 ± 0.9 (15)	1.22 ± 0.2 (15)
21d. 18L-6D	64.2 ± 6.4 (9)	28.9 ± 4.9 (9)	4.09 ± 0.47 (9)
21d. 18L-6D T. O. N.	136.0 ± 9.0 (3)	21.8 ± 5.2 (3)	3.97 ± 0.76 (3)
21d. 18L-6D (-15°)	50.5 ± 6.2 (8)	13.3 ± 3.1[a] (8)	5.30 ± 1.0 (11)
21d. 18L-6D 17d. Starvation	16.7 ± 6.0[a] (4)	2.0 ± 1.2[b] (4)	1.27 ± 0.35[b] (4)

T. O. N.: Bilateral transection of optic nerve.
[a] $p < 0.05$; [b] < 0.01 vs 21 d. 18L-6D.

Table 1 shows the classical stimulating effect of artificial "long days" (18L-6D) on all sexual parameters of Pekin Ducks. In a similar experiment on Japanese Quail NICHOLLS et al. (1973) have demonstrated that plasma LH begins to increase as soon as three days after exposure to "long days." On the other hand, it can be seen from the table that two other external factors, namely severe cold and deprivation of solid food, can interfere, as limiting depressing factors, with the stimulatory photogonadal response. The modulatory role of temperature or food availability on the very strong stimulatory effect of the vernal increase in day length may explain the occurrence of moderate phase shifts in the annual recurrence of sexual cycles in various natural field conditions (ASSENMACHER, 1973).

Neuroendocrine Mechanisms. The strong photogonadotropic response that persists in experimentally blinded ducks (Table 1) illustrates the occurrence and effective role of extra-retinal photoreceptors. Although a fine comparative exploration of photogonadal responses in intact vs blinded birds could establish that the kinetics of the response were significantly slower in blinded ducks (BENOIT and ASSENMACHER, 1953) and Japanese Quail (BONS et al., 1975), the respective role of both the retinal and extra-retinal photoreceptors in photogonadal responses of intact birds in still a matter of controversy. However the decisive demonstration of a specific retinohypothalamic tract with synaptic endings within the suprachiasmatic nucleus of the anterior hypothalamus (BONS and ASSENMACHER, 1973) affords a strong support of the thesis of an active participation of the eye as a receptor for photoneuroendocrine responses.

On the other hand the irreplaceable role of the median eminence and of the hypophysial portal vessels in these regulations has been verified by the blocking effect of their respective surgical suppresion in ducks (ASSENMACHER, 1958) domestic fowls (GRABER et al., 1967), pigeon and Japanese Quail (BAYLÉ, 1970). The recent cytoimmunochemical identification of LH-RH containing nerve terminals on the basement membrane of the portal capillaries in the rostral and caudal median eminence of ducks (CALAS et al., 1974) points undoubtedly to this neurohemal organ as the final route for the photogonadotropic response.

Although the problem of the nature and location of the hypothalamic machinery that integrates the photoperiodical information, and ultimately provides the median eminence with LH-RH still awaits a final clarification, certain facts have at least gained consistent support.

In the duck two hypothalamic areas seem to be involved in the photogonadotropic response (1) the tubero-infundibular region with its neurons extending down to the internal layer of the median eminence, and (2) the dorsal anterior hypothalamus. As a matter of fact large freehand surgical lesions (ASSENMACHER, 1958), as well as testosterone implants (KORDON and GOGAN, 1970) in both of these hypothalamic areas impaired the photogonadal response. The recent location of immunoreactive LH-RH producing neurons in the preoptic periventricular nucleus of ducks (BONS et al., 1977), in addition to the termination of the retino-hypothalamic pathway in the suprachiasmatic nuclei, bring rather strong support to the participation of the anterior hypothalamus, together with the tubero-infundibular region, in this regulation.

The hypothalamic regulation does not seem basically different in Japanese Quail. While stereotaxic destruction of the tubero-infundibular area constantly blocked the photogonadal response (SHARP and FOLLET, 1969; STETSON, 1969; OLIVER and BAYLÉ, 1973), the response was also inhibited by more dorsal lesions including the dorso-medial hypothalamus and the paraventricular organ (FOLLETT, 1973), or by lesions extending more rostrally up to the suprachiasmatic area (OLIVER and BAYLÉ, 1973).

A further basic component of the neuroendocrine machinery that controls the gonadotropic function of birds may involve the abundant catecholaminergic (CA) innervation of the hypothalamus (FOLLETT, 1973; CALAS, 1975). As a matter of fact the depletion of CA by reserpine blocks photogonadal stimulation in ducks (ASSENMACHER, 1973) and depresses plasma LH levels in domestic fowl (SHARP, 1975); whereas the inhibition of CA synthesis by 6-OH dopamine reduces by 75% the light-induced testicular growth in Japanese Quail (ASSENMACHER, 1973).

Cessation of the Reproductive Phase. Gonadothyroid Interactions

Although the depressing effect of the transfer from "long days" to "short days" on an experimentally induced cycle of plasma LH has been very clearly demonstrated in intact (NICHOLLS et al., 1973) and in gonadectomized Japanese Quail (GIBSON et al., 1975), emphasis has been laid on the termination of the annual reproductive phase in outdoor living ducks (see above) and Red Grouse (SHARP et al., 1975) prior to the summer solstice i.e., in late May or early June. Under natural conditions the seasonal decrease in day length cannot therefore be considered as the primary factor that initiates the cessation of the reproductive phase. Nor can a simple mechanism provide any explanation for the transient sexual rebound that occurs in late summer months. At the present state of knowledge, at least two different mechanisms seem to contribute to the complex events that immediately follow the reproductive phase, namely (1) negative testis-thyroid interactions, and (2) modifications of threshold levels of negative-feedback sites at the central, hypothalamo-hypophysial level.

Interference of Reciprocal Negative Testis-Thyroid Interactions in the Sexual and Thyroid Cycle. It has already been stressed that the almost complete phase-inversion between the annual cycle of plasma testosterone and thyroxin in ducks and teal may reflect a reciprocal antagonism between high levels of these hormones. This hypothesis was strengthened by a series of experiments in ducks with hormonal treatments that mimicked the seasonal peak levels of either testosterone or thyroxin. And indeed high levels in testosterone used to depress the thyroxine levels and vice versa (ASSENMACHER et al., 1975). Curiously enough, however, the thyroxine treatments that suppressed the high plasma testosterone levels may be almost ineffective on plasma LH. This may indicate a possible direct inhibitory effect of thyroxin at the peripheral level, and an electron-microscopic investigation of the interstitial cells indeed revealed that in this case thyroxine supplementation led to a complete disorganization of the cell organelles and especially of the endoplasmic reticulum (JALLAGEAS et al., 1977).

The assumption of a very close interference between the sexual and the thyroid cycles gained further support from the exploration of the modification of the annual cycles in ducks submitted to either castration or surgical thyroidectomy. Castration (Fig. 1.3) modified the thyroid cycle by raising the plasma thyroxine levels to the annual maximum levels from December through July, thus indicating that the increasing testosterone secretion during the spring months inhibits thyroid function until late May. On the other hand, the annual decline in plasma T4 beginning by August in castrated, as in intact, animals appears unrelated to testis-thyroid interactions. Thyroidectomy (Fig. 1.4) induced a striking increase in plasma LH and testosterone from June to October, which points to an inhibitory effect of the high T4 levels of summer on sexual function. Strangely enough the plasma testosterone levels retained in thyroidectomized as in intact ducks a significant, though dampened biphasic profile. The temporary dissociation between high LH and decreased testosterone titers, that can be observed in intact (ASSENMACHER et al., 1975) and in thyroidectomized ducks may therefore result only partially from a direct insensitizing effect of T4 on the endocrine testis.

Summarizing these results, it can be stated that reciprocal inhibitory interactions between seasonally elevated plasma concentrations in testosterone and thyroxine seem to play a significant role in both profiles of the sexual and thyroid cycles in male ducks.

Seasonal Modifications at the Central Hypothalamo-Hypophysial Level. The inevitable occurrence of an autumnal decline in plasma LH beginning in September, in intact, gonadectomized and thyroidectomized ducks (Fig. 1) may indicate a seasonal depression of the central control machinery to the gonadotropic system. Among the possible origins of this depression, the steady decrease in day length may play a limited and tardy role. It is, however, very unlikely that the cause of the reduced activity of the hypothalamic-hypophysial unit in fall be merely exogenous. In addition to a cycling decay in the central neurogenic oscillator that is presumed to drive the endogenous sexual rhythm, as measured in constant darkness (ASSENMACHER, 1974), variations in sensitivity thresholds may also intervene at various levels of the neuroendocrine machinery.

As a matter of fact, cyclic modifications in the pituitary responsiveness to LH-RH have been postulated in Japanese Quail (DAVIES and BICKNELL, 1976). Moreover the hypothalamic neurons that have been shown to react to the negative feedback of testosterone implants may undergo seasonal variations in their responsiveness to steroids, which could explain the compatibility of high testosterone levels with elevated LH levels in ducks (JALLAGEAS et al., 1976a) and Japanese Quail (DAVIES et al., 1976) during the sole annual reproductive period.

In addition to environmental factors and to endogenous multihormonal interactions, annually cyclic variations in the sensitivity of the hypothalamohypophysial system to testosterone could, therefore, be a basic functional component of sexual rhythmicity.

References

ASSENMACHER, I.: Recherches sur le contrôle hypothalamique de la fonction gonadotrope prêhypophysaire chez le Canard. Arch. Anat. Micr. Morphol. Exp. 47, 447-572 (1958)

ASSENMACHER, I.: Reproductive endocrinology: The hypothalamo-hypophysial axis. In: Breeding Biology of Birds. Farner, D.S. (ed.). Washington, D.C.: Nat. Acad. Sci., 1973, pp. 158-191

ASSENMACHER, I.: External and internal components of the mechanisms controlling reproductive cycles in drakes. In: Circannual Clocks. Pengelley, E.T. (ed.). New York: Academic Press, 1974, pp. 197-248

ASSENMACHER, I., ASTIER, H., DANIEL, J.Y., JALLAGEAS, M.: Experimental studies on the annual cycles of thyroid and adrenocortical functions in relation to the reproductive cycle of drakes. J. Physiol. 70, 507-520 (1975)

BALTHAZART, J., HENDRICK, J.: Annual variations in reproductive behaviour, testosterone and plasma FSH levels in the Rouen duck, *Anas Platyrhynchos*. Gen. Comp. Endocrinol. 28, 171-183 (1976)

BAYLÉ, J.D.: Activité de l'adéno-hypophyse déconnectée chez les Oiseaux. In: Neuroendocrinologie. Benoit, J., Kordon, C. (eds.). Paris: Edit. CNRS, 1970, pp. 261-283

BENOIT, J., ASSENMACHER, I.: Rôle des photorécepteurs superficiels et profonds dans la gonadostimulation par la lumière chez les oiseaux. J. Physiol. 45, 34-37 (1953)

BONS, N., ASSENMACHER, I.: Nouvelles recherches sur la voie nerveuse rétinohypothalamique chez les Oiseaux. C.R. Acad. Sci. (Paris) 277, 2529-2532 (1973)

BONS, N., JALLAGEAS, M., ASSENMACHER, I.: Influence des photorécepteurs rétiniens et extra-rétiniens dans la stimulation testiculaire de la Caille par les "jours longs". J. Physiol. 71, 265A-266A (1975)

BONS, K., KERDELHUÉ, B., ASSENMACHER, I.: Evidence for LH-RH containing neurons in the anterior hypothalamus of the duck (*Anas platyrhynchos*): an immunofluorescence study. Proc. 9th Congr. Eur. Compar. Endocrinol. Giessen, 1977, Abstr. 13 (1977)

CALAS, A.: The avian median eminence as a model for diversified neuroendocrine routes. In: Brain-Endocrine Interactions II. Knigge K.M. et al. (eds.). Basel: Karger, 1975, pp. 54-69

CALAS, A., KERDELHUÉ, B., ASSENMACHER, I., JUTISZ, M.: Les axones à LH-RH de l'éminence médiane. Etude ultrastructurale chez le Canard par une technique immunocytochimique. C.R. Acad. Sci. (Paris) 178, 2557-2560 (1974)

DANIEL, J.Y., ASSENMACHER, I.: Hormonal effects on plasma binding capacity of transcortine in ducks. J. Ster. Biochem. 5, 399 (1974)

DAVIES, D.T., BICKNELL, R.J.: The effect of testosterone on the responsiveness of the quail's pituitary to luteinizing hormone releasing hormone (LH-RH) during photoperiodically induced testicular growth. Gen. Comp. Endocrinol. 30, 487-499 (1976a)

DAVIES, D.T., GOULDEN, L.P., FOLLETT, B.K., BROWN, N.L.: Testosterone feedback on luteinizing hormone (LH) secretion during a photoperiodically induced breeding cycle in japanese quail. Gen. Comp. Endocrinol. 30, 477-486 (1976b)

FOLLETT, B.K.: The neuroendocrine regulation of gonadotropin secretion in avian reproduction. In: Breeding Biology of Birds. Farner, D.S. (ed.). Washington, D.C.: Nat. Acad. Sci., 1973, pp. 209-243

GARNIER, D.H.: Variations de la testostérone du plasma périphérique chez le Canard Pékin au cours du cycle annuel. C.R. Acad. Sci. (Paris) 272, 1665-1668 (1971)

GIBSON, W.R., FOLLETT, B.K., GLEDHILL, B.: Plasma levels of luteinizing hormone in gonadectomized Japanese quail exposed to short or long daylength. J. Endocrinol. 64, 87-101 (1975)

GOURDJI, D., TIXIER-VIDAL, A.: Variations du contenu hypophysaire en prolactine chez le Canard Pékin mâle au cours des cycles sexuels et de la photostimulation. C.R. Acad. Sci. (Paris) 262, 1746-1749 (1966)

GRABER, J.W., FRANKEL, A.I., NALBANDOV, A.V.: Hypothalamic center influencing the release of LH in the cockerel. Gen. Comp. Endocrinol. 9, 187-192 (1967)

HAASE, E., SHARP, P.J., PAULKE, E.: Seasonal changes in plasma LH levels in domestic ducks. J. Reprod. Fert. 44, 591-594 (1975)

HÖHN, O.E.: Seasonal changes in the thyroid gland and effects of thyroidectomy in the Mallard in relation to molt. Am. J. Physiol. 158, 337 (1949)

JALLAGEAS, M., ASTIER, H., ASSENMACHER, I.: Thyroid-gonadal interactions during the postnuptial phase of the sexual cycle in male ducks. Proc. 9th Conf. Europ. Compar. Endocrinol. Giessen 1977. Abstr. 15 (1977)

JALLAGEAS, M., FOLLETT, B.K., ASSENMACHER, I.: Testosterone secretion and plasma luteinizing hormone concentration during a seasonal cycle in the Pekin duck, and after thyroxine treatment. Gen. Comp. Endocrinol. 23, 472-475 (1974)

JALLAGEAS, M., FOLLETT, B.K., ASSENMACHER, I.: Effects of castration and/or testosterone administration on plasma LH and testosterone concentrations in the duck. Gen. Comp. Endocrinol. 29, 272 (1976a)

JALLAGEAS, M., TAMISIER, A., DURIEUX, A., ASSENMACHER, I.: Etude comparée du cycle sexuel chez le Canard domestique et chez la Sarcelle d'hiver (*Anas crecca*). Bull. Soc. Ecophysiol. 2, 52-53 (1976b)

KORDON, C., GOGAN, F.: Interaction du feed-back et de la photostimulation dans les régulations gonadotropes chez les Mammifères et les Oiseaux. In: La Photoregulation de la Reproduction chez les Oiseaux et les Mammifères. Benoit, J., Assenmacher, I. (eds.). Paris: Edit. CNRS, 1970, pp. 325-346

NICHOLLS, T.J., SCANES, C.G., FOLLETT, B.K.: Plasma and pituitary luteinizing hormone in Japanse quail during photoperiodically induced gonadal growth and regression. Gen. Comp. Endocrinol. 21, 84-98 (1973)

OLIVER, J., BAYLÉ, J.D.: Photically evoked potentials in the gonadotropic areas of the quail hypothalamus. Brain Res. 64, 103-121 (1973)

SHARP, P.J.: The effects of reserpine on plasma LH concentrations in intact and gonadectomized domestic fowl. Brit. Poult. Sci. 16, 79-82 (1975)

SHARP, P.J., FOLLETT, B.K.: The effect of hypothalamic lesions on gonadotrophin release in Japanese quail, *Coturnix coturnix japonica*. Neuroendocrinology 5, 205-218 (1969)

SHARP, P.J., MOSS, R., WATSON, A.: Seasonal variations in plasma luteinizing hormone levels in male Red Grouse (*Lagopus lagopus scoticus*). J. Endocrinol. 64, 44 P (1975)

STETSON, M.H.: Hypothalamic regulation of TSH and LH secretion in male and female Japanese quail. Am. Zool. 9, 104 (1969)

8. Regulation of Reproductive Cycles of Tropical Spotted Munia and Weaverbird

A. CHANDOLA and J. P. THAPLIYAL

The Spotted munia, *Lonchura punctulata*, and the weaverbird, *Ploceus philippinus*, are seasonally breeding nonmigratory birds distributed all over the Indian sub-continent. In nature (Varanasi, 25°18' N, 83°01' E) the gonads of the Spotted munia begin to develop immediately after the summer solstice, are fully active upto October to November and collapse before the winter solstice (Fig. 1). Gonads of the weaverbird begin to

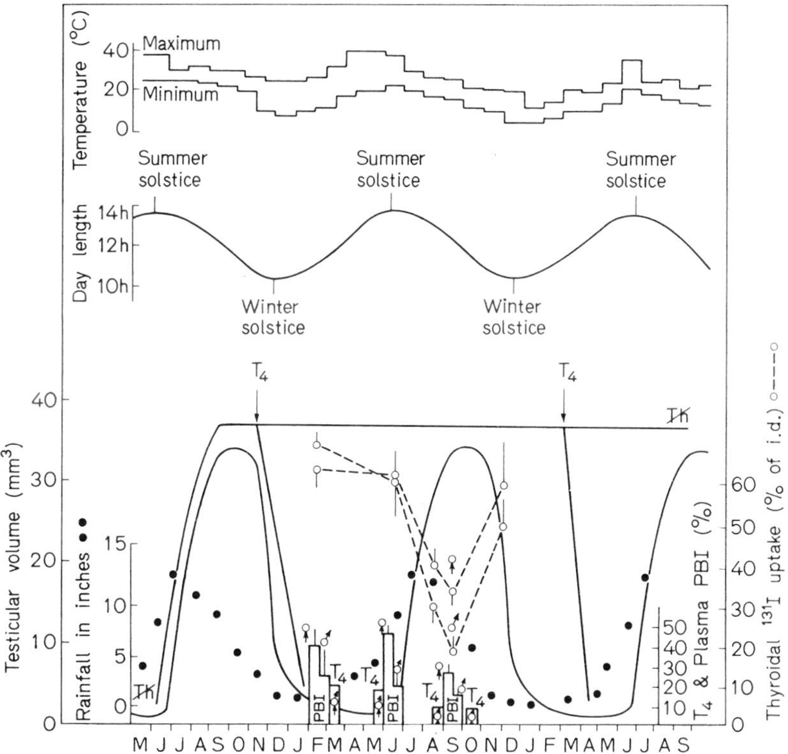

Fig. 1. Testicular cycle and thyroid/gonad association in Spotted Munia. Data based on references cited in text

develop earlier, in March to April, attain maximal size in June to July and regress thereafter (Fig. 2). It is interesting that these two species occupying similar habitats, and sharing the same food habits

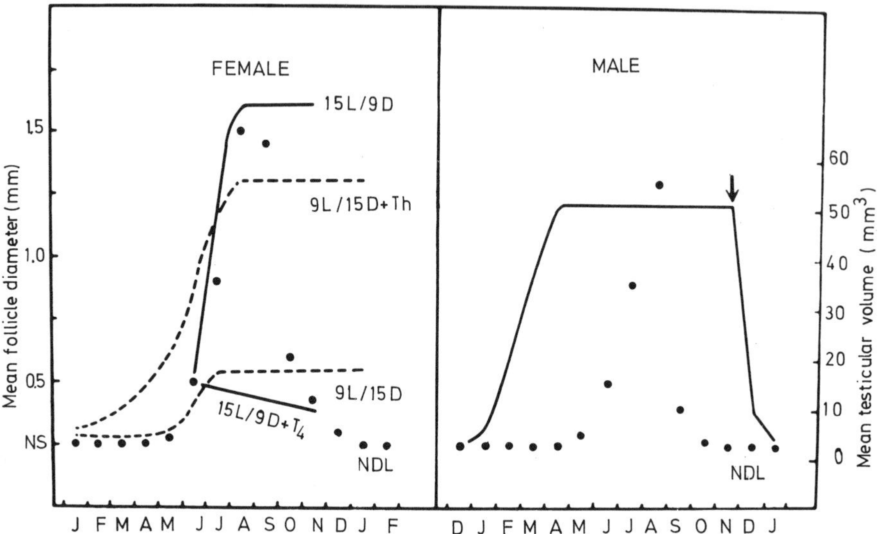

Fig. 2. Gonadal cycle (solid circles) and effects of short day length (---) vs thyroidectomy and long day length (——) vs exogenous thyroxine in weaverbird. Data based on references cited in text

and environment should enter breeding cycles at different times, thus, perhaps reflecting synchronization by different environmental factors.

Artificial long days are gonadostimulatory and short days gonadoinhibitory in weaverbird. This species thus appears to use day length as information for the timing of its breeding cycle. Results of asymmetric skeleton photophases are also in agreement with this supposition (CHANDOLA et al., 1976). The Spotted Munia is not photperiodic. Customary long and short day lengths have no effect on its gonadal cycle, and the tendency to an endogenous rhythm of reproduction is indicated, for references see CHANDOLA and THAPLIYAL (1977). How far the monsoon, which coincides with the gonadal development, and which is fairly predictable each year, and other environmental factors influence the cycle of this bird is not known.

Among the internal factors, on the other hand, there is strong evidence for the involvement of the thyroid gland in the regulation of the gonadal cycle in both these species (see reviews THAPLIYAL, 1969; THAPLIYAL and CHANDOLA, 1972). Thyroidectomy causes precocious gonadal development and abolishes seasonal regression, while mild hyperthyroidism precipitates regression any time of the year (Fig. 1). Even the photoperiodic responses can be completely overridden by thyroidal manipulations (THAPLIYAL and GARG, 1969; THAPLIYAL and BAGESHWAR, 1970; CHANDOLA et al., 1974, 1976; Fig. 2). These effects may be induced by the mediation of hypothalamo-hypophysial system, since the sensitivity of the gonads to gonadotrophins is not altered by thyroidectomy (THAPLIYAL, 1969). Further, exogenous thyroxine in the weaverbird inhibits the appearance of the characteristic LH-specific yellow pigmentation in the regenerating feathers (CHANDOLA, unpublished). Thyroid activity has also been shown to be inversely related to the reproductive cycle, in Spotted Munia, atleast (CHANDOLA and THAPLIYAL, 1974). Similar observations were made in the Pekin Duck recently (see Chap. I.7, this vol.). This kind of thyrogonad association may gain greater significance in photoperiodic birds especially in those that lack a photo-refractory phase (e.g., weaverbird) in that it may be of adaptive value ensuring against unseasonal gonadal growth in the greatly insolated tropics.

References

CHANDOLA, A., SINGH, R., THAPLIYAL, J.P.: Evidence for a circadian oscillation in the gonadal response of the tropical weaver bird to photoperiod. Chronobiologia 3, 219-227 (1976)

CHANDOLA, A., THAPLIYAL, J.P.: Iodine metabolism in spotted munia. Gen. Comp. Endocrinol. 22, 184-194 (1974)

CHANDOLA, A., THAPLIYAL, J.P.: Photoperiodic responses of Indian birds. Proc. 1st. Int. Symp. Avian Endocrinol. Calcutta, January 1977, pp. 60-62

CHANDOLA, A., THAPLIYAL, J.P., PAVNASKAR, J.: The effects of thyroidal hormones on the ovarian response to photoperiod in a tropical finch. Gen. Comp. Endocrinol. 24, 437-441 (1974)

THAPLIYAL, J.P.: Thyroid in avian reproduction. Gen. Comp. Endocrinol. Suppl. 2, 111-122 (1969)

THAPLIYAL, J.P., Bageshwar, K.: Light response of thyroidectomised common weaver bird. Condor 72, 190-195 (1970)

THAPLIYAL, J.P., CHANDOLA, A.: Thyroid in wild finches. Proc. Natl. Acad. Sci. India 42(B) Part I, 76-90 (1972)

THAPLIYAL, J.P., GARG, R.K.: Relation of thyroid to gonadal and body weight cycles in male weaver bird. Arch. Anat. Histol. Embryol. Norm. Exp. 516, 689-695 (1969)

THAPLIYAL, J.P., SAXENA, R.N.: Absence of refractory period in the common weaver bird, *Ploceus philippinus*. Condor 66, 199-208 (1969)

9. Breeding Cycles in Three Species of African Ungulates

J. D. Skinner

It is nearly a decade since the Symposium of Comparative Biology of Reproduction in Mammals (PERRY and ROWLANDS, 1969) was held in Nairobi to stimulate research in this important field in Africa. Yet there has been no great increase in knowledge since then. Moreover, much of the endocrinologic research has been of an indirect nature, and hormone levels are only infrequently determined. This is first because research is carried out under difficult climatic conditions at great distances from modern facilities, and second because endemic diseases frequently preclude the collection and assaying of fresh material because of the veterinary restrictions imposed. It has therefore been decided to restrict this paper to three species of ungulates. Moreover, unlike domesticated ungulates where ambient temperature can have a marked detrimental influence on reproduction, no results have been reported for reproductive failure in indigenous wild African ungulates. The substance of this paper is devoted to rhythms dependent on day length, and the influence of nutrition in the reproductive cycle, as there has been little research on other aspects of mammalian endocrinology.

At the equator, day-length-dependent rhythms are masked by other environmental factors such as rainfall and nutrition. For example, FIELD and BLANKENSHIP (1973) found that in four species of wild ungulates in Kenya, conception rate was related to rainfall, biomass of vegetation, and crude protein content of the vegetation. This is also true for southern Africa, which has a pattern of summer rainfall, rain falling from spring (September) until autumn (April), after which the nutritional quality of the vegetation, particularly the grasslands, declines to reach a low point just before the spring rains occur. The nutritional levels of the grasses cycle according to day length, and many of the favored trees for browse are deciduous. As will be seen later, this also tends to influence the annual endocrine rhythm. On the other hand in the sub-desert regions, rainfall is sporadic, and species which have evolved there tend to be opportunistic breeders, reacting to nutritional stimuli.

BAKER (1938) suggested that the optimal conditions that occur at birth are the ultimate cause for the timing of breeding. However, all phases of reproduction are subject to selective pressures; and the final selection of the breeding pattern will ensure the temporal pattern of mating, gestation, parturition, lactation, and weaning in a way that will be most beneficial to the survival of a species. The timing of the breeding season therefore seems to be related to the length of gestation, which is closely correlated to the size of the adult animal.

In areas with a fixed summer rainfall pattern, it is advantageous for the lambing or calving to occur only after the first spring rains. If the duration of pregnancy is six months, then mating will take place in autumn; if nine months, then the peak of mating will take place three months earlier. The young are then born just before or when green grass is abundant, and milk secretion is stimulated.

In seasonally breeding animals the mating season could be classified in three ways. First, a continual optimal season as found, for example, in equatorial regions, although this may be influenced by fluctuating nutritional levels in the herbage. Secondly, an unpredictable season, as in certain deserts and semi-deserts where the optimal season can occur at any time depending on climatic factors. Thirdly, a fixed optimal season, determined primarily by day length and perhaps other factors, usually occurring in late summer and autumn.

Species and Localities

The species discussed are the giraffe *Giraffa camelopardalis*, springbok *Antidorcas marsupialis*, and impala *Aepyceros melampus*. The data for the latter two species are from the S.A. Lombard Nature Reserve (27° 35' S, 25° 30' E) in the west, and for impala also from the Kruger National Park, while those for the giraffe are largely from reserves adjoining the Kruger National Park in the east centerd on 24° 24' S, 31° 21' E. Additional data for giraffe are from the Langjan Nature Reserve (22° 52' S, 29° 30' E), the Nairobi National Park (01° 18' S, 36° 45' E) and Taronga Park Zoological Gardens in Sydney Australia (33° 51' S, 151° 13' E). Standard laboratory procedures were used for all analyses (FAIRALL, 1972; SKINNER et al., 1974; HALL-MARTIN et al., 1975).

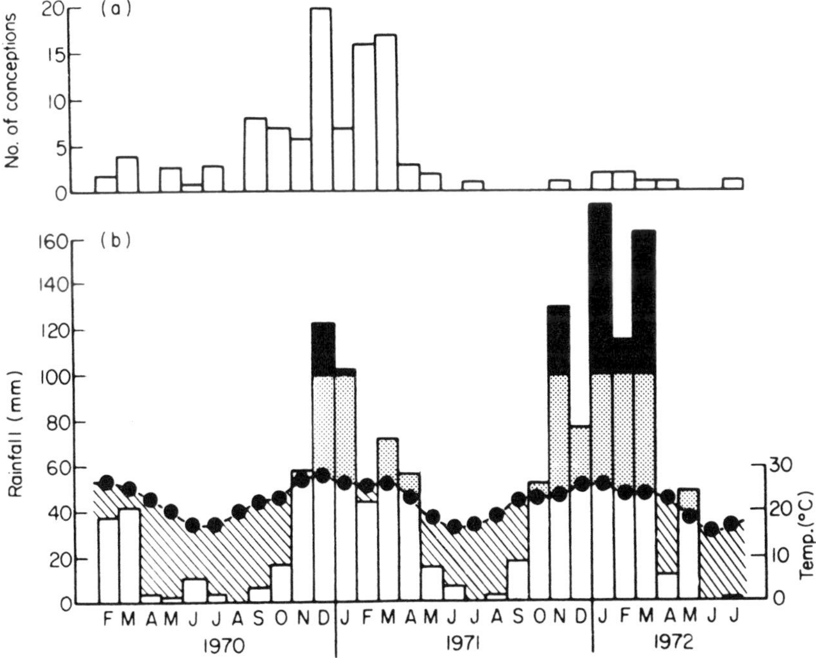

Fig. 1. (a) Histograms showing the number of conceptions per month. Data from the Timbavati Private Nature Reserve for the period February 1970-July 1972. (b) Climatograms showing rainfall (histograms) and temperature (●) (with humid periods indicated by light stippling, perhumid periods shown in black and arid periods indicated by cross hatching). (From HALL-MARTIN et al., 1975)

The Giraffe

The giraffe is an interesting example because it is the only ungulate species with a gestation period longer than a year, namely 457 days (SKINNER and HALL-MARTIN, 1975). When the frequency of conceptions of all available birth and fetus records are plotted against the humid periods of the year (HALL-MARTIN et al., 1975; see Figs. 1 and 2) it is apparent that there is a positive relationship between humid months and conception peaks for all areas except Langjan, where the data are scanty. Moreover, HALL-MARTIN et al. (1975) found a positive correla-

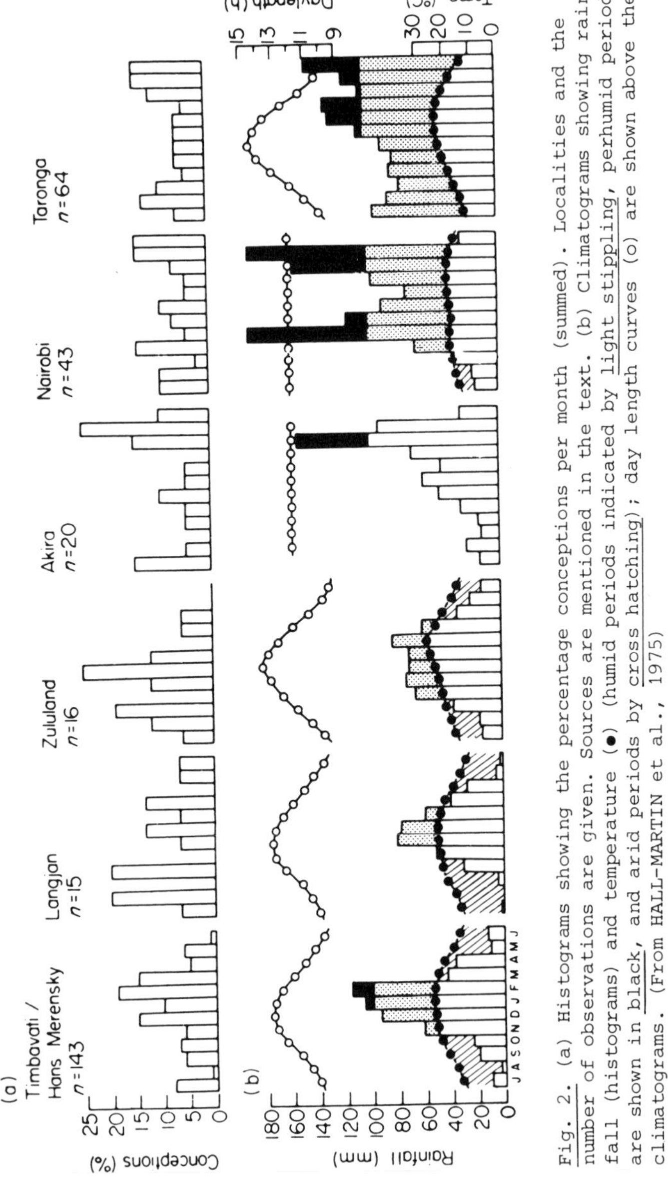

Fig. 2. (a) Histograms showing the percentage conceptions per month (summed). Localities and the number of observations are given. Sources are mentioned in the text. (b) Climatograms showing rainfall (histograms) and temperature (●) (humid periods indicated by light stippling, perhumid periods are shown in black, and arid periods by cross hatching); day length curves (o) are shown above the climatograms. (From HALL-MARTIN et al., 1975)

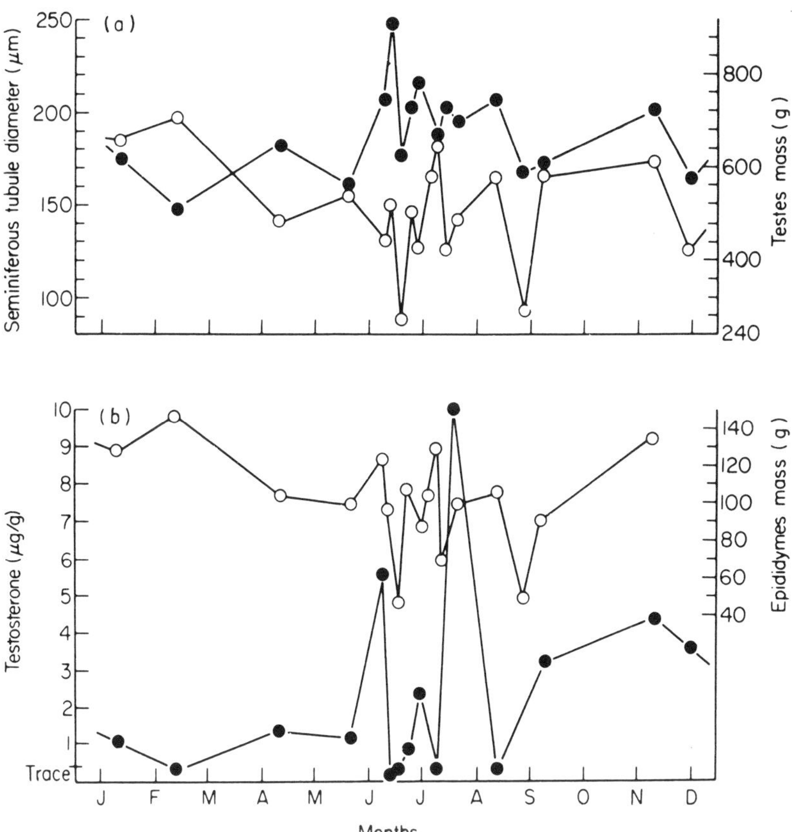

Fig. 3. (a) Graphs showing seminiferous tubule diameter (•) (n = 17) and testes mass (o) n = 18). Data from adult giraffe collected in the Timbavati Private Nature Reserve from June 1971 to July 1972. (b) Graphs showing testosterone concentrations (•) (n = 15); and epididymes mass (o) (n = 17). (From HALL-MARTIN et al., 1975)

tion between rainfall one month before conception and conception at Akira (r = 0.720 $p < 0.01$) and Timbavati/Hans Merensky (r = 0.766 $p < 0.001$). No significant correlations were found between rainfall and conception at Nairobi. The correlation between temperature and conception was clearcut, but there was a significant correlation for both the month of conception and the previous month at Timbavati/Hans Merensky (r = 0.695 $p < 0.02$ and r = 0.661 $p < 0.02$).

Day length for the 17th day of each month (from LIST, 1951) was plotted for six areas (Fig. 2) by HALL-MARTIN et al. (1975), and the correlations with time of conception determined. As expected, there was no correlation at the equator apart from a probably spurious positive correlation at Nairobi (r = 0.637 $p < 0.02$). Highly significant correlations between day length and conception were found for the Timbavati/ Hans Merensky data for both one (r = 0.750 $p < 0.01$) and two (r = 0.719 $p < 0.01$) months preceding conception (HALL-MARTIN et al., 1975), but only significant at the 5% probability level for the month of conception.

Day length strongly influences the appearance of new leaves and flowers (KOZLOWSKI, 1971; LONGMAN and JENIK, 1974), and it is probably more realistic to conclude that the stimulus exerted by day length is indirect via the nutritional status of the vegetation, particularly as there is no seasonal effect on male fertility, despite a marked drop in body condition during late winter (Fig. 3). Nor is there a seasonal cycle in male behavior, although this is difficult to determine as no detailed behavioral studies have been made on male giraffe.

The Springbok

This is an example of an opportunistic breeder that has apparently evolved in arid regions, inhabits the desert and sub-desert areas but may also inhabit the grassland plains. There is no clearly defined

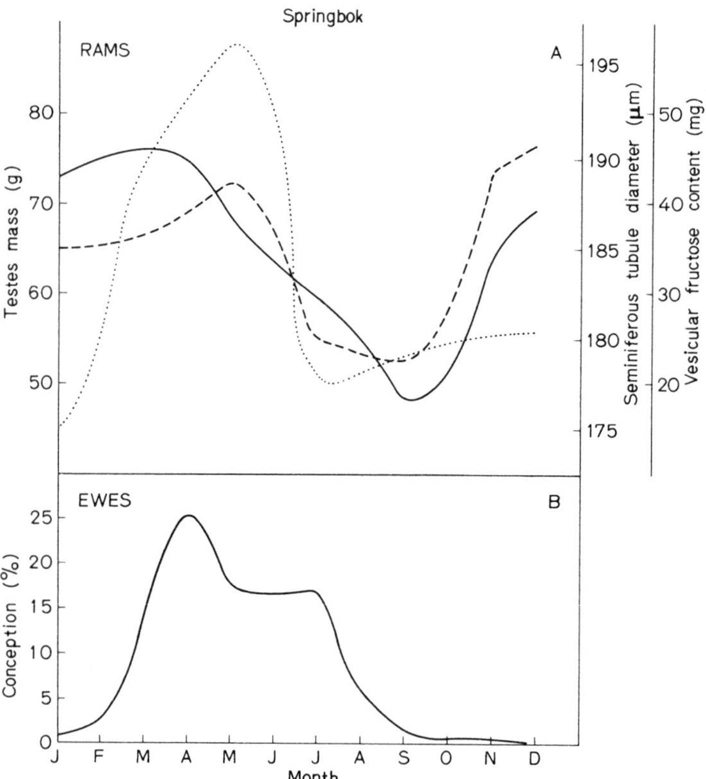

Fig. 4. The breeding pattern in springbok showing (A) Testes mass (---), seminiferous tubule diameter (....) and vesicular fructose content (——) in the ram, and (B) conception rate in the ewe. (Adapted from SKINNER et al., 1974)

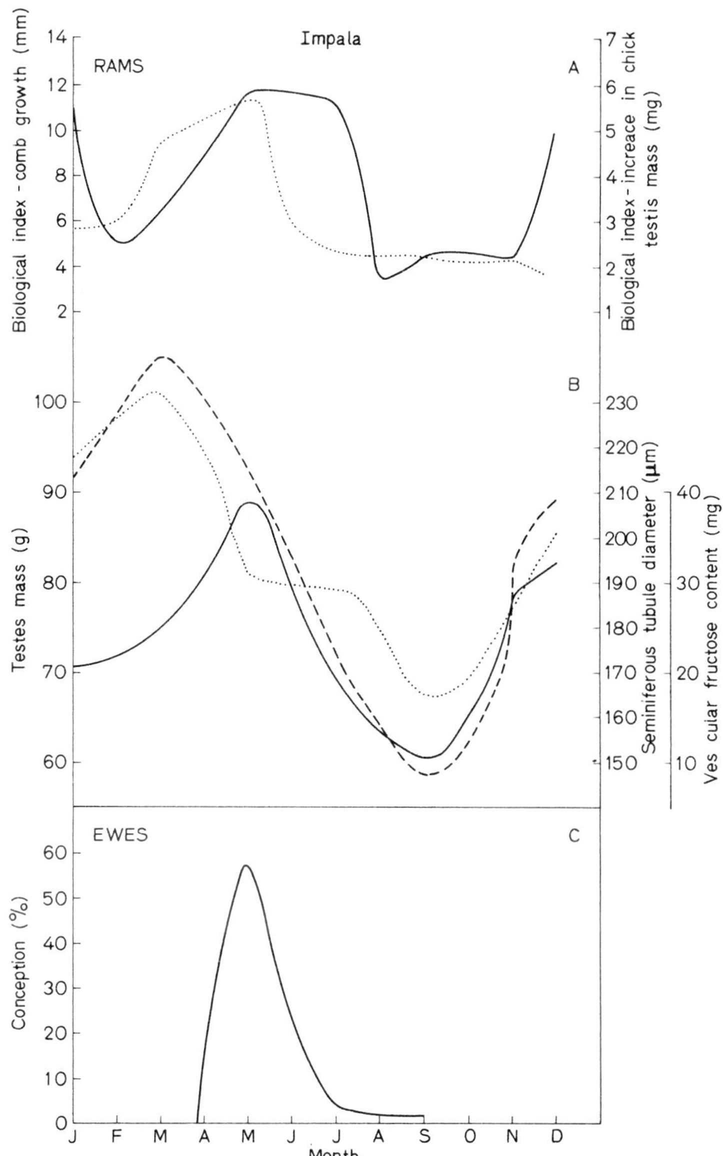

Fig. 5. The breeding cycle in the impala showing (A) Biological index, chick testis growth (———) and comb growth (....). (From FAIRALL, 1972). (B) Testes mass (----), seminiferous tubule diameter (....) and vesicular fructose content (———) in the ram and (C) conception rate in the ewe. (Adapted from SKINNER et al., 1974)

breeding season, but in the grassland plains of western Transvaal there is a maximum in breeding that enables parturition to occur at a favorable time of the year. The time of conception at the S.A. Lombard Nature Reserve is illustrated in Figure 4 with the peak in April. In the ewe, lactation anestrus lasts between four and six months and, as a result, influences the entire endocrine cycle. Ewes show no marked annual cycle in follicular development, and puberty can occur at any time under favorable conditions (SKINNER and VAN ZYL, 1970a).

Springbok rams are territorial, maintaining territories and being capable of breeding at any time of the year, but they do show an annual cycle on the grassland plains (SKINNER and VAN ZYL, 1979b) that is related to the nutritive cycle of the available forage (WEINMANN, 1959), and capacity for reproduction would be lower at times when the nutritive value of the pasture is low.

There is little doubt that the springbok responds to nutritional cues in breeding, as shown in Figure 6, where breeding is related to nutritional levels in the forage compared with the constant cycle of the impala.

The Impala

This is an example of a South-African species with a clearly defined breeding season (Fig. 5). SPINAGE (1973) has demonstrated that breeding becomes earlier as the equator is approached until at the equator there is a typical bimodal pattern (KAYANJA, 1969). It is tempting to suggest that the impala evolved on the eastern, moister side of Africa as it is more "water dependent" than, for example, the springbok. This dependence on moisture and the summer rainfall pattern and its influence on vegetation induced the evolution of a fixed annual breeding cycle, so that young are born at the most favorable time of the year for survival. Moreover, the onset of puberty in this species, in contrast to the springbok, is also seasonally limited, and usually occurs at a later age than in an opportunistic breeder of similar size. FAIRALL (1972) found that in nonpregnant ewes, the number of developing ovarian follicles and the diameter of the largest follicle declined steadily from a peak of 13 and 3.7 μm in March/May to 5 and 1.8 μm in September/ December. This was related to the monthly variation in gonadotrophin production. During estrus ewes show an active interest in seeking the ram (FAIRALL, 1972).

Impala rams show a seasonal pattern in their "territoriality", becoming much more aggressive just prior to the breeding season (FAIRALL, 1972), and herding and other sex-related behavior attain maximum intensity at the height of the breeding season. Six weeks after the breeding season, this distinctive male behavior is no longer apparent. Rams show a marked physiologic cycle that matches this pattern of behavior and are incapable of breeding throughout the year (SKINNER, 1971; FAIRALL, 1972; SKINNER et al., 1974; HANKS et al., 1976), reaching a low point in spring just prior to the onset of the rains (Fig. 5). This cycle in the male may be influenced by the considerable loss in body condition.

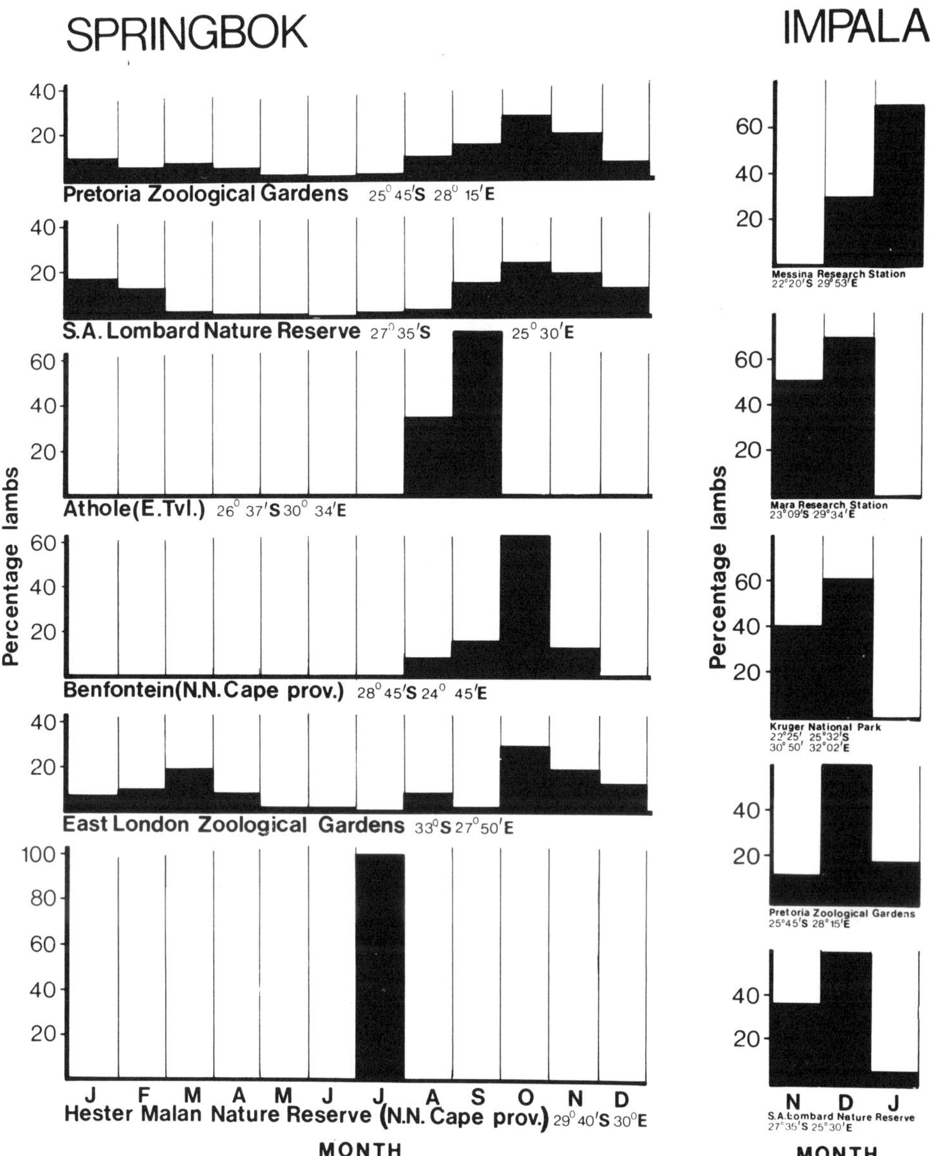

Fig. 6. Distribution of births for springbok and impala in different localities in South Africa. The histograms for springbok were compiled from data supplied as follows: Pretoria (245 lambs 1923-1975 BRAND, 1963 and pers. comm.), S.A. Lombard (1655 lambs 1949-1973 SKINNER, VAN ZYL and OATES, 1974), Athole (Standard annual pattern D. FORBES, pers. comm.), Benfontein (717 fetuses 1972-1973 - birth dates calculated by D.A. ELS from the formula of HUGGETT and WIDAS, 1951) East London (55 lambs 1962-1975 H. VON KETELHODT, pers. comm.), Hester Malan (18 lambs - total crop 1976 R. DIECKMANN, pers. comm.); those for impala as follows: Messina and Mara standard pattern 1960-1963, own records), Kruger Park (FAIRALL, 1968), Pretoria (233 lambs 1917-1975 BRAND, 1963 and pers. comm.; 7% were born in Feb./March and 1% in each of April, May and June), S.A. Lombard (568 lambs 1949-1974 SKINNER et al., 1974 and OATES, pers. comm.). (From SKINNER et al., 1977)

Conclusion

Breeding cycles have evolved in different regions and respond to different cues. That of the giraffe is dependent on the nutritional status of the vegetation, which is markedly influenced by the prime species browsed, *Acacia* spp., which are deciduous in late winter. That of the springbok is also greatly influenced by the "flushing" effect following rain in arid regions, and is also related to the nomadic behavior of this species which treks to areas of more abundant grazing thereby ensuring its survival. That of the impala, which is nonmigratory, has evolved in an area of fixed rainfall pattern that ensures survival of the lambs after birth.

References

BAKER, J.R.: Evolution of breeding seasons. In: Evolution: Essays on Aspects of Evolutionary Biology Presented to Professor E.S. Goodrich. D Beer, G.R. (ed.). Oxford: Clarendon Press, 1938, 350 pp

FAIRALL, N.: Behavioural aspects of the reproductive physiology of the impala, *Aepyceros melampus* (Licht). Zool. Afr. 7, 167-174 (1972)

FIELD, C.R., BLANKENSHIP, L.H.: Nutrition and reproduction of Grant's and Thomson's gazelles, Coke's hartebeest and giraffe in Kenya. J. Reprod. Fert. Suppl. 19, 187-301 (1973)

HALL-MARTIN, A.J., SKINNER, J.D., VAN DYK, J.M.: Reproduction in the giraffe in relation to some environmental factors. E. Afr. Wildl. J. 13, 237-248 (1975)

HANKS, J., CUMMING, D.H.M., ORPEN, J.L., PARRY, D.F., WARREN, H.B.: Growth, condition and reproduction in the impala ram (*Aepyceros melampus*). J. Zool. 170, 421-435 (1976)

KAYANJA, F.I.B.: The ovary of the impala, *Aepyceros melampus* (Lichtenstein, 1812) J. Reprod. Fert. Suppl. 6, 311-317 (1969)

KOZLOWSKI, T.T.: Growth and Development of Trees. New York: Academic Press, 1971

LIST, R.J. (ed.): Smithsonian Meteorological Tables. Publ. No. 4014. Washington, D.C.: Smithsonian Institute, 1951

LONGMAN, K.A., JENIK, J.: Tropical Forest and its Environment. London: Longman, 1974

PERRY, J., ROWLANDS, I.W.: Biology of reproduction in mammals. J. Reprod. Fert. Suppl. 6, 531 pp. (1969)

SKINNER, J.D.: The sexual cycle of the impala ram *Aepyceros melampus* Lichtenstein. Zool. Afr. 6, 75-84 (1971)

SKINNER, J.D., HALL-MARTIN, A.J.: A note on foetal growth and development in the giraffe *Giraffe comelopardalis giraffa*. J. Zool. 177, 73-76 (1975)

SKINNER, J.D., NEL, J.A.J., MILLAR, R.P.: Evolution of time of parturition and differing litter sizes as an adaptation to changes in environmental conditions. Proc. 4th Int. Symp. Comp. Reprod. Sydney: Aust. Acad. Science, 1977, pp. 39-44

SKINNER, J.D., VAN ZYL, J.H.M.: A study of growth in springbok ewes. Afr. Wildl. 24, 149-154 (1970a)

SKINNER, J.D., VAN ZYL, J.H.M.: The sexual cycle of the springbok ram (*Antidorcas marsupialis* Zimm.). Proc. S. Afr. Soc. Anim. Prod. 9, 197-202 (1970b)

SKINNER, J.D., VAN ZYL, J.H.M., OATES, L.G.: The effect of season on the breeding cycle of plains antelope of the western Transvaal Highveld. J. S. Afr. Wildl. Mgmt. Ass. 4, 15-23 (1974)

SPINAGE, C.A.: The rôle of photoperiodism in the seasonal breeding of tropical African ungulates. Mammal. Rev. 3, 71-84 (1973)

WEINMANN, H.: The chemistry and physiology of grasses. In: The Grasses and Pastures of South Africa. Meredith, D. (ed.). Johannesburg: Central News Agency, 1959, pp. 571-600

10. The Annual Cycle of Plasma Testosterone and Territorial Behavior in the Roe Deer

A. SEMPERE

The annual cycle of plasma testosterone in the European Roe Deer (*Capreolus capreolus* L.) exhibits pronounced seasonal variations. There appears to be a clear relationship between the plasma testosterone levels and the annual cycle in day length and ambient temperature (Fig. 1).

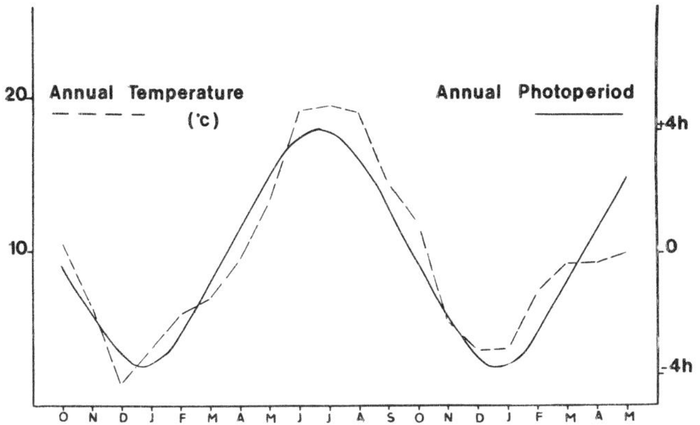

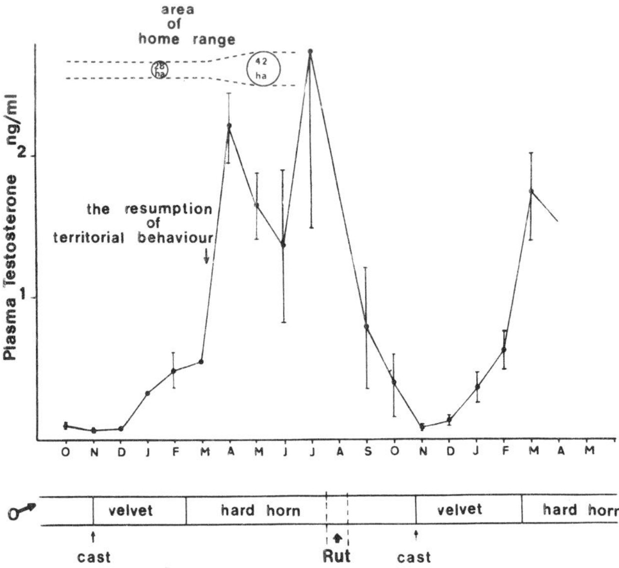

Fig. 1. Annual pattern of plasma testosterone cycle in relation with environment and territorial behavior in the Roe Deer

Extremely low testosterone levels are associated with low temperatures and short days. In summer the concentration of testosterone is markedly higher. An increase in plasma testosterone levels is evident at the beginning of January, followed by a highly significant increase in April (1976) or March (1977).

This major increase in testosterone coincides with the appearance of territorial behavior in the buck as determined by radio-tracking in the Forêt de Chizé. This behavior is characterized by frequent visits to the periphery of the territory, resulting in marked increase in the size of the home range from 28 to 42 ha.

In summer, this testosterone curve seems to follow a biphasic pattern with maxima in May and July, the latter corresponding with the beginning of rut. In September, the plasma testosterone concentration is low, and continues to decline until November (when the antlers are cast). Active spermatogenesis has been demonstrated to occur from the beginning of May (SHORT and MANN, 1966; CADARIU, 1976).

References

CADARIU, M., POPOVICI, N., GOTEA, I.: Activitatea tiroidei la Capriorul (*Capreolus capreolus* L.) mascul in decursul cicluliu anual. Stud. Univ. Babes - Bolyai, Biol. Rouman 21, 57-64 (1976)

SHORT, R.V., MANN, T.: The sexual cycle of a seasonally breeding mammal, the roebuck (*Capreolus capreolus* L.). J. Reprod. Fertil. 12, 337 (1966)

11. Annual Cyclic Variations in Prolactin in Sheep

R. ORTAVANT, J. PELLETIER, J. P. RAVAULT, and J. THIMONIER

It is well known that reproductive activity of many breeds of domestic sheep in temperate climates is restricted to certain months of the year. These seasonal variations in reproductive activity occur in both males and females. Gonadotropic hormones are involved in regulation of male and female reproductive processes; thus, it is possible to observe seasonal variations in their secretion by studying the plasma levels of each of them. Variations in the secretion in LH, FSH, PRL have been studied; in this paper, only fluctuations in plasma levels of PRL are reported.

Seasonal variations in plasma prolactin have been described in male sheep (RAVAULT, 1976; Fig. 1). From 15 weeks of age, variations in prolactin are parallel with day length, showing a regular increase

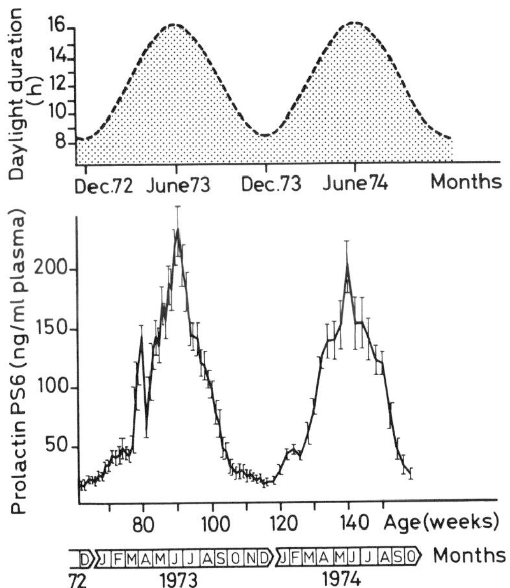

Fig. 1. Seasonal variations of plasma prolactin levels in Ile de France rams (RAVAULT, 1976)

until June, followed by a decline to a minimum in December. Similar variations were observed in the second and in the third years, but with an increased amplitude. These results indicate that prolactin secretion is maximum in summer (long days, high temperature) and minimum in winter (short days, low temperature). Ewes also show a similar pattern (THIMONIER et al., 1977).

As has been shown in cattle (TUCKER and WETTEMAN, 1976) temperature can play a role in the secretion of prolactin associated with day length.

PELLETIER (1973) and ALBERIO (1976) have studied this effect in sheep. For instance, PELLETIER (1973) has submitted intact or castrated rams to an "annual" photoperiodic cycle shortened to six months while temperature remained constant. The results show the parallelism between variations in the light period and the plasma prolactin level in both intact and castrated animals ($r = 0.88$; $P < 0.001$). Maximum prolactin values were found when animals were exposed to light for 16 h per day.

ALBERIO and RAVAULT (cited by RAVAULT and ORTAVANT, 1977) also subjected rams to either constant temperature (between 19°and 21°C) or to variable temperature (between 1° and 24°C), according to the season. The results show that temperature did not significantly affect the level of prolactin. It seems that the variations of temperature are not responsible for the pattern of prolactin secretion, and that day length appears to be the external factor in the control of prolactin secretion.

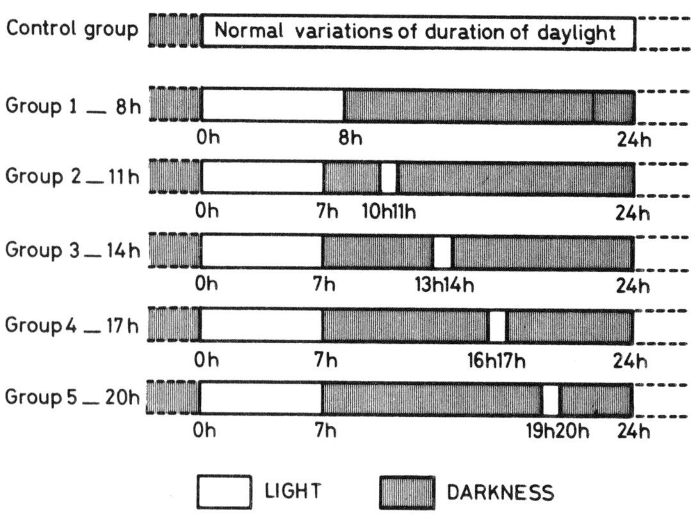

Fig. 2. Protocol of the experiment

To elucidate the mechanism of the effect of day length, RAVAULT and ORTAVANT (1977), using skeleton light treatment (main photophase : 7 h + 1 h light pulse given at various times of the scotophase) (Fig. 2), have shown that plasma prolactin levels were higher when the light pulse was given during hour 17 after dawn than for all other light treatment. Thus, when the light pulse is given at hour 17 after dawn (Fig. 3), prolactin levels were maximal, and comparable to those observed with long (16 h daily photophases) even though the total daily illumination was only 8 h.

The same type of photoperiodic treatments was given to ewes. Again the plasma prolactin levels were influenced largely by the time at which the scotophase was interrupted by the light pulse (Fig. 4). The group that received the light pulse during the 17th h after dawn had significantly higher levels of prolactin than all other groups, results similar to those obtained with rams.

However, even under these constant conditions of light treatment, an annual variation in plasma prolactin levels was observed. Although the

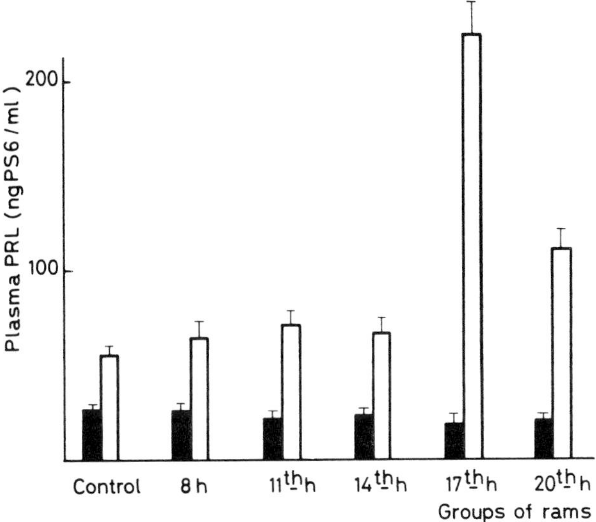

Fig. 3. Daily mean plasma prolactin level before treatment ■, and 5 weeks after the beginning of light treatment □

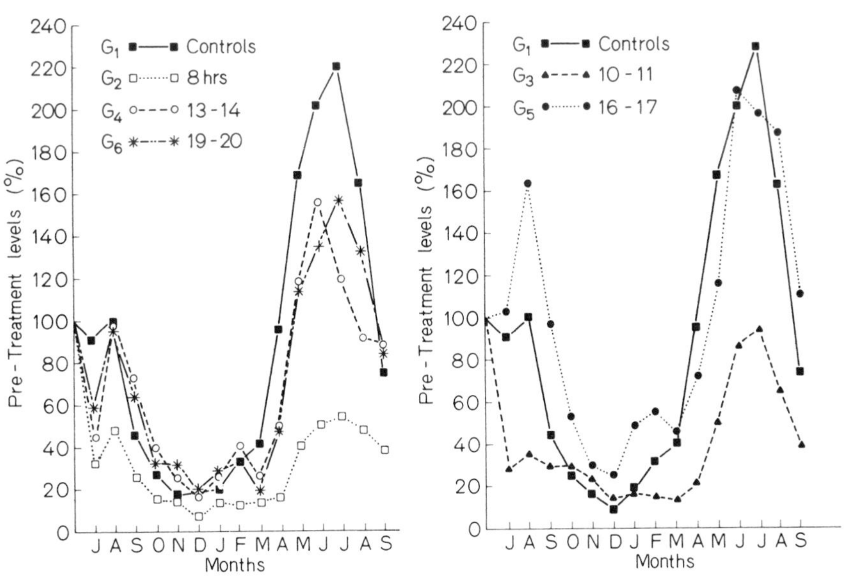

Fig. 4. Variations of prolactin levels in light treated ewes (expressed as % of pre-treatment levels)

levels of secretion are different among the various groups, the same pattern of variations was observed: during May, June, and July, the levels of prolactin were higher than in December and January, as in the control group subjected to the normal cycles of day length.

It is difficult to explain such a result, since feeding and light regimes were constant. It was not related to the sexual season and estrogen secretion. Only ambient temperature variations were observed. Thus it seems necessary to investigate the action of temperature on prolactin secretion in sheep in relationship with the annual cycle.

References

ALBERIO, R.: Role de la photopériode dans le dévelopment de la fonction de reproduction chez l'agneau Ile-de-France. Thèse de 3ème Cycle. Université Paris VI, 1976

PELLETIER, J.: Evidence for photoperiodic control of prolactin release in rams. J. Reprod. Fert. 35, 143-147 (1973)

RAVAULT, J.P.: Prolactin in the ram: seasonal variations in the concentration of blood plasma from birth until three years old. Acta. Endocrinol. 83, 720-725 (1976)

RAVAULT, J.P., ORTAVANT, R.: Light control of prolactin secretion in sheep. Evidence for a photoinductible phase during a diurnal rhythm. Ann. Biol. Anim. Bioch. Biophys. 17, 459-473 (1972)

THIMONIER, J., RAVAULT, J.P., ORTAVANT, R.: Influence of light on cyclic ovarian activity and prolactin secretion in the ewe (abstract). Dublin: Society for Study of Fertility. 11-15 July 1977

TUCKER, H.A., WETTEMAN, R.P.: Effects of ambient temperature and relative humidity on serum prolactin and growth hormone in heifers. Proc. Soc. Biol. Med. 151, 623-628 (1976)

12. Seasonal Reproductive Activity of the European Wild Boar. Comparison with the Domestic Sow

R. MAUGET

The domestic pig is known to be reproductive all around the year. There is, however, a trend toward a seasonal activity, or more exactly, a seasonal decrease in reproductive efficiency (CORTEEL et al., 1964; STORK, 1977). An excessive inefficiency occurs in animals served during the summer months.

In the wild boar, reproduction appears to be clearly seasonal. Two peaks of farrowing, and consequently of estrus, can be observed. These peaks occur in late fall-early winter and in late spring. The animals involved in those two main periods are females reaching puberty at one of those peaks, and females farrowing twice a year. The second litter per year is obtained by the separation of the sow from her young three weeks after parturition. The sow returns to estrus in April or May. In a natural environment, without any human management, as can be observed in the Chizé forest (midwestern France), there is often only one estrus peak in winter. The possibility that a female wild boar may produce two litters per year seems correlated with earliness of the winter estrus and consequently with the end of suckling. If the end of lactation occurs in May, there is a possibility of estrus returning; a further pregnancy is then established. When, after a later farrowing, the lactation extends to late June-July, a post-weaning estrus does not occur. The suppression of lactation three weeks after parturition in May, in rearing or in accidental natural conditions, is accompanied by a return to estrus.

There appears to be a critical period during the summer months. Comparing the domestic sow with the wild boar in a natural environment, there is, in the former, a tendency to a seasonal decrease in reproductive efficiency, and, in the latter, a cessation of reproduction. This summer anestrus coincides with high environmental temperature, long days and restricted food.

References

CORTEEL, J.M., SIGNORET, J.P., DU MESNIL DU BUISSON, F.: Variations saisonnières de la reproduction de la Truie et facteurs favorisant l'anoestrus temporel. 5th Cong. Int. Reprod. Anim. Insem. Artif. Trente 3, 1964, pp. 536-546

STORK, M.G.: Seasonal reproductive inefficiency in the pig. Proc. Pig Vet. Soc. U.K., 1, pp. 55-66

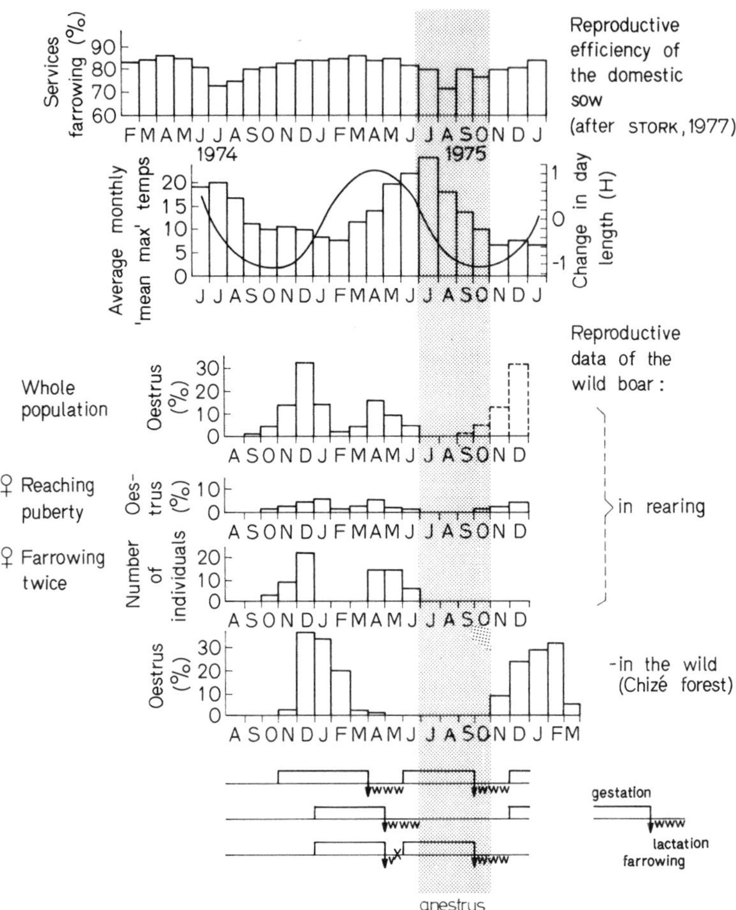

Fig. 1. Seasonal reproductive activity of the European Wild Boar compared with the domestic sow

13. Field Studies in Southern Tunisia on Water Turnover and Thyroid Activity in Two Species of Meriones

F. LACHIVER, T. CHENITI, D. BRADSHAW, J. L. BERTHIER, and F. PETTER

Meriones libycus and *Meriones shawii* are nocturnal burrowing rodents. The former is typically xerophilic; the latter is more hygrophilic. The populations studied were found to occur sympatrically in a dry wadis south of Foum Tatahouine at approximately the 120-150 mm H_2O per year isohyet (LE HOUEROU, 1969).

Investigations were carried out in June to July 1975 and in November to December 1976. The mean values for climatic variables were: maximum and minima for temperature in summer - 42.3°C and 16.4°C, respectively, and in winter 15.8°C and 5.8°C; relative humidity in summer, 55.4% and 8.4% and in winter 88% and 51.5%. The soil temperature at a depth of 50 cm was 25°-27°C in summer and 15°-17°C in winter. Temperatures of occupied burrows varied by 13°C between summer (30°C) and winter (17°C). The food of the rodents consisted primarily of leaves of the succulent halophytic plant *Haloxylon schmittianum*, the water content of which averaged 55%-60%. Capture methods and the techniques used for the measurement of water turnover of free-ranging animals has been described by BRADSHAW et al. (1976). The activity of the thyroid gland was studied both histologically and by the metabolism of iodine (^{127}I, ^{131}I, and ^{125}I).

Results

The body weight of animals captured in the field was significantly lower in winter (*M. shawii* 78 g, *M. libycus* 59.6 g) than in summer (108.4 g and 85 g, respectively).

1. Thyroid Gland

Histologically the thyroid of the two species is very active in winter and somewhat less active in summer. From summer to winter the height of the thyroidal epithelium increases from 7.5 to 11 μ for *M. shawii* and from 8.4 to 9.3 μ for *M. libycus*. The total amount of iodine in the thyroid gland averaged approximately 1 μg per gland showed neither seasonal nor sexual variation. For both species the PBI^{127}I is significantly high in summer (in μg ^{127}I/dl *M. shawii*, 3.7 and *M. libycus* 3.7) than in winter (1.2 and 1.5, respectively). The rate of turnover of thyroidal iodine in winter was determined by double iotopic marking of each animal with I^{131}I (sampled at 2, 4 and 8 h after injection) and ^{125}I (sampled at 30, 48, 96 and 108 h). Maximal fixation is obtained 8 h after injection of ^{131}I. The biological half life of ^{125}I released from the thyroid is 1.4 days, which corresponds to an apparent secretion rate of 0.45 μg of iodine per day in the form of thyroxine. PBI ^{125}I reaches a maximum 28-34 h after injection of radioiodine and averaged 57.1% for *M. libycus* in summer and 58.5% in winter. The maximum value attained for *M. shawii* in winter was 61.6%. The concentration of iodine in the urine collected in metabolic cages was 0.16 μg ^{127}I/ml in both

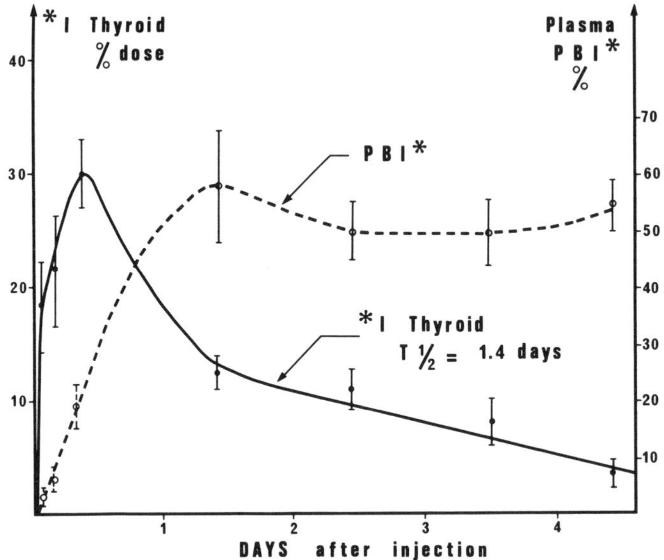

Fig. 1. *Meriones libycus* (December 1976) uptake and release of radioactive iodine from the thyroid gland (solid line). Plasma-labeled protein-bound iodine (PBI*) (dashed line). T 1/2, Biological halflife

species. The daily excretion of iodine as micrograms ^{127}I/100 g averaged 0.4 for *M. libycus* 0.42 for *M. shawii* in winter.

2. Water Turnover

Total body water was significantly lower in winter than in summer in *M. libycus* (72.1 ml/100 g and 80.4 ml/100 g, respectively). Values for *M. shawii* in summer and winter were 73.3 ml/100 g and 71.1 ml/100 g, respectively. In both seasons the influx was not significantly different from outflux, and the animals were thus in water equilibrium in their natural biotope. Although fractional turnover of water did not differ significantly in *M. shawii* between summer and winter, the efflux expressed either per kg or per $kg^{0.82}$ were elevated in winter due to the smaller average body size of the animals. The same trend was evident with *M. libycus*, but in this species fractional turnover expressed as a percentage of the body water exchanged per 24 h was significantly higher in winter than in summer for both influx and efflux.

Discussion

Recent studies have shown that thyroid activity is reduced in desert rodents. This has been correlated with their reduced metabolic rates, considered to be an adaptation to high environmental temperatures. Lower half lives for thyroidal iodine have been measured in a number of desert rodents from North America *Dipodomys deserti* and *Dipodomys merriari* (HUDSON and WANG, 1969) and in various species of *Citellus* (HUDSON and DEAVERS, 1976). It has also shown that the rate of secretion of thyroxin by the thyroid gland of desert rodents of the genus *Dipodomys* and *Peroganthus* is lower than that of rodents of temperate regions. In addition SCOTT et al. (1976) have shown in various heteromyids, sciurids, and cricetids that the circulating level of thyroxin increases with the basal metabolic rate, and is lower in desert rodents than those from montane regions.

In general these data have been collected in the laboratory with rodents that have been held captive for a number of weeks, and under experimental conditions that are very different from those of their natural environment. Our results obtained in the field show that the thyroid gland of *Meriones shawii* and *libycus* is very active both in summer and in winter in southern Tunisia. Amongst those factors likely to influence the activity of the thyroid glands of *Meriones*, the nutritional intake of iodine is certain to play a large role. In fact, the combination of factors of a low amount of iodine in the thyroid gland, a low rate of urinary excretion of iodine and an elevated rate of turnover of iodine in the thyroid gland are all reminiscent of laboratory rats maintained on an iodine-deficient diet. This conclusion has already been reached for *M. shawii* in the north of Tunisia (LACHIVER and CHENITI, 1974), and it would appear that the thyroid of *Meriones* both in the north and the south of Tunisia are adapted biochemically to a diet that is extremely poor in iodine. In contrast, the activity of the thyroid gland of the gerboise (*Jaculus orientalis*), which lives sympatrically with *M. shawii* in northern Tunisia, presents all the characteristics of a hypofunctional gland comparable with that of *Dipodomys* (LACHIVER and CHENITI, 1974). Hypoactivity of the thyroid gland is therefore not a general characteristic of desert rodents, but it would appear to vary depending upon the species and upon the conditions of their desert existence. The decrease in total body water is probably due to an increase in body lipids with the onset of winter. Similarly, the increased rate of water turnover in winter is probably related to an increased consumption of food and water and may also be in response to decreased environmental temperatures and increased rates of metabolism.

Table 1. Water turnover of free-living *Meriones shawii* and *M. libycus* in June 1975 and December 1976

Species	Month (N°)	Body weight g	Total body Water ml/100 g	Water Intake and Output ml/24 h		ml/kg/24 h		ml/kg$^{0.82}$/24 h		%Body water/24 h	
				In	Out	In	Out	In	Out	In	Out
Meriones shawii	June (7)	108.4	73.3	17.5	14.2	155	131	108	88	21.8	17.5
	December (3)	78	71.1	11.1	12.2	145	156	90	100	20.4	21.9
Meriones libycus	June (13)	85	80.4	11.0	12.1	127	141	83	91	15.3	16.4
	December (30)	59.6	72.1	8.7	8.7	150	165	86	87	20.9	20.6

References

BRADSHAW, D., CHENITI, T., LACHIVER, F.: Taux de renouvellement d'eau et balance hydrique chez deux rongeurs désertiques, *Meriones shawii* et *Meriones libycus*, étudiés dans leur environment naturel en Tunisie. C.R. Acad. Sci. (Paris) 282, 481-484 (1976)

CHENITI-LAMINE, T.: Etude écophysiologique et biochimique de la thyroide d'un rongeur de Tunisie: *Meriones shawii*. Thèse de doctorat des sciences, Tunis (1976)

HOUEROU, H.N. LE: La végétation de la Tunisie steppique. Int. Nat. Rech. Agr. Tunisie, Ariana, 1969

HUDSON, J.W., DEAVERS, D.R.: Thyroid function and basal metabolism in the ground squirrels: *Ammospermophilus leucurus* and *Spermophilus* spp. Physiol. Zool. 49, 425-444 (1976)

HUDSON, J.W., WANG, L.C.H.: Thyroid function in desert ground squirrels. In: Physiological Systems in Semiarid Environments. Hoff and Riedesel (eds.). Albuquerque: University of New Mexico Press, 1969, pp. 17-33

LACHIVER, F., CHENITI, T.: Activité thyroidienne comparée chez deux rongeurs de Tunisie: la mérione (*Meriones shawii*) et la gerboise (*Jaculus orientalis*) Colloque sur les problèmes endocriniens chez les mammifères sauvages. Entretien de Chizè. 1974

LACHIVER, F., CHENITI-LAMINE, T.: Cinétique d'iodation de la thyroglobuline dans la thyroide d'un rongeur de Tunisie: *Meriones shawii*. J. Physiol. 69, 201A (1974)

SCOTT, I.M., YOUSEF, M.K., JOHNSON, H.D.: Plasma thyroxine levels of mammals desert and mountain. Life Sci. 19, 807-812 (1976)

YOUSEF, M.K., JOHNSON, H.D.: Thyroid activity in desert rodents: a mechanism for lowered metabolic rate. Am. J. Physiol. 229, 427-431 (1976)

14. Seasonal Changes of the Testicular and Thyroid Functions in the Badger, *Meles meles* L.

D. MAUREL

The european Badger is a nocturnal underground mammal with a reduced general locomotor activity during winter. The plasma testosterone and

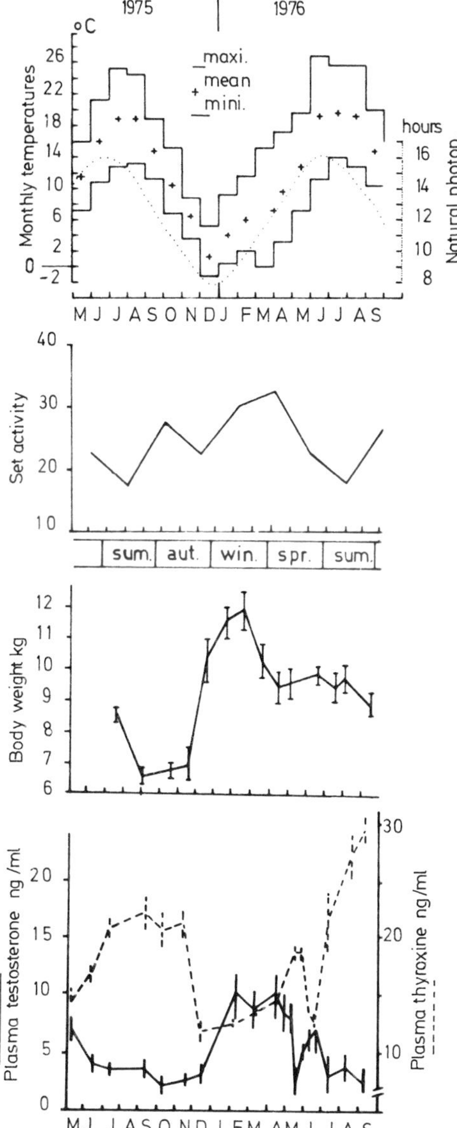

Fig.1

thyroxine levels present marked seasonal variations (MAUREL et al., 1977). At the end of summer and in autumn, plasma testosterone concentrations are low, while the plasma thyroxine level is high. The resumption of testicular activity takes place in December at the beginning of the phase of hypoactivity of the thyroid gland. From February to May, the plasma testosterone concentration remains at a high level; then after a rapid decrease there is an other peak in June. In summer, the plasma testosterone level decreases continuously, while thyroid activity is more pronounced. The biphasic annual rhythms occur annually, although in the location of the maximal testicular and thyroid activity.

Physiologic and bioclimatic experiments will allow us to determine if there is a causal inverse relationship between thyroidal and testicular activity. However, preliminary results have shown that in castrated animals testosterone injections provoke a highly significant decrease in plasma thyroxine concentration in comparison to nontreated castrated animals.

References

MAUREL, D., JOFFRE, J., BOISSIN, J.: Cycle annuel de la testosteronémie et de la thyroxinémie chez le Blaireau européen (*Meles meles* L.). C. R. Acad. Sci. (Paris) 284, 1577-1580 (1977)

15. Day Length and the Annual Reproductive Cycle in the Ferret *(Mustela furo)*: the Role of the Pineal Body

J. HERBERT and M. KLINOWSKA

Introduction

Information about the relations between day length and the breeding season of the female ferret has been accumulating for almost fifty years. Here we take stock of the present state of knowledge, discuss the way in which changing day lengths control or modify the annual cycle of the ferret, how much is known about the neuroendocrine mechanisms by which the reproductive system responds to these changes, how the ferret compares with other species, and whether any basic relationships between annual and other rhythms can be detected. We pay particular attention to the pineal gland, since its role in seasonal breeding is being established, and it is time to consider whether such a role is securely based on experimental evidence.

Light and the Breeding Season in Ferrets

The Reproductive Cycle. The basic features of the ferret cycle are well known, though there is still comparatively little information available about hormone levels in this species. Under natural lighting, estrus starts in the spring (March and April in England) and is signalled by the unmistakable appearance of vulval edema. Estrus continues without interruption for a variable period (20-25 weeks), usually ending between July and September. Ovulation is provoked by coitus and seldom occurs otherwise. In unmated animals, therefore, one can study an annual breeding rhythm separately from an ovulatory cycle.

Recent reports (DONOVAN and TER HAAR, 1977) show that the female ferret has higher, strongly fluctuating levels of plasma follicle-stimulating hormone (FSH) and luteinizing hormone (LH) during anestrus and lower, stable levels during estrus; prolactin levels hardly change.

Progestin levels are low and similar in estrus and anestrus (BLATCHLEY and DONOVAN, 1972): estrogen levels are higher during estrus, low in anestrus (TER HAAR, M.B.: GLENCROSS, R., personal communications). These findings are consistent with those for other induced ovulators, e.g., voles (GRAY et al., 1974), and rabbits (SCARAMUZZI et al., 1972).

Onset of Estrus. The ferret was one of the first mammals in which the stimulating effect of artificial illumination was shown (BISSONETTE, 1932). Anestrous ferrets exposed to extra light during winter came into premature estrus after 6-8 weeks, that is, several months before controls kept in natural daylight.

The physical parameters of the light necessary to evoke this response have received some attention. The neuroendocrine system seems exceedingly sensitive to light and illumination above 0.42 foot candles given for 14 h a day will induce estrus (VINCENT, 1970). The only attempt to define an action spectrum for induction of estrus (MARSHALL and BOWDEN, 1934) showed 365 nm to be highly effective, followed by 520, 650 and 577 nm; 436.8 and 750 were ineffective.

There is now considerable experimental support for one and possibly two photosensitive phases each 24 h (PITTENDRIGH and DAAN, 1976). This can be demonstrated by giving animals skeleton (interrupted) light treatments, so that the animals are exposed only to a brief pulse of light, but at various times during the postulated photosensitive cycle. Systematic studies have not been carried out on ferrets, though estrus is not advanced by exposure to 7L:17D, whereas the same amount of light given as 3 1/2L:5D:3 1/2L:5D is effective (HAMMOND, 1951).

There is a latent interval between exposing anestrous ferrets to light and the response - a minimum of 35 days' exposure is necessary. Evidence from the ram suggests a comparatively gradual change in gonadotrophin levels when day lengths are altered (LINCOLN, 1976), but our unpublished results show that in the ferret the transition from anestrus to estrus is abrupt in this respect, coinciding with the vulval response to estrogen, which also takes place rapidly. It would appear that the inertia does not lie in the response to gonadotrophins.

A critical question in whether, although increasing day length may induce early estrus, this change in the light environment is <u>necessary</u> for estrus to occur. The evidence in ferrets is strongly against this being the case. Ferrets kept in short days (e.g., 8L:16D) during winter and spring nevertheless come into estrus at the usual time. Subsequently, such animals fail to show an annual estrous rhythm, though they do come into estrus from time to time, suggesting that changes in day length are necessary only for <u>timing</u> the breeding season (HERBERT and VINCENT, 1972).

<u>Duration of the Breeding Season.</u> Ferrets can be made to go out of breeding condition by exposing them to short day length (e.g. 8L:16D) during the summer (THORPE and HERBERT, 1976b). Under natural daylight, however, they may end their estrus when the day lengths are as long, or even longer than those prevailing when they began. Either, therefore, there is a mechanism determining the duration of estrus which does not depend on light, or the animals are defining the day length of autumn as "short" with reference to the midsummer maximum, or they are becoming photorefractory.

The evidence from animals kept entirely in short days suggests that a change in day length is not required for estrus to end. Animals kept in long days (e.g., 14L:10D) eventually end their estrus (though it may be far longer than normal) and subsequently remain permamently anestrus, which suggests the existence of photorefractoriness. This was confirmed by transferring such animals to short days for 7 to 8 weeks and returning them to long days, whereupon they returned to estrus within 6 to 8 weeks (THORPE and HERBERT, 1976b). Since at least three factors could determine the duration of estrus, individual sensitivities to them may differ and thus be responsible for the relative asynchrony in the ending of estrus.

<u>Periodicity of Breeding.</u> Artificial light cycles can change the periodicity of the ferret breeding rhythm. In regimes of 6, 4, or 2 months' exposure to long days followed by the same period in short days, ferrets come into estrus at corresponding 12-, 8-, or 4-month intervals. There is a limit to this effect, since a 1-month alternating regime results in a breakdown of the rhythm, and estrus occurs irregularly (HERBERT and VINCENT, 1972).

Neuroendocrine Mechanisms

Receptors. Sectioning the optic nerves, or removal of the eyes, prevents the effect of long days on the ferret's breeding season (THOMPSON, 1954). Blind ferrets also show recurrent estrous seasons, initially in concert, but subsequently becoming asynchronous, both with respect to each other and to the prevailing seasons. There is no evidence for regular circannual rhythms in these animals, although they have been followed for up to three years after operation, neither do they seem to show a characteristic "free running" frequency (HERBERT, STACEY and THORPE, unpublished). While we conclude that the receptors for photoperiodic information lie in the retina, their nature is unknown.

The Pineal Gland. To put it simply, removing the ferret pineal or interrupting its autonomic nerve supply, which derives from the superior cervical ganglia, blocks the effects of light on the annual rhythm (HERBERT, 1969). Recurrent breeding seasons still occur, as they do in blind animals, but no longer in phase with each other or with the environment. Thus the entraining effects of the photoperiod are prevented by pinealectomy, whereas the underlying recurrent nature of the breeding cycle remains. We can conclude firstly, that the two are separable, and secondly, that the pineal must be an essential component if receptors in the retina are to pass information about the photoperiod to the mechanism regulating the timing of breeding (HERBERT, 1972).

Comparison of animals pinealectomized at different times of the year reveals that, if the operation is carried out in early anestrus, estrus occurs at the normal time the following season; pinealectomy in early estrus results in a delay in onset of the next season.

Pathways to the Pineal. Attempts to implicate the accessory optic tracts in the response of the ferret pineal have proved negative (THORPE and HERBERT, 1976a). There is no anterior accessory optic tract, but a posterior tract, containing only crossed fibers, leaves the branchium of the superior colliculus and ends in the two terminal nuclei lying either side of the cerebral peduncle. Thus enucleation, combined with lesions of the ipsilateral nuclei, should prevent access to the system. Ferrets so treated still respond to long days by showing premature estrus. A predominantly crossed retinohypothalamic pathway, terminating in the ventral portion of the suprachiasmatic nucleus, was found (THORPE, 1975).

The essential role of the pineal autonomic nerve supply has been mentioned above. In the ferret, autonomic terminals lie in the pineal perivascular space adjacent to the terminals from pinealocytes, and it is presumably there that their regulatory action is exerted (JOHNSON et al., 1974). It seems unlikely that signals could reach the pineal from the habenula (DAVID and HERBERT, 1973; HERBERT, unpublished).

Signals from the Pineal. Melatonin is a pineal substance that has attracted a great deal of attention in recent years. It seems to be secreted from the pineal, since it is found in the cerebrospinal fluid, and its concentration in plasma shows a marked circadian rhythm with a peak during the night; this is in phase with changes in pineal n-acetyltransferase, the rate-limiting enzyme for melatonin production (HEDLUND et al., 1977).

MOORE (1974) found that the circadian component in the activity of this enzyme is abolished by section of the retinohypothalamic tract. He also found that section of the anterior accessory optic tract abolished the rhythm in pineal hydroxyindole-O-methyltransferase (HIOMT), the second enzyme concerned with melatonin synthesis. HIOMT will only show a diurnal rhythm in alternating light/dark cycles and does not free-run in constant conditions - that is to say it does not contain an endogenous circadian component. In rats, which MOORE used for these investigations, HIOMT remains at high levels in constant dark, low levels in constant light.

Thus melatonin production, in the rat at least, is under very subtle photoperiodic control, both enzymes reacting in different ways to environmental light.

Melatonin does not appear to be concerned with the activating effect of long days on the ferret's estrus. It does not enable pinealectomized ferrets to respond to long days, nor does it induce early estrus by itself. On the contrary, it delays the onset of estrus induced by long days (HERBERT, 1969). Melatonin does cause premature termination of estrus, as do short days. Melatonin given to photorefractory ferrets kept in long days restores their photosensitivity, just as if they had been exposed to short days (THORPE and HERBERT, 1976b). The action of melatonin on 5-hydroxytryptamine (5HT) rhythms is discussed below.

The Pineal and Cerebral 5HT Rhythms. 5HT is found in high concentration in the pineal itself, and also in the suprachiasmatic nuclei, which probably play an essential part in the photoperiodic response. We know that circadian rhythms in 5HT in certain parts of the brain are different if ovariectomized ferrets are kept either in long or short days. In long days, this differential rhythm occurs in only two of the areas examined - the pineal and the hypothalamus, which are considered to be involved in the photoperiodic response; but it does not take place in three other areas - hippocampus, cortex, and midbrain. All these five regions show rather similar daily rhythms in short days, where 5HT levels decrease during the first 6 h of light. Pinealectomy or ganglionectomy prevent this differential effect of day length (YATES and HERBERT, 1976). Exposure to constant levels of estrogen from implants suppresses the rhythms (YATES and HERBERT, unpublished).

Melatonin, given 8 h after the onset of light in animals kept in long days - that is when the dark phase would have begun had they been exposed to short days - caused 5HT rhythms in the pineal and hypothalamus to assume the short-day form. The same dose given 14 h after the onset of light - that is, just as the lights were turned off - had no effect, and the animals maintained their long-day 5HT pattern (YATES and HERBERT, 1976).

We suspect, therefore, that the 5HT neural system is concerned in transmitting or effecting information on day length in ferrets. This cannot be the whole story, however, since we have recently found that gonadotrophin levels in a similar group of animals do not reflect day length, nor do they respond to melatonin (KLINOWSKA et al., unpublished).

Relations between Rhythms

Reproduction in Other Species. Which features of reproduction are organized by environmental light and which photoperiodic component involves the pineal? Taking examples from several species, it seems that reproduction can take place autonomously, i.e., using only internal cues, but that photoperiodic information has been exploited in various ways to ensure that reproduction takes place at a favorable time.

Let us first consider control of LH release during the ovulatory cycle. In, for example, the rat and the hamster, LH discharge results from the combination of two factors: a circadian photically determined estrogen-sensitive phase, and adequate levels of estrogen at that time. Pinealectomy does not disturb this relationship (REITER, 1974) because, in our view, the pineal of mammals is not concerned with such photically determined circadian rhythms. In a second group, including sheep and monkey, the photic component is lacking, so that LH surges occur whenever estrogen levels are sufficient. In a third group, including the ferret, the first component, i.e., changes of sensitivity to estrogen, may be induced by coitus. Pinealectomy would not be expected to disturb this either, though direct evidence is lacking.

Considering now annual reproductive cycles, we see again that two components are involved. The first is a circadian system, independent of the pineal, but the second involves the action of light during a light-sensitive phase. Light acts during this phase to induce (or prevent) estrus just as estrogen acts during its sensitive phase to induce LH secretion. It is this second component which, we believe, is prevented by pinealectomy. Thus pinealectomy will only disturb the timing of reproductive processes that depend upon changes in the day length, and this excludes, for example, the timing of ovulation in the rat.

In the ferret and hamster, pinealectomy prevents the photoperiodically dependent changes in the breeding season, though we might expect that other parameters, e.g., the timing of ovulation by the daily photocycle in the hamster, would not be altered.

Integration of Reproductive Rhythms. It appears from the points made above, that in annual reproduction we may be studying the interactions of three phenomena, which can be facultatively coupled. These are a circadian system, the ovarian (estrogen) system and a pineal photosystem. How do they communicate?

Recent evidence suggests that the suprachiasmatic nuclei may be responsible for the first system (MORIN et al., 1977). Thus destruction of these structures will disrupt all three, since circadian mechanisms underlie them all. We still do not know what determines the timing of the estrogen surge, the second component of the ovulation system, nor do we really know the site of the estrogen-sensitive mechanism, though the anterior hypothalamus is a possibility. The site must be separate from that concerned with photoperiodic mechanisms, since some species show one, but not the other (e.g., rat, the first; sheep, the second; hamster, both).

Though we postulate that the pineal is concerned with the second component of the mechanism regulating seasonal breeding, we do not know whether it determines the occurrence of the light-sensitive phase, or the access that light has to it. The same proviso applies to melatonin, which may be the way the pineal signals a "short" day in the ferret.

Summary

The breeding season of the female ferret is controlled by light. The pineal gland is essential for timing estrus in daylight and for the response of the animals to artificial day lengths. Estrus can occur in the absence of the pineal, eyes, superior cervical ganglion, main optic tracts, or changes in the day length, but seems in these cases to show no circannual or other periodicity. Timed injections of melatonin can drive ferrets out of estrus, break photorefractoriness, antagonize the stimulating effects of artificial long days, and drive pineal and hypothalamic 5HT rhythms.

In comparing the ferret and other species, we conclude that seasonal breeding may involve two components: a circadian signal and a photoperiodic component, which is pineal-dependent. Photically controlled ovulatory mechanisms involve also two systems, a circadian mechanism, but a separate estrogen-dependent one. Other work suggests that the site of the integration of the circadian systems may be the suprachiasmatic nuclei.

Acknowledgments. This work and MK were supported by a grant from the Agricultural Research Council.

References

BISSONETTE, T.H.: Modification of mammalian sexual cycles: reactions of ferrets (*Putoris vulgaris*) of both sexes to electic light added after dark in November and December. Proc. Roy. Soc. (London) Ser. B. 110, 322-336 (1932)

BLATCHLEY, F.R., DONOVAN, B.T.: Peripheral plasma progestin levels during anoestrus, oestrus and pseudopregnancy and following hypophysectomy in ferrets. J. Reprod. Fert. 31, 331-333 (1972)

DAVID, G.F.X., HERBERT, J.: Experimental evidence for a synaptic connection between habenula and pineal ganglion in the ferret. Brain Res. 64, 327-343 (1973)

DONOVAN, B.T., TER HAAR, M.B.: Effects of luteinizing hormone releasing hormone on plasma follicle-stimulating hormone and luteinizing hormone levels in the ferret. J. Endocrinol. 73, 37-52 (1977)

GRAY, G.D., DAVIS, H.N., KENNEY, A.MCM., DEWSBURY, D.A.: Effect of mating on plasma levels of progesterone in montane voles (*Microtus montanus*). J. Reprod. Fert. 47, 89-91 (1974)

HAMMOND, J.: Control by light of reproduction in ferrets and minks. Nature (London) 167, 150-151 (1951)

HEDLUND, L., LISCHKO, M.M., ROLLAY, M.D., NISWENDER, G.D.: Melatonin: daily cycle in plasma and cerebrospinal fluid of calves. Science 195, 686-687 (1977)

HERBERT, J.: The pineal gland and light induced oestrus in ferrets. J. Endocrinol. 43, 625-636 (1969)

HERBERT, J.: Initial observations on pinealectomized ferrets kept for long periods in either daylight or artificial illumination. J. Endocrinol. 55, 591-597 (1972)

HERBERT, J., VINCENT, D.S.: Light and the breeding season in mammals. Proceedings of the Fourth International Congress of Endocrinology. Int. Congr. Ser. No. 273. Excerpta Mecica, Amsterdam. 875-879 (1972)

JOHNSON, J.R., MEYER, P.A.R., WESTABY, D.A., HERBERT, J.: The autonomic nerve supply to the ferret pineal gland studied by electron microscopy. J. Anat. 119, 491-506 (1974)

LINCOLN, G.A.: Seasonal variation in the episodic secretion of luteinizing hormone and testosterone in the ram. J. Endocrinol. 69, 213-226 (1976)

MARSHALL, F.H.A., BOWDEN, F.P.: The effect of irradiation with different wavelengths on the oestrus cycle of ferrets, with remarks on the factors controlling sexual periodicity. J. Exp. Biol. 11, 409-422 (1934)

MOORE, R.Y.: Visual pathways and the central neural control of diurnal rhythms. In: The Neurosciences. 3rd Study Program. Schmitt, F.O., Worden, F.G. (eds.). Cambridge: MIT Press, 1974, pp. 537-542

MORIN, L.P., FITZGERALD, K.M., RUSAK, B., ZUCKER, I.: Circadian organization and neural mediation of hamster reproductive rhythms. Psychoneuroendocrinology 2, 73-98 (1977)

PITTENDRIGH, C.S., DAAN, S.A.: A Functional analysis of circadian pacemakers in nocturnal rodents. J. Comp. Physiol. 106, 223-355 (1976)

REITER, R.J.: Circannual reproductive rhythms in mammals related to photoperiod and pineal function: a review. Chronobiologia 1, 365-395 (1974)

SCARAMUZZI, R.J., BLAKE, C.A., PAPKOFF, H., HILLIARD, J., SAWYER, C.H.: Radioimmunoassay of rabbit luteinizing hormone; serum levels during various reproductive states. Endocrinology 90, 1285-1291 (1972)

THOMPSON, A.P.D.: The onset of oestrus in normal and blinded ferrets. Proc. Roy. Soc. London Ser. B. 142, 126-135 (1954)

THORPE, P.A.: The presence of a retinohypothalamic projection in the ferret. Brain Res. 85, 343-346 (1975)

THORPE, P.A., HERBERT, J.: The accessory optic system of the ferret. J. Comp. Neurol. 170, 3, 295-310 (1976a)

THORPE, P.A., HERBERT, J.: Studies on the duration of the breeding season and photorefractoriness in female ferrets pinealectomised or treated with melatonin. J. Endocrinol. 70, 255-262 (1976b)

VINCENT, D.S.: Modification of the annual oestrous cycle of the ferret by various regimes of artificial light. J. Endocrinol. 48, iii (1970)

YATES, C.A., HERBERT, J.: Differential circadian rhythms in pineal and hypothalamic 5HT induced by artificial photoperiods or melatonin. Nature (London) 262, 219-220 (1976)

16. Photoperiodic Mechanism in Hamsters: the Participation of the Pineal Gland

K. HOFFMANN

For many mammalian species there are now descriptions of marked annual cycles in reproductive activity which are usually accompanied by distinct changes in size and functional state of gonads and accessory glands. Among the external factors that regulate these seasonal cycles day length, and its seasonal variations play a major role. Considerable experimental effort has been made to analyze the underlying mechanism; and many of these investigations have been conducted on hamsters.

The Photoperiodic Phenomena

In two species of true hamsters (Cricetinae), the Golden Hamster (*Mesocricetus auratus*) and the Djungarian Hamster (*Phodopus sungorus*), short daily photophases lead to rapid regression of gonads and accessory glands, while long daily photophases induce recrudescence (GASTON and MENAKER, 1967; HOFFMANN, 1973, 1974). In *Phodopus* changes in body weight and pelage color can also be brought about by manipulating day length (FIGALA et al., 1973; HOFFMANN, 1973, 1978a). The critical day length, dividing long-day and short-day effects, is about 12 1/2 h in the Golden Hamster.

It has been shown in the Golden Hamster that the underlying principle of photoperiodic time measurement is based on a circadian rhythm of photosensitivity, and not upon measuring the length of the light or the dark portion of the cycle of illumination (ELLIOT et al., 1972). In an elegant set of experiments, ELLIOT (1974) was able to demonstrate, using principles of circadian entrainment, that 1 h of light only, if administered daily in the same phase of the animals' circadian cycle, may have the effect of either long or short photophases, depending upon the phase of the circadian cycle as determined by simultaneous recording of locomotor activity. When the light pulse fell within the time span from just prior to onset of activity to 12 h thereafter, long-day effects were observed. These findings must be taken into consideration when the underlying physiologic mechanisms are analyzed.

When gonadal regression is instigated by short photophases this state is not maintained indefinitely. After several months, spontaneous recrudescence occurs (REITER, 1972a; HOFFMANN, 1973; TUREK et al., 1975b). The same holds for pelage color in the Djungarian Hamster (FIGALA et al., 1973; HOFFMANN, 1978b). These findings show that stimulation by long photophases only induces prematurely, or accelerates, a process that will occur anyway. Under natural conditions gonadal recrudescence in spring may be largely due to such an endogenous process (REITER, 1972a). On the other hand, spontaneous regression has never been observed, in spite of extended times of observation. Thus a true endogenous circannual cycle appears to be lacking.

No refractoriness to the stimulatory effect of long photophases has been detected. Not only can recrudescence be stimulated immediately after involution is completed, but we have also observed that regression initiated by short photophases can be interrupted and reversed at practically any stage by exposure to long photophases. On the other hand, photorefractoriness to the effects of short photophases has been demonstrated in the Golden Hamster (REITER, 1972a; STETSON et al., 1976). After gonads recrudesce, a prolonged exposure to long daily photophases is necessary to again render the animals sensitive to the antigonadotrophic effects of short photophases. Hence refractoriness is the exact opposite to that observed in several species of birds in which testicular development is stimulated by long days, regression occurs spontaneously after some time, and development can only be stimulated again by long days if a prolonged treatment with short days has terminated refractoriness (FARNER and FOLLET, 1966).

In adult *Mesocricetus* and *Phodopus*, all comparable experiments on the photoperiodic mechanism gave identical results, but marked differences were observed in prepubertal animals of both species. The gonadal development in the Golden Hamster is independent of day length, and photoperiodic sensitivity is only observed after puberty (GASTON and MENAKER, 1967; REITER et al., 1970; STETSON et al., 1976). In the Djungarian Hamster sexual development is strictly controlled by day length (HOFFMANN, 1978b). Figure 1 shows testis weight of young males that were

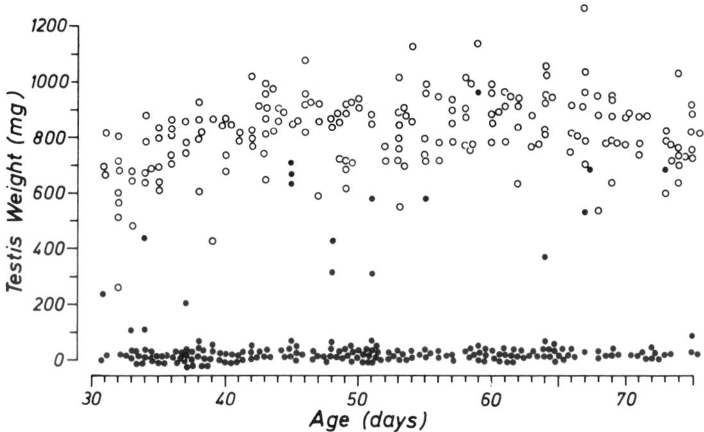

Fig. 1. Testis weight of Djungarian Hamsters raised from birth in long (16L 8D, open circles) or short (8L 16D, closed circles) days, and sacrificed at ages between 31 and 75 days. (From HOFFMANN, 1978b)

raised in either long or short photoperiods from birth, and were sacrificed at ages between 31 and 75 days. While large and functional testes were found in hamsters maintained in long days, in short days testes remained small and undeveloped, and closely resembled those of adult males after regression. These differences in the photoperiodic reaction of juveniles of both species should warn against broad generalizations. It must be mentioned that in young *Phodopus* sexual maturation finally ensues even in short days (HOFFMANN, 1978b). At about 120 days of age, first indications of further testicular development can be observed, and full maturation is reached between 160 and 200 days. This spontaneous maturation is comparable to the spontaneous recrudescence observed in adults of both species.

Photoreception and the Role of the Suprachiasmatic Nuclei

In the photoperiodic response light stimulates retinal receptors. In numerous experiments with golden hamsters, after bilateral enucleation, effects corresponding to those of exposure to short days were found, regardless of the conditions of illumination (e.g., REITER, 1974; RUSAK and MORIN, 1976). Recent experiments suggest strongly that the neural pathway involves the retino-hypothalamic tract which projects to the suprachiasmatic nuclei (RUSAK and MORIN, 1976). Destruction of other known retinal efferents does not interfere with the photoperiodic response. Selective transection of the retino-hypothalamic tract without severe damage to the suprachiasmatic nuclei has so far not been feasible.

The suprachiasmatic nuclei are also involved in processing photoperiodic information. In the Golden Hamster their destruction abolishes the effect of short daily photophases (RUSAK and MORIN, 1976; STETSON and WATSON-WHITMYRE, 1976). This result cannot be explained by the simultaneous interruption of the retinohypothalamic tract, since blinding leads to regression. The functional significance of the suprachiasmatic nuclei in the photoperiodic mechanism is not fully understood. After their destruction a large number of circadian cycles are abolished (ZUCKER et al., 1976) including that of N-acetyltransferase activity in the pineal gland (see below). Since photoperiodic effects are based on a circadian cycle of sensitivity, it seems likely that the suprachiasmatic nuclei participate in the generation and regulation of this cycle.

The Pineal Gland

It has long been known that the pineal gland is involved in the photoperiodic mechanism of mammals, and considerable experimental effort has been made to characterize its function in this mechanism. In both species of hamsters it has been consistently found that pinealectomy prevents gonadal regression after exposure to short days (e.g., HOFFMAN and REITER, 1965; HOFFMANN, 1974). Similar effects ensue if the pineal is left intact but is deprived of its nervous input by superior cervical ganglionectomy, by decentralization of the ganglia, or by anterior hypothalamic denervation (REITER, 1972b). Based on these and numerous other observations, the assumption prevails that the pineal conveys antigonadotrophic effects that are suppressed by light or long days, and intensified by darkness or short days. It should be mentioned in this context that pinealectomy in *Phodopus* not only prevents gonadal regression, but also the changes into winter pelage which are normally induced by short days (see Fig. 2).

However, in some instances it has also been observed that pinealectomy may interfere with the stimulatory effects of long days (HOFFMANN and KÜDERLING, 1975). Figure 3 shows three replicates of an experiment in which male *Phodopus* were first exposed to natural or artificial daily photophases. When testes had regressed, some of the hamsters were pinealectomized, and then exposed to either long or short days. In all cases there was a slight but significant retardation in development of testes and accessory glands in the pinealectomized animals exposed to long days, as compared to controls. Comparable results have been obtained in juvenile *Phodopus* (BRACKMANN and HOFFMANN, 1977). These results suggest that the pineal is at least partially involved also in the transduction of the stimulatory effects of long days.

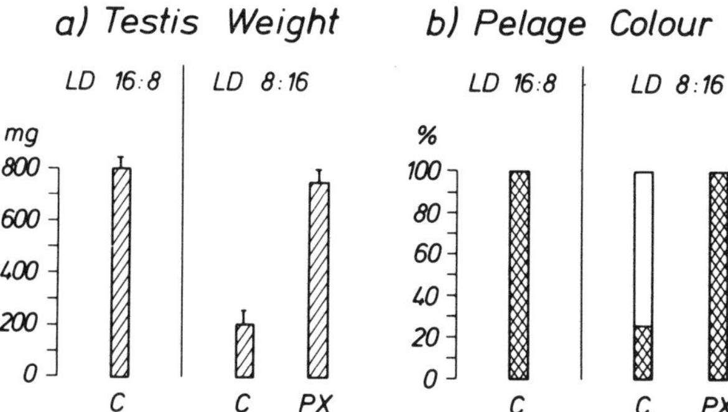

Fig. 2. Effect of pinealectomy in *Phodopus*. Inhibition of testicular regression (a) and molt into winter pelage (b) by short daily photophases. Exposure to 16L 8D or 8L 16D for 2 months. In b, crosshatching indicates summer pelage; open bar winter pelage. (From HOFFMANN, 1974, 1978a)

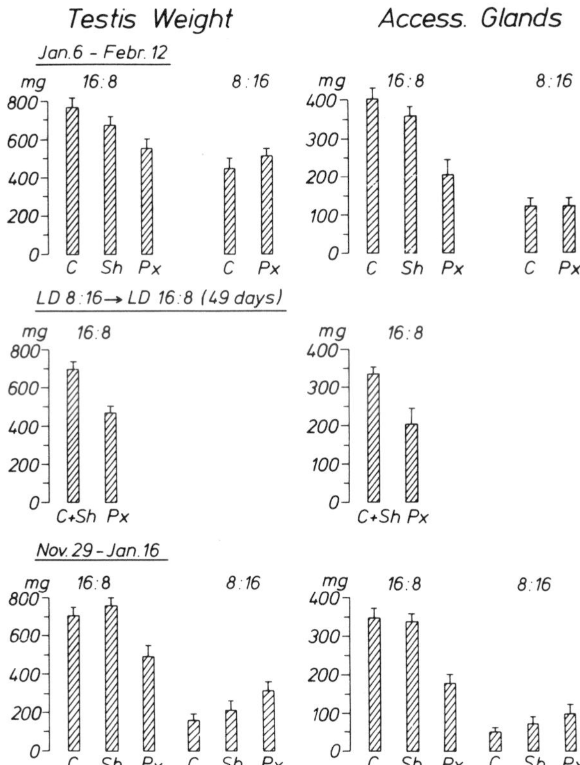

Fig. 3. Weight of testes and accessory glands in Djungarian Hamsters after exposure to long or short days. Animals were pinealectomized (*Px*), sham-operated (*Sh*), or untreated (*C*) before the beginning of the experiment. Note that development of testes and accessory glands was significantly delayed in pinealectomized animals in 16L 8D. Development in short days is due to spontaneous recrudescence. (Data for uppermost part of diagram are from HOFFMANN and KÜDERLING, 1975)

Melatonin

Two groups of pineal compounds, 5-methoxyindoles and polypeptides, have been discussed in conjunction with the role of the pineal gland in the photoperiodic regulation of gonadal activity. Especially melatonin (5-methoxy-N-acetyltryptamine) and the mechanism of its synthesis have been studied, and marked influences of the light schedule on melatonin formation have been found, albeit in the rat (KLEIN, 1973; AXELROD, 1974). Melatonin is synthesized from serotonin in two steps. Serotonin is acetylated to N-acetyl-serotonin by N-acetyltransferase (NAT) which seems to be the rate-limiting step in melatonin synthesis. N-acetyl-serotonin is then O-methylated by hydroxyindole O-methyltransferase to form melatonin. Serotonin, NAT activity, and melatonin in the pineal show marked circadian rhythms that persist in constant darkness or after blinding, but are abolished by constant light. Serotonin content is high during the day and low during the night, while high values for NAT activity and melatonin content have been found at night, exceeding the low daytime values by factors of 15 to 70 and 7 to 10, respectively. Light during the normal night time suppresses NAT activity to the low day-time values; a brief exposure to light during the night lowers NAT activity to less than 10% within 10 min, and the previous value is attained after about 3 h. Exposure to darkness during normal day-time does not cause an elevation of NAT activity. It has also been shown that LD cycles with very short photophases (2 h or less) may double the nocturnal maximum of NAT activity as compared to the value found in 12L 12D (RUDEEN and REITER, 1977). Pineal NAT activity is dependent on the presence of norepinephrine released from the sympathetic nerve fibers that terminate in the pineal gland. Denervation of the pineal by extirpation of the superior cervical ganglia, preganglionic denervation, and destruction of the suprachiasmatic nuclei all prevent the nocturnal increase in NAT activity, and thus in melatonin synthesis.

It is evident that all of the manipulations effective in the photoperiodic mechanism also influence melatonin synthesis in the pineal. Surgical procedures or light pulses that prevent short-day effects also interfere with the nocturnal rise in NAT activity. This parallelism suggests that melatonin has an important function in transducing environmental light signals into biochemical messages that influence the neuroendocrine-gonadal axis. It should be borne in mind, however, that all the reported observations on NAT activity and its modification by light or surgery have been made in the laboratory rat, a species that shows little or no photoperiodic reactions. In the Golden Hamster a daily rhythm of NAT activity qualitatively similar to that in the rat has been described, but the nocturnal maximum was only three-fold as compared to a 60-fold nocturnal increase in parallel experiments with rats (RUDEEN et al., 1975).

Many investigations of the effects of melatonin administration have been performed. In hamsters, chronic application by implanting melatonin in silastic tubing or in beeswax often produced drastic effects (e.g., HOFFMANN, 1973; REITER et al., 1974). Figure 4 shows that testicular development in juvenile *Phodopus* held on long days was inhibited by implantation of melatonin. Such findings might suggest that melatonin mimics the effect of short daily photophases, as was also indicated by experiments in adults (HOFFMANN, 1973; see also Fig. 5). However, in other experiments, exactly the opposite action of melatonin was reported; implantation was able to suppress the effects of short days that normally lead to regression (HOFFMANN, 1974; REITER et al., 1974). Though the effects of melatonin implantation in hamsters were fairly consistent when comparable experiments were performed, no clear picture

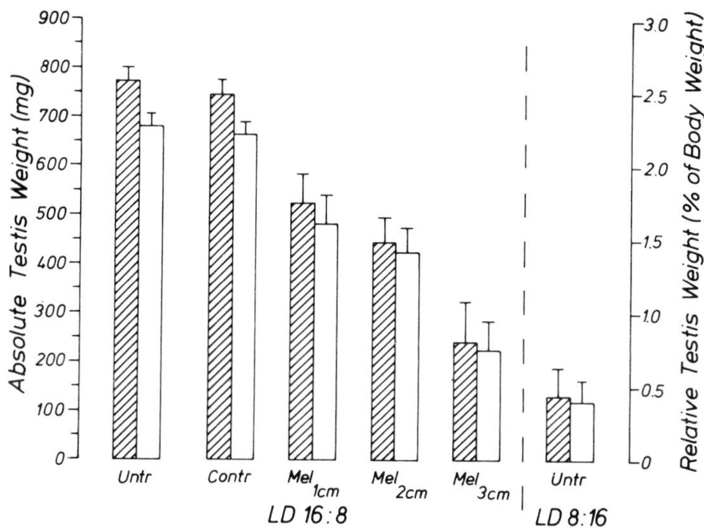

Fig. 4. Testis weight in young *Phodopus* maintained on long days from birth. At 6 days they received implants of silastic tubing of 1, 2, or 3 cm length filled with melatonin (Mel); empty tubes (Contr); no implants (Untr.). Right, values for untreated animals raised on short days. Hatched bars, absolute weight; open bars, relative weight. From BRACKMANN (1977)

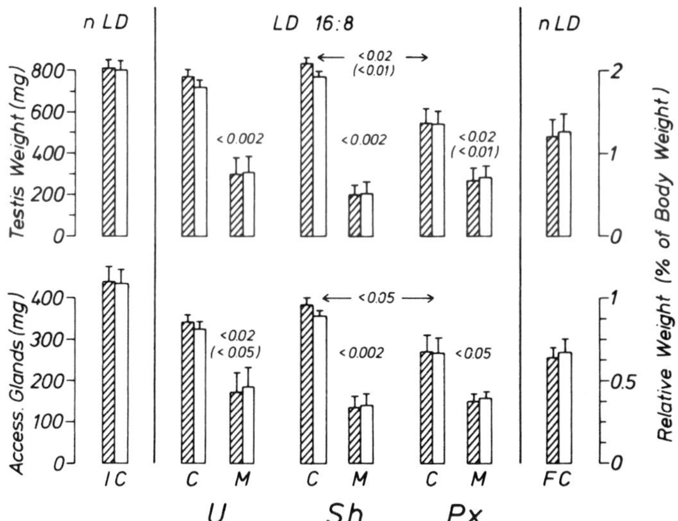

Fig. 5. Weight of testes and accessory glands of Djungarian Hamsters exposed to long days for 36 days (beginning on 21. August). *U*, untreated; *Sh*, sham operated; *Px*, pinealectomized. *C*, empty implant; *M*, melatonin implant. Initial (*IC*) and final (*FC*) controls were held under natural day length (*n LD*) throughout, as were the experimental animals before the beginning of the experiment. (From HOFFMANN and KÜDERLING, 1977)

as to the underlying physiologic mechanism of melatonin action has evolved from such experiments. Effects varied with dosage, physiologic state of the hamsters (active or regressing or regressed gonads) and with the photoperiodic schedule to which they were exposed (e.g., TUREK et al., 1975a; HOFFMANN, 1978a).

One generalization seems possible. In all cases in which gonadal development does not depend upon day length, it was not affected by implantation of melatonin. Spontaneous recrudescence in short days cannot be depressed in either species (HOFFMANN, 1973; TUREK and LOSEE, 1977). Melatonin fails to influence development towards puberty in the Golden Hamster in which sexual maturation is independent of day length (TUREK and LOSEE, 1978). On the other hand, in the Djungarian Hamster in which sexual maturation is under photoperiodic control, implantation of melatonin caused drastic effects (Fig. 4). When TUREK et al. (1976) compared the effects of the same treatment with melatonin in two photoperiodic and two nonphotoperiodic species of rodents, no demonstrable effect was found in the latter two species, whereas in the photoperiodic species gonadal regression was observed. Taken together, these findings suggest that implantation of melatonin interferes with the transduction of photoperiodic information in an as yet unspecified way, but does not cause direct antigonadotrophic effects, as has often been assumed.

Synthesis of melatonin in the pineal, and its release, show a marked light-dependent rhythm. Therefore, chronic administration by implantation is rather unphysiologic. Recent findings show that the effects of injection of melatonin depend on the time of day of application (TAMARKIN et al., 1976, 1977a; REITER et al., 1976b). In Golden Hamsters maintained on 14L 10D, injection of melatonin towards the end of the photophase, or towards the end of the scotophase, led to testicular regression in males, and to cessation of estrus cyclicity in females when the treatment was repeated daily for several weeks. Daily administration of the same dosage of melatonin in the early light period or at about the middle of the dark period failed to have an effect. The data suggest that these injections supplemented the endogenous production of melatonin in such a way that a pattern of melatonin release similar to that found in short days resulted, and that this pattern is the physiologic mechanism of transduction of photic information into humoral information that is transmitted finally to the neuroendocrine-gonadal axis.

The site of action of melatonin is unknown. Since antigonadotrophic effects of pineal constituents other than melatonin have been found, the hypothesis was advanced that melatonin might regulate the synthesis and/or release of such substances within the pineal (QUAY, 1974; REITER et al., 1976a). The observation that daily injections of melatonin in the afternoon induce gonadal regression only if the pineal and its innervation were intact (TAMARKIN et al., 1976; REITER et al., 1976b) has been considered supporting evidence for such an assumption (REITER et al., 1976b). However, experiments on Djungarian Hamsters demonstrated that testicular regression occurs in pinealectomized animals, as well as in controls after implantation of melatonin (HOFFMANN and KÜDERLING, 1977; see Fig. 5), and similar results have been obtained with the Golden Hamster (TUREK, 1977). In addition TAMARKIN et al. (1977b) have recently found that a repeated daily pattern of several injections of melatonin per day causes testicular regression in pinealectomized Golden Hamsters. Thus the assumption that the pineal is the primary site of the effect of melatonin in relaying photoperiodic information can hardly be maintained. It seems that the rhythmic release of melatonin has an effect on some area of the brain, and that this is the information that finally influences the neuroendocrine-gonadal axis. It should also be recalled that not only gonadal activity, but also other functions reacting to day length, might be so regulated.

Concluding Remarks

This paper deals nearly exclusively with data obtained in hamsters, since in these species much progress in the analysis of the photoperiodic mechanism has been made. It must be stressed, however, that a number of the results mentioned here have also been obtained, not only in other rodents, but also in two mustelid species (HERBERT, this volume; RUST and MEYER, 1969). This suggests that the mechanism discussed here is not restricted to hamsters but is probably valid in many more mammals that are spring breeders. Only manipulation of day lengths and/or of the pineal gland and the gonadal reaction have been considered here. It should be mentioned that in many experiments also LH, FSH, and prolactin were measured. Restriction on space does not allow a discussion of the hypothalamo-hypophysial aspects of photoperiodic effects.

Acknowledgment. Investigations on *Phodopus* cited in this paper were supported by grants from the Deutsche Forschungsgemeinschaft, Schwerpunktprogramm "Biologie der Zeitmessung."

References

AXELROD, J.: The pineal gland: A neurochemical transducer. Science 184, 1341-1348 (1974)

BRACKMANN, M.: Melatonin delays puberty in the Djungarian hamster (*Phodopus sungorus*). Naturwissenschaften 64, 642-643 (1977)

BRACKMANN, M., HOFFMANN, K.: Pinealectomy and photoperiod influence testicular development in the Djungarian hamster. Naturwissenschaften 64, 341-342 (1977)

ELLIOT, J.A.: Photoperiodic regulation of testis function in the golden hamster: relation to the circadian system. Ph.D. thesis, Univ. of Texas at Austin 1974

ELLIOT, J.A., STETSON, M.J., MENAKER, M.: Regulation of testis function in golden hamsters: A circadian clock measures photoperiodic time. Science 178, 771-773 (1972)

FARNER, D.S., FOLLET, B.K.: Light and other environmental factors affecting avian reproduction. J. Anim. Sci. (Suppl.) 25, 90-115 (1966)

FIGALA, J., HOFFMANN, K., GOLDAU, G.: Zur Jahresperiodik beim Dsungarischen Zwerghamster *Phodopus sungorus* Pallas. Oecologia 12, 89-118 (1973)

GASTON, S., MENAKER, M.: Photoperiodic control of hamster testis. Science 167, 925-928 (1967)

HOFFMAN, R.A., REITER, R.J.: Pineal gland: influences on gonads of male hamsters. Science 148, 1609-1611 (1965)

HOFFMANN, K.: The influence of photoperiod and melatonin on testis size, body weight, and pelage colour in the Djungarian Hamster (*Phodopus sungorus*). J. Comp. Physiol. 95, 267-282 (1973)

HOFFMANN, K.: Testicular involution in short photoperiods inhibited by melatonin. Naturwissenschaften 61, 364-365 (1974)

HOFFMANN, K.: Die Funktion des Pineals bei der Jahresperiodik der Säuger. Nova Acta Leopoldina (1978a, in press)

HOFFMANN, K.: Short photoperiods delay puberty and growth, and induce molt into winter pelage in the Djungarian hamster. J. Reprod. Fert. (1978b, in press)

HOFFMANN, K., KÜDERLING, I.: Pinealectomy inhibits stimulation of testicular development by long photoperiods in a hamster. Experientia 31, 122-123 (1975)

HOFFMANN, K., KÜDERLING, I.: Antigonadal effects of melatonin in pinealectomized Djungarian hamsters. Naturwissenschaften 64, 339-340 (1977)
KLEIN, D.C.: The role of serotonin N-acetyltransferase in the adrenergic regulation of indole metabolism in the pineal gland. In: Serotonin and Behavior. Barchas, J., Usdin, E. (eds.). New York-London: Academic Press, 1973, pp. 109-119
QUAY, W.B.: Pineal Chemistry. Springfield: C.C. Thomas, 1974, p. 430
REITER, R.J.: Evidence for refractoriness of the pituitarygonadal axis to the pineal gland in golden hamsters and its possible implications in annual reproductive rhythms. Anat. Rec. 173, 365-371 (1972a)
REITER, R.J.: Surgical procedures involving the pineal gland which prevent gonadal degeneration in adult male hamsters. Ann. Endocrinol. (Paris) 33, 571-581 (1972b)
REITER, R.J.: Circannual reproductive rhythms in mammals related to photoperiod and pineal function: a review. Chronobiologia 1, 365-395 (1974)
REITER, R.J., BLASK, D.E., JOHNSON, L.Y., RUDEEN, P.K., VAUGHAN, M.K., WARING, P.J.: Melatonin inhibition of reproduction in the male hamster: its dependence on time of day of administration and on an intact and sympathetically innervated pineal gland. Neuroendocrinology 22, 107-116 (1976b)
REITER, R.J., LUKASZYK, A.J., VAUGHAN, M.K., BLASK, D.E.: New horizons of pineal research. Am. Zool. 16, 93-101 (1976a)
REITER, R.J., SORRENTINO, S., HOFFMAN, R.A.: Early photoperiodic conditions and pineal antigonadal function in male hamsters. Int. J. Fertil. 15, 163-170 (1970)
REITER, R.J., VAUGHAN, M.K., BLASK, D.E., JOHNSON, I.Y.: Melatonin: its inhibition of pineal antigonadotrophic activity in male hamsters. Science 185, 1169-1171 (1974)
RUDEEN, P.K., REITER, R.J.: Effect of shortened photoperiods on pineal serotonin N-acetyltransferase activity and rhythmicity. J. Interdiscipl. Cycle Res. 8, 47-54 (1977)
RUDEEN, P.K., REITER, R.J., VAUGHAN, M.K.: Pineal serotonin N-acetyltransferase activity in four mammalian species. Neurosci. Lett. 1, 225-230 (1975)
RUSAK, B., MORIN, L.P.: Testicular responses to photoperiod are blocked by lesions of the suprachiasmatic nuclei in golden hamsters. Biol. Reprod. 15, 366-374 (1976)
RUST, C.C., MEYER, R.K.: Hair color, molt, and testis size in male short-tailed weasels treated with melatonin. Science 165, 921-922 (1969)
STETSON, M.H., MATT, K.S., WATSON-WHITMYRE, M.: Photoperiodism and reproduction in golden hamsters: circadian organization and the termination of photorefractoriness. Biol. Reprod. 14, 531-537 (1976)
STETSON, M.H., WATSON-WHITMYRE, M.: Nucleus suprachiasmaticus: the biological clock in the hamster? Science 191, 197-199 (1976)
TAMARKIN, L., HOLLISTER, C.W., LEVEBVRE, N.G., GOLDMAN, B.D.: Melatonin induction of gonadal quiescence in pineal-ectomized Syrian hamsters. Science 198, 953-955 (1977b)
TAMARKIN, L., LEFEBVRE, N.G., HOLLISTER, C.W., GOLDMAN, B.D.: Effect of melatonin adminstered during the night on reproductive function in the Syrian hamster. Endocrinology 101, 631-634 (1977a)
TAMARKIN, L., WESTROM, W.K., HAMILL, A.I., GOLDMAN, B.D.: Effect of melatonin on the reproductive systems of male and female Syrian hamsters: a diurnal rhythm in sensitivity to melatonin. Endocrinology 99, 1534-1541 (1976)
TUREK, F.W.: Antigonadal effect of melatonin in pinealectomized and intact male hamsters. Proc. Soc. Exp. Biol. Med. 155, 31-34 (1977)
TUREK, F.W., DESJARDINS, C., MENAKER, M.: Melatonin: antigonadal and progonadal effects in male golden hamsters. Science 190, 280-282 (1975a)
TUREK, F.W., DESJARDINS, C., MENAKER, M.: Differential effects of melatonin on the testes of photoperiodic and nonphotoperiodic rodents. Biol. Reprod. 15, 94-97 (1976)
TUREK, F.W., ELLIOT, J.A., ALVIS, J.D., MENAKER, M.: Effects of prolonged exposure to nonstimulatory photoperiods on the activity of the neuroendocrine-testicular axis of golden hamsters. Biol. Reprod. 13, 475-481 (1975b)
TUREK, F.W., LOSEE, S.H.: Melatonin-induced testicular growth in golden hamsters maintained on short days. Biol. Reprod. (1978, in press)
ZUCKER, I., RUSAK, B., KING, R.G.: Neural basis for circadian rhythms in rodent behavior. In: Advances in Psychobiology, Vol. III, Riesen, A., Rhompson, R.F. (eds.). New York: Wiley-Interscience, 1976, pp. 35-74

17. Seasonal Variations in the Endocrine System of Hibernators

B. W. JOHANSSON

The term hibernation is often used in a loose sense to signify any state of torpor. However, it should be confined to homeotherms that, at certain times and under natural conditions, abandon homeothermia and permit body temperature to fall as low as the environmental temperature, with a low limit of about $0^{o}C$ - and are able to regain the homeothermia at any time regardless of environmental temperature. Thus defined, hibernation occurs in some species of bats, birch mouse, chipmunks, dormice, ground squirrels, hamsters, hedgehogs, marmots, pigmy possums and humming-birds, whereas bears and badgers are not true hibernators.

Considerable differences exist among the species of mammalian hibernators, that fall among such diverse orders as insectivores, rodents, and carnivores. Certainly one cause of conflict in the literature can be ascribed to interspecific differences. The proneness to enter hibernation differs greatly from the Golden Hamster, which can be forced into hibernation only after prolonged exposure to a cold environment and lack of food and water, to some species of bats, which enter hibernation easily during a cool summer night. In between are the "typical" hibernators, such as the hedgehog and the marmot, with strict annual rhythms.

Although hibernation is one way of coping with a thermally or trophically stressful environment, the hibernators do not maintain low body temperature persistently, but become active periodically. The cause of such arousals is unknown, but it has been speculated that the accumulation of metabolic end products constitutes the stimulus (PENGELLEY and FISCHER, 1961).

Although a cool environment is a prerequisite for hibernation, it is only one of several factors necessary. These are external such as temperature and light; internal such as inhibition of temperature regulation, increase of fat depots, hypertrophy of brown fat, and polyendocrine involution; as well as innate qualities, such as an ability of the tissues to function at temperatures just above $0^{o}C$.

Some animals "test" their preparation for hibernation; the body temperature is decreased to a certain level and then returns to prehibernation level. Such "test drops" have been described for a ground squirrel, *Citellus beecheyi* (STRUMWASSER, 1959) and a similar pattern was found in the Asian chipmunk, *Eutamias sibiricus* (JAEGER, 1974).

The endogenous preparation for hibernation is not due solely to environmental changes in day length and ambient temperature. PENGELLEY and ASMUNDSON (1974) kept Golden Mantled Ground Squirrels, *Citellus lateralis*, in constant conditions of light and ambient temperature and observed annual changes in weight, food consumption and hibernation pattern. The existence of a circannual clock has been confirmed by HELLER and POULSON (1970) in the same species, by AMBID (1971); in the garden dormouse, *Eliomys quercinus*, and by CANGUILHEM (1973) in the hamster, *Cricetus cricetus*.

Islets of Langerhans. Because there is a marked reduction of the blood glucose level in the hedgehog during hibernation, it has been claimed that the regulation of glucose plays a central role in the induction of the hibernating state, and that insulin is the agent that induces hibernation. This has been supported by reports of successful induction of hibernation by the administration of insulin (LAUFBERGER, 1924 and SUOMALAINEN, 1938). In other laboratories, however, this technique has not been successful (KAYSER, 1955 and JOHANSSON, 1973, unpublished). In our unpublished investigations a state of hypothermia could be induced, but no true hibernation.

In order to test this hypothesis further we determined the fasting serum insulin activity during different parts of the year as follows:

Season I : October 25-November 14, just prior to hibernation
Season II : January 10-31, during hibernation
Season III: March 19-April 9, just after arousal from hibernation
Season IV : June 10-26, during nonhibernating season

In general, each sample consisted of six male and six female hedgehogs, and except during season II, the animals were anesthetized with 3.3 ml/kg of chloral hydrate-urethane solution (18.75 g urethane, 2.25 g chloral hydrate, sterile water qs to 100 ml; JOHANSSON and SENTURIA, 1972).

Our studies failed to detect any immunoreactive insulin activity at all in any of the four seasons. The method used was a modification of the radioimmunoassay method of YALOW and BERSON (1960). In assays of extract of the pancreas, high concentrations of immunoreactive insulin were consistantly found. In the organs collected in November and January, mean concentration of insulin in the pancreas was 156 and 173 mU/g, respectively. This difference was not significant. In the animals in which the pancreas was collected in July, the insulin content was significantly ($p < 0.001$) higher, the average being 762 mU/g.

These results do not support the insulin theory, but they show that there is assayable insulin in the hedgehog pancreas. After the administration of glucose intravenously to three nonhibernating hedgehogs, the blood glucose increased to a level of 230-270 mg/100 ml. The effect on plasma insulin was irregular, but immunoreactive material was found in plasma from two of the three animals tested. The absence of demonstrable insulin in plasma in the basal state may depend on lower rate of release or higher rate of disappearance than in other species studied. It may also be caused by a low immunoreactivity of the hedgehog insulin in this assay as compared to the homologous antigen.

The irregular effect of hyperglycemia on insulin release could be an effect of anesthesia and operative procedure during the test, with stress-induced release of adrenaline blocking the release of insulin from the pancreas. The observation that blockade of the α-receptors with phentolamine abolished this influence suggests that such a mechanism might be in effect during stress. The insulin results show the difficulties that can be encountered. Anesthesia necessary for the collection of blood or tissue sample may profoundly alter the "milieu intérieur", thus concealing possible circannual changes.

It should also be pointed out that although the blood glucose levels drop during hibernation in the hedgehog, this is not true for all hibernators (KAYSER, 1961), and the glucose levels in hibernating animals are not as low as during insulin-induced hypothermia (DISCHE et al., 1931).

Thyroid Gland. The thyroid gland of hibernators has been of interest for many years. However, its exact importance is not known (JOHANSSON, 1973; LACHIVER, 1969). In comparison with nonhibernating animals, we observed lower protein-bound iodine levels in hedgehogs during hibernation, probably a result and not a cause of hibernation, but perhaps instrumental in maintaining the metabolic depression in hibernation. FONTAINE and LACHIVER (1955) found a very low and slow ^{131}I uptake in the thyroid of hibernating marmots. The thyroid activity of the woodchuck increases prior to arousal, but while the animal is still in deep hibernation.

In investigations with fluorescence microscopy, it was found that the thyroid gland of the hedgehog has a small number of adrenergic nerves, most of which accompany blood vessels, although it could not be excluded that some fibers also ran in close association with the (nonfluorescent) follicular epithelium. No seasonal changes were observed in the adrenergic innervation. The calcitonin cells (C cell, light cell, parafollicular cell) showed no formaldehyde-induced fluorescence. In another hibernator, the bat *Myotis lucifugus*, the thyroid gland has been found to contain C cells that store a fluorogenic compound that has been interpreted as 5-HT. Electron microscopy has shown striking changes in the number and fine structure of C cells during the course of the annual hibernation cycle (NUNEZ and GERSHON, 1972).

Parathyroid Gland. The annual rhythm of the parathyroid gland has scarcely been investigated. SKOWRON and ZAJACZEK (1947) reported a maximal activity in October with lowest activity in summer. KAYSER (1961) also reported an increased activity during hibernation in the hamster. These reports conform with the annual changes in serum calcium in hedgehogs with highest values in the winter (JOHANSSON and SENTURIA, 1972). KAYSER et al. (1964) observed decalcification of bones and teeth during hibernation, and a decreasing mineral content of bone as hibernation progresses has been described in bats (BRUCE and WIEBERS, 1970). In addition to seasonal changes in the activity of the parathyroids, BRUCE and WIEBERS (1970) discuss the importance of enforced immobility of hibernation in the demineralization of bone in *Myotis lucifugus*.

Adrenal Glands. Weights of adrenal glands in the hedgehog vary seasonally, being lowest in winter during hibernation. Beginning as early as the observations of CUSHING and GOETSCH (1915) most investigators have observed an annual cycle of the adrenal cortex, characterized by a reduction in winter of the thickness of the cortex and its ascorbic acid content (KAYSER, 1961). The increased adrenocortical activity in the prehibernating stage has been interpreted by SUOMALAINEN and NYHOLM as the first step of SELYE'S adaptation syndrome (SUOMALAINEN and NYHOLM, 1956). ROMAGNOLI (1972) observed marked increase in the number of intramitochondrial dense granules during hibernation, while the mitochondria of the zona fasciculata decreased in number and in length of cristae. During arousal the mitochondria first appear to undergo degeneration; later a regeneration pattern appears. These microscopic observations conform well with the corticosteroid determinations in the hedgehog and garden dormouse (BOULOUARD, 1964). The seasonal changes of the adrenals persist when hamsters are kept at a temperature of 23°C (CANGUILHEM and BLOCH, 1967).

The adrenaline concentration was much higher than that of noradrenaline in the right adrenal gland of the hedgehog (OWMAN and STUDNITZ, 1972). The adrenaline level was remarkably constant throughout the year, whereas noradrenaline was high during fall and summer and low during winter and spring. The highest values of monoamine oxidase (MAO) and catechol-O-methyltransferase (COMT) were found in the winter and spring periods, respectively; the lowest values were measured at fall and summer. The phenylethanolamine-N-methyltransferase (PNMT) activity decreased continuously from high levels during fall to a minimum in the summer period. The low summer activity of COMT in the adrenals, corresponding to maximal catecholamine levels, may indicate the presence of an increased amount of noradrenaline in the large cellular storage pool, which would agree with an enhanced sympathetic tone during the summer period. MAO is responsible for the continuous inactivation of the excess of catecholamines stored in the cells. Therefore, the combination of a minimal MAO activity and low catecholamine levels during the prehibernating period are consistent with a relatively low turnover rate of stored catecholamines during this period. The low adrenal PNMT activity in combination with high catecholamine concentrations may be a result of the known substrate-product inhibition of this enzyme (FULLER and HUNT, 1967). A high adrenal PNMT activity was observed concomitant with a maximal ratio of adrenaline to noradrenaline, which may reflect a particularly high synthesis of adrenaline from noradrenaline.

The Reproductive Organs. In the hedgehog the weight of the testes is strikingly seasonal (JOHANSSON and SENTURIA, 1972), being lowest in the fall and highest in the spring and summer. The increase in weight during winter is similar to that in the Mexican Ground Squirrel (SENTURIA et al., 1970). These data suggest a continued activity of the hypothalamo-hypophysial-pineal axis during hibernation. Despite the difference in latitude (Malmö, Sweden 55° 35'N compared with Austin, Texas 30° 18'N), and diverse phylogenetic origin, the two species show similar patterns in testis weight.

The ovary weight is highest in the fall, and uterine weight lowest in winter. This reflects a seasonal breeding cycle in the hedgehog. No immediate explanation is available for the high weight of ovaries in the fall.

The changes in gonads occur independently of hibernation. European hamsters kept at 27°C throughout the year still show a seasonal variation of the testes (KAYSER, 1961). When WELLS (1935-1936) attempted to modify the testicular cycle of the thirteen-lined Ground Squirrel by restriction for 3-7 weeks in a refrigerator during the breeding period, he failed to elicit an involution of the testes and this low temperature also was unable to induce earlier activity, when they were exposed to cold during the involution period. On the other hand, other authors stress the importance of hibernation, and conclude that the influence of hibernation itself, and not an independent seasonal cycle, must be regarded as the cause for the strong testicular involution of the hibernating European hamster (REZNIK-SCHÜLLER, 1973). SMIT-VIS (1972) concluded from studies on Golden Hamsters, which were kept sexually active either by pinealectomy or administration of testosterone, that hibernation occurred only in animals with atrophy of the reproductive organs.

In our studies on the seasonal variations in the hedgehogs (JOHANSSON and SENTURIA, 1972) the uterus was found to be the only organ with distinct seasonal variation in the adrenergic innervation. The network of varicose nerve terminals was well developed. During spring and summer, the entire wall of the uterus had increased in thickness. The number of nerves in the outer longitudinal layer had increased. In the circular layer, the adrenergic nerve plexus had the same density as during fall and winter, in spite of the marked increase in volume of the smooth musculature. This would mean that the total number of fluorescent nerves had increased during spring and summer.

The Pineal Gland. Despite the efforts of Descartes to stress the importance of the pineal gland, this was a neglected organ until a few years ago, when functional relationships between the environmental photoperiod and pineal activity were demonstrated (QUAY, 1963; WURTMAN et al., 1963). The absence of light seems to exaggerate at least certain aspects of pineal function. When Golden Hamsters are deprived of light, reproductive activity ceases (HOFFMAN and REITER, 1965). This cessation is prevented by removal of the pineal gland. Interestingly enough, the pineal body can hold the gonads in inactive state for only 20-25 weeks, after which they "spontaneously" regenerate (REITER, 1975). If the hamsters are then exposed to long daily photophases simulating summer, their return to darkness is followed by regression of the sexual organs. For this to occur, however, the simulated summer must be about 22 weeks in length. If pinealectomized females are caged with pinealectomized male hamsters in late December in natural photoperiodic environments, the females become pregnant and deliver young during January and February. Intact hamsters, however, were not capable of reproducing until March, the time at which their gonads regenerate (HOFFMAN and REITER, 1965).

One important function of the pineal gland seems to be to synchronize the reproductive periods of seasonal breeding species at the season of the year that ensures maximal chances of survival of the young, thereby permitting perpetuation of the species. In pinealectomized animals, day length exerts no influence on reproductive physiology, and either no seasonal rhythm in reproduction occurs, e.g., in hamsters, or else the rhythm free-runs. In the latter case, the breeding period comes out of phase with the appropriate season of the year.

The Pituitary Gland. Annual variations in the structure of the master gland were described as early as 1906 by GEMELLI (1906) in the marmot, although some later studies were unable to confirm these early findings. On the basis of previous findings and his own experiments, including intratesticular grafts of the anterior pituitary, KAYSER (1961) concluded that there is a seasonal cycle in the gonadotropic and thyrotropic hormones of hibernators.

Studies of the function of testes in the European hamster suggest complete lack of gonadotropins, as after a hypophysectomy, in hibernating animals, whereas the nonhibernating hamsters only show signs of a slight reduction in hormone synthesis during winter (REZNIK-SCHÜLLER and REZNIK, 1973). Hypophysectomy carried out in summer or fall allows the induction of a state of hibernation, but the animals die in a few days. Injection of anterior pituitary extracts delays hibernation (LACHIVER, 1969). The fluorescence microscopic distribution of serotonin and catecholamines by the formaldehyde method of FALCK and HILLARP revealed no seasonal variations in the hedgehog.

Brown Adipose Tissue. Brown adipose tissue (BAT) was first described more than 400 years ago (JOHANSSON, 1959) and was originally believed to be thymus tissue. Later it was regarded as an endocrine gland, and was often called the "hibernating gland". In the middle of the last century it was viewed only as a specialized adipose tissue (JOHANSSON, 1975). Some years ago the importance of BAT in nonshivering thermogenesis became obvious and recently LINCK and PETROVIC (1972) have claimed that BAT is able to synthesize from ^{14}C-acetate cholesterol a steroid-type material.

In our investigations of the hedgehog (JOHANSSON and SENTURIA, 1972) we observed pronounced seasonal variations. The tissue is largest in fall and smallest in summer. The number of mitochondria in this tissue is greatest in winter, coordinating well with its thermogenic role.

Although gas-chromatographic analysis revealed some changes of the fatty acid composition of BAT from hedgehogs during different seasons, these changes had little effect on the degree of unsaturation (ÅKESSON, 1972). Lactic dehydrogenase was maximally active during hibernation, whereas a different pattern was observed for the activities of glucose-6-phosphate dehydrogenase and α-glycerophosphate dehydrogenase (OLSSON, 1972). Due to the greater amount of BAT, the amount of cytochrome C in brown fat from hibernating hedgehogs was higher when compared to nonhibernating animals, but the concentration remained essentially unchanged (PALÉUS and JOHANSSON, 1968).

Although the brown adipose tissue was once confused with the thymus, the hibernators of course do have a true thymus, which has been described in the marmot as undergoing seasonal variations, perhaps secondary to changes in adrenal activity. The thymic involution during the winter has been considered a spontaneous, natural, seasonal thymectomy (GALETTI and CAVALLARI, 1972).

It is clear that annual endocrine rhythms occur in hibernators. This does not mean, however, that these are circannual endogenous rhythms in the sense of PENGELLEY and ASMUNDSON (1974). Furthermore, the relationship of a seasonal change in the microscopical picture of an endocrine gland to its secretory activity can only be elucidated by determination of the concentration of its hormone in the circulation.

Other factors of importance are the sensitivity of the hormonal receptors, which might also undergo seasonal variations and perhaps in an opposite direction, which means that the net result may differ only slightly or remain unchanged. There is no doubt, however, about the importance of recognition of circannual rhythms. Awareness of the existance of these rhythms may explain unclear or conflicting experimental results and should be taken into consideration, when planning long-term biologic studies.

References

ÅKESSON, B.: Fat metabolism II Fatty acid composition of adipose tissue. In: Seasonal variations in the physiology and biochemistry of the European hedgehog (*Erinaceus europaeus*) including comparisons with non-hibernators, guinea-pig and man. Acta Physiol. Scand. Suppl. 380, 62-95 (1972)

AMBID, L.: Modifications metaboliques en relation avec l'hibernation et les reveils periodiques du Lérot (*Eliomys quercinus* L.). Thèse Sci. Nat. Toulouse, 1971

BOULOUARD, R.: Activité cortico-surrenalienne durant la phase léthargique et le reveil chez deux hibernants: Le Lerot (*Eliomys quercinus*) et le Hérisson (*Erinaceus europaeus*). J. Physiol. 56, 304-305 (1964)

BRUCE, D.S., WIEBERS, J.E.: Calcium and phosphate levels in bats (*Myotis lucifugus*) as function of season and activity. Experientia 26/6, 625-627 (1970)

CANGUILHEM, B., BLOCH, R.: Evolution saisonnière de l'élimination des hormones surrénaliennes chez un hibernant, *Cricetus cricetus*. Arch. des Sciences Physiol. XXI/1, 27-44 (1967)

CANGUILHEM, B., SCHIEBER, J.-P., KOCH, A.: Rhythme circannuel pondéral du hamster d'Europe (*Cricetus cricetus*). Influences respectives de la photopériode et de la température externe sur son déroulement. Arch. Sci. Physiol. 27, 67-90 (1973)

CUSHING, H., GOETSCH, H.: Hibernation and the pituitary body. J. Exp. Med. 22, 25-47 (1915)

DISCHE, Z., FLEISCHMANN, W., TREVANI, E.: Zur Frage des Zusammenhanges zwischen Winterschlaf und Hypoglykämie. Pflüg. Archiv Ges. Physiol. 227, 235-238 (1931)

FONTAINE, M., LACHIVER, F.: Thyroide et thermorégulation chimique. Arch. Sci. Physiol. 9, 63-81 (1955)

FULLER, R.W., HUNT, J.M.: Inhibition of phenylethanolamine-N-methyltransferase by its product, epinephrine. Life Sci. 6, 1107 (1967)

GALETTI, G., CAVALLARI, A.: The thymus of marmots: spontaneous, natural, seasonal thymectomy? Acta Anat. 83, 593-605 (1972)

GEMELLI, A.: Sur l'ipofisi della marmotta durante il lethargo e nella stagione estiva. Arch. Sci. Med. 30, 341-349 (1906)

HELLER, H.C., POULSON, TH.L.: Circannian rhythms-II. Endogenous and exogenous factors controlling reproduction and hibernation in chipmunks (Eutamias) and ground squirrels (*Spermophilus*). Comp. Biochem. Physiol. 33, 357-383 (1970)

HOFFMAN, R.A., REITER, R.J.: Pineal gland: Influence on gonads of male hamsters. Science 148, 1609-1611 (1965)

JAEGER, R.: Die unterschiedliche Dauer von Schlaf- und Wachphasen während einer Winterschlafperiode des Burunduk, *Tamias (Eutamias) sibiricus* Laxmann. Z. Säugetierk. 39/1, 10-15 (1974)

JOHANSSON, B.W.: Brown fat: A review. Metabolism 8, 221-240 (1959)

JOHANSSON, B.W.: Effects of durgs on hibernation. In: The Pharmacology of Thermoregulation. San Francisco, 1972. Basel: Karger, 1973, pp. 364-381

JOHANSSON, B.W.: The B.A.T. Saga eller sagan om vintersömnkörteln. Observanda Medica 3, 78-83 (1975)

JOHANSSON, B.W., BIÖRCK, G., VEIGE, S.: Some laboratory data on hedgehogs, hibernating and non-hibernating. Acta Physiol. Scand. 37, 281-294 (1956)

JOHANSSON, B.W., SENTURIA, J.B.: Seasonal variations in the physiology and biochemistry of the European hedgehog (*Erinaceus europaeus*) including comparisons with non-hibernators, guinea pig and man. Acta Physiol. Scand. Suppl. 380 (1972)

KAYSER, C.: Hibernation et hibernation artificelle. Rev. Pathol. Gen. Comp. 668, 704 (1955)

KAYSER, C.: The Physiology of Natural Hibernation. Oxford: Pergamon Press, 1961

KAYSER, C., VINCENDON, G., FRANK, R., PORTE, A.: Some external (climatic) and internal (endocrine) factors in relation to production of hibernation. Ann. Acad. Sci. Fenn. Ser. AIV 71, 269 (1964)

LACHIVER, F.: Seasonal hormonal effect of states of depressed metabolism. In: Depressed Metabolism. Musacchia, X.J., Saunders, J.F. (eds.). New York: Elsevier, 1969, pp. 199-230

LAUFBERGER, V.: Versuche über die Insulinwirkung. Z. Ges. Exp. Med. 42, 570 (1924)

LINCK, G., PETROVIC, A.: Does brown adipose tissue of the European hamster (*Cricetus cricetus*) store and synthesize corticosteroids? The isolation of a cortico-steroid-like compound. Arch. Sci. Physiol. 26, 85-100 (1972)

NUNEZ, E.A., GERSHON, M.D.: Synthesis and storage of serotonin by parafollicular (C) cells of the thyroid gland of active, prehibernating and hibernating bats. Endocrinology 90, 1008-1024 (1972)

OLSSON, S.-O.: Dehydrogenases (LDH, MDH, G-6-PDH, and alpha-GPDH) in the heart, liver, white and brown fat. In: Seasonal variations in the physiology and biochemistry of the European hedgehog (*Erinaceus europaeus*) including comparisons with non-hibernators, guinea-pig and man. Acta Physiol. Scand. Suppl. 380, 62-95 (1972)

OWMAN, CH., VON STUDNITZ, W.: Sympathetic nervous system. I. Metabolism. In: Seasonal variations in the physiology and biochemistry of the European hedgehog (*Erinaceus europaeus*) including comparisons with non-hibernators, guinea-pig and man. Acta Physiol. Scand. Suppl. 380, 96-105 (1972)

PALÉUS, S., JOHANSSON, B.W.: Seasonal variations in cytochrome C content of hedgehog brown adipose tissue. Acta Chem. Scand. 22, 342-344 (1968)

PENGELLEY, E.T., ASMUNDSON, S.J.: Circannual rhythmicity in hibernating mammals. In: Circannual Clocks. Annual Biological Rhythms. Pengelley, E.T. (ed.). London: Academic Press, 1974

PENGELLEY, E.T., FISCHER, K.C.: Rhythmical arousal from hibernation in the golden-mantled ground squirrel, *Citellus lateralis tescorum*. Can. J. Zool. 39, 105-120 (1961)

QUAY, W.B.: Circadian rhythm in rat pineal serotonin and its modifications by estrous cycle and photoperiod. Gen. Comp. Endocrinol. 3, 473-479 (1963)

REITER, R.J.: Endocrine rhythms associated with pineal gland function: In: Biological Rhythms and Endocrine Function. Hedlund, L.W., Franz, J.M., Kenny, A.D. (eds.). Advances in Experimental Medicine and Biology. 54. New York: Plenum Press, 1975, pp. 43-78

REZNIK-SCHÜLLER, H., REZNIK, G.: Comparative histometric investigations of the testicular function of European hamsters (*Cricetus cricetus*) with and without hibernation. Fertility and Sterility 24/9, 698-705 (1973)

ROMAGNOLI, P.: Il corticosurrene di riccio (*Erinaceus europaeus*) con particulare riferimento alle modificazione mitocondriali durante le varie tappe del ciclo annuale. Arch. Ital. Anat. Embriol. 77/1, 87-110 (1972)

SENTURIA, J.B., STEWART, S., MENAKER, M.: Rate temperature relationships in the isolated hearts of ground squirrels. Comp. Biochem. Physiol. 33, 43-50 (1970)

SKOWRON, S., ZAJACZEK, S.: Modifications histologiques des glandes endocrines durant le cycle annuel chez le hérisson. C.R. Soc. Biol. 141, 173-188 (1947)

SMIT-VIS, J.H.: The effect of pinealectomy and of testosterone administration on the occurrence of hibernation in adult male golden hamsters. Acta Morphol. Neerl. Scand. 10, 269-282 (1972)

STRUMWASSER, F.: Factors in the pattern, timing and predictability of hibernation in the squirrel, *Citellus beechyi*. Am. J. Physiol. 196, 8-14 (1959)

SUOMALAINEN, P.: Production of artificial hibernation. Nature (London) 142, 1157 (1938)

SOUMALAINEN, P., NYHOLM, P.: Neurosecretion in hibernating hedgehog. In: Zool. Papers in Honour of Bertil Hanströms 65th Birthday. Lund: Wingstrand, 1956, pp. 269-277

WELLS, L.J.: Prolongation of breeding capacity in males of an annual breeding wild rodent (*Citellus tridecimlineatus*) by constant low temperature. Anat. Rec. 64, Suppl. 1, 138-139 (1935-1936)

WURTMAN, R.J., AXELROD, J., PHILLIPS, L.S.: Melatonin synthesis in the pineal gland: control by light. Science 142, 1071-1072 (1963)

YALOW, R.S., BERSON, S.A.: Immunoassay of endogenous plasma insulin in man. J. Clin. Invest. 39, 1157 (1960)

18. Seasonal Changes and Environmental Control of Testicular Function in the Hedgehog, *Erinaceus europaeus* L.

M. SABOUREAU and J. BOISSIN

Hedgehogs captured in the wild in the west of France were bred in semi-captivity under natural conditions of light and temperature, with free access to food throughout the year.

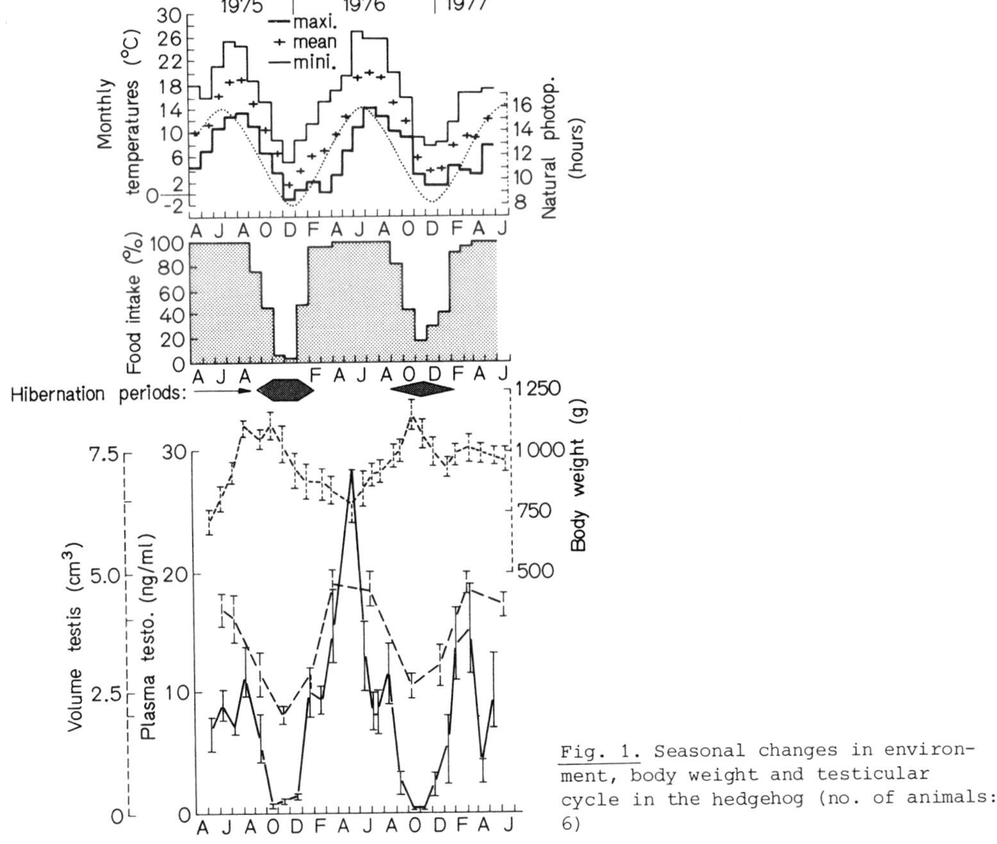

Fig. 1. Seasonal changes in environment, body weight and testicular cycle in the hedgehog (no. of animals: 6)

Hedgehogs exhibit a marked cycle in body weight (Fig. 1), the most elevated weights occurring at the end of summer and in autumn. Thereafter there is a regular decrease during winter. In the first year the minimum was reached in May; in the second, the cycle exhibited an unusual profile on account of the mild winter conditions. The animals gained some weight in January, but this was not statistically significant.

The biology of reproduction of the hedgehog in the West of France is characterized by two unequal periods of birth: the most important is in May to June, and the other in September to October. In the male, there is an annual cycle in testis volume (Fig. 1) with a minimum in winter and a maximum from the beginning of spring to the middle of summer. Testicular development starts in winter. This cycle presents a monophasic profile with a maximum during spring and summer, at which time the mean volume of the testis is twice that observed in winter. The endocrine function is very depressed from October to December. This function increases again between December to January while the animals are still hibernating. The importance and the position of the spring peak are undoubtedly ecodependent. In fact in 1976 hormonal levels increased from December to April-May, and after a peak in March the hormonal level fell in April. It is possible to attribute this pattern to the particular climatic conditions of spring. If we consider the individual seasonal variations, we note that there is always a decline during the increase period at the end of winter. After the spring peak the hormonal level fell and then increased again to reach a second maximum, distinct from the first, in August. This biphasic pattern is often described in vertebrates with a seasonal testicular cycle. In nonhibernating mammals, the winter resumption is controlled by the increase in day length after the winter solstice. It is quite possible that the same process is involved in hibernating mammals, although the perception of the change in day length is difficult to explain. Possibly this change was detected during the periodic arousals that characterized hibernation.

In order to test the sensibility of the neuroendocrine axis towards external factors we subjected hedgehogs, from early December, to different conditions of light and temperatures. The animals in each case were fed ad libitum.

We observed: (1) Whatever environmental change was invoked, testicular function starts again, as indicated by testis volume and plasma testosterone level. (2) The resumption of testicular activity occurs more quickly when ambient temperatures are high. (3) The level of the peak is higher in animals subjected to a temperature of 20°C, whatever conditions of light were used.

These results show that the resumption of testicular function may be an endogenous process. It seems that the environmental factors are only able to modify the rapidity of the response and the level of the stimulation.

19. Annual Endocrine Rhythms in Healthy Young Adult Men: Their Implication in Human Biology and Medicine

A. REINBERG and M. LAGOGUEY

Circadian and circannual rhythms in morbidity and mortality (SMOLENSKY et al., 1972; REINBERG et al., 1973), in feeding behavior (SARGENT, 1954; DEBRY et al., 1975), as well as in sexual behavior (UDRY and MORRIS, 1967; REINBERG and LAGOGUEY, 1978) have been objectively described in men. To seek a better understanding of these rhythmic phenomena, endocrine components, among others, were investigated. In animal experiments both temporal and causal relationships were demonstrated, or suspected to exist, between changes in endocrine activities and reproductive functions, behavioral processes, inter alia. Against this background several studies were performed to document endocrine bioperiodicities in men.

Three preliminary remarks may be useful:

a) Circadian and circannual rhythms must be investigated in the same experiment. The fact that bioperiodicity of a given physiologic variable can be expressed in several frequency domains has been documented in various animal species, including mice (HAUS and HALBERG, 1970), and men (REINBERG, 1974). When sampling once daily (e.g., every other month) at different or even at the same clock hour(s), collected data may reflect circadian rather than circannual rhythmicity. Moreover, not only the 24 h mean level M, but also the circadian crest time Θ of a physiologic variable can be the subject of a circannual rhythm.

b) The location (city and/or state) of the study must be given. The circannual acrophase can be geographically dependent in men, as demonstrated for certain variables by BATSCHELET et al. (1973) and by SIMPSON and BOHLEN (1973). Annual changes in the day length with respect to the latitude, seem to be some of the major environmental factors (signals) to be considered in various species. Most of the results summarized in this paper were obtained from subjects living in the northern hemisphere.

c) A temporal relationship between changes of two variables does not demonstrate in itself a direct causal relationship. This latter can be suspected if, in addition to the temporal relationship, a set of other arguments can be given. From this point of view, studies of circannual rhythms in humans are somewhat frustating, since experimental manipulations (e.g., isolation for one year, etc.) cannot be realized for obvious reasons.

Endocrine Circadian and Circannual Changes in Five Healthy Parisian Males

For 14 months, five mature, apparently healthy (routine clinical examinations and biologic tests) young males (medical student and biochemists) living in Paris, volunteered to document circadian change. At the beginning of the study they were 26, 26, 28, 29 and 31 years old. Their respective height and weight were: 168 cm 64 kg; 183 cm 70 kg; 180 cm 78 kg; 178 cm 63 kg; 171 cm 64 kg.

At the time of the 28-h tests (every other month for plasma sampling; monthly for urine sampling) the subjects were not taking any medication and had no sexual activity. Food and water intake was not controlled; meals were taken at about 07.00, 13.00 and 20.00. The subjects' circadian periodicity was synchronized with light-on at 07.00 (7 a.m.) + 1 h and light-off at 23.00 (11 p.m.) ± 1.5 h during the year.

Circadian rhythms in levels of plasma hormone were explored simultaneously in the five subjects during the same two days in January, March, May, July, September, November 1973 and again in February 1974. On test days, venous blood samples were withdrawn in a EDTA vacutainer (BECTON and DICKINSON) at fixed 4-h intervals for 28 h, starting at 08.00 on day 1.

Plasma (after centrifugation) and urine samples were stored at -25°C, ten tubes per sample to facilitate control and multiple determinations, each tube being defrozen only once. Determinations were performed in large series, at the end of the entire study. Radioimmunoassay procedures were used for plasma variables and urinary aldosterone determinations. Specificity, sensitivity, and precision were tested according to the best current methodology.

Both conventional and single cosinor (HALBERG et al., 1972) methods were used for the statistical analysis of time series thus obtained. In a first step, data were plotted as a function of time (mean $\bar{X}$ ± 1 SE). Rhythmic changes can be visualized when the curve is roughly sinudoidal and associated with a statistically significant creast-trough difference. Thereafter, detection and quantification of rhythms were achieved by fitting a sine curve of 24 h or 365 days, by the method of least squares, to each time series of respectively one day or one year in duration. With this cosinor method, a rhythm is validated when its amplitude differs from zero with $p < 0.05$. The rhythm, when detected, can be characterized by several parameters: the acrophase, Θ, circadian or circannual crest time (more precisely, crest time - clock hour of day, or day of a specified month - of the sine function approximating all data); the amplitude, A (equal to 1/2 the within daily or yearly rhythmic variability) and the mesor, M, or rhythm-adjusted mean. Θ and A are given as mean values with their 95% confidence limits and M as mean ± 1 SE.

Circadian Rhythms (Table 1). No circadian rhythm in plasma FSH is detected in any monthly time series or in pooled data. Circadian rhythm in LH is detected only from July to November and in pooled data, with a small amplitude. Other documented variables exhibit statistically significant circadian rhythms.

Annual Changes of Circadian Acrophase (when rhythms are validated in most if not all documented months; Table 1). Plasma prolactin has a remarkably fixed acrophase, located in the vicinity of 04.00 throughout the year. Circadian Θ's of sexual activity and urinary 17-OHCS do not exhibit detectable annual change, in contrast with circadian Θ's of plasma testosterone and plasma cortisol, respectively.

Both circadian Θ's of plasma testosterone and thyroxin have an early location in spring and a late location in autumn. On the contrary, Θ's of circadian rhythms related to the adrenal activity (plasma cortisol, urinary aldosterone, etc.) occur earlier in autumn (first half) winter and later in (second half) winter-spring. The fixation of circadian Θ of 17-OHCS could be due to noisy data.

Annual Changes of Circadian 24-h Mean M. The single sodinor method was used to summarize all findings in Figure 1. Prolactin has no circannual periodicity. Statistically significant circannual rhythms are observed in the other documented variables. Both FSH and LH reach their

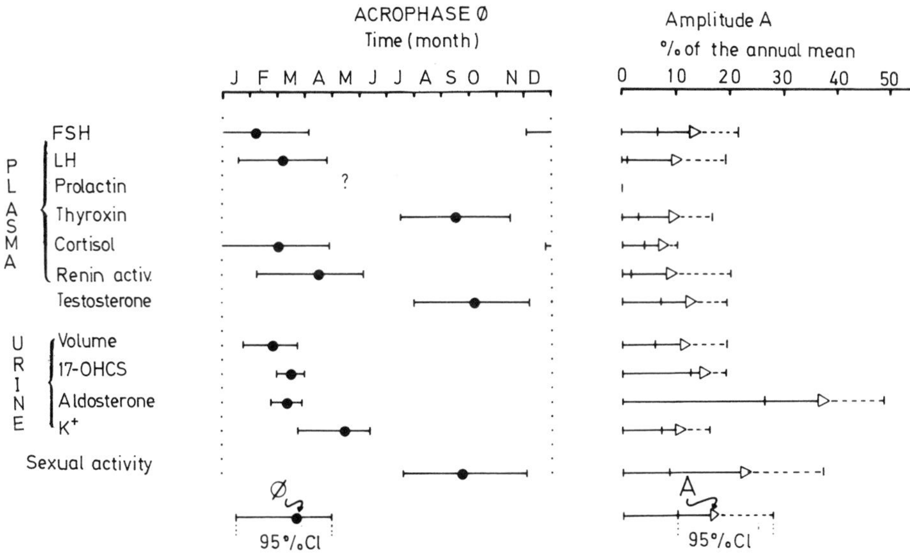

Fig. 1. Circannual rhythms of five healthy young Parisian males: single cosinor summary. Annual acrophase, Θ (crest time) and amplitude A (1/2 of the total variability/year) are given with their 95% confidence limits. A is in percent of the annual 24 h mean M (Table 1). Θ's of FSH, LH and variables related to adrenocortical activity occur from early winter to early spring, while Θ's of thyroxin, testosterone and sexual activity occur from mid summer to late fall. The annual A is large for urinary aldosterone, small for plasma cortisol. A does not differ from zero for plasma prolactin (no annual rhythm detected in the latter)

crest in winter (February-March). Adrenal activity (plasma cortisol, urinary 17-OHCS and aldosterone) has also its crest time in February to March. Respective acrophases of plasa-renin activity and urinary potassium are located somewhat later, in April to May. The annual Θ's for thyroxin occurs in September in phase with annual Θ's of both plasma testosterone and sexual activity. Individual changes of the considered variables were similar to those depicted for the group.

A set of circannual rhythms have been already reported, in healthy men, for the following variables: urinary 17-ketosteroids, HAMBURGER (1954), crest in November, Copenhagen, Denmark; 17-OHCS, WATANABE (1964), crest in February, Niigata, Japan, AHUJA and SHARMA (1971), in January, New Delhi, India; plasma cortisol, WEITZMAN (1974), crest in autumn-winter. Tromsø, Norway; plasma ACTH, COPINSCHI et al. (1977), crest in winter, Belgium - only 2 time points/year. Annual changes in sexual activity (intercourse) of married North American couples shows a Θ location in July, extending from June to August. A circannual rhythm in plasma testosterone of healthy males in Holland has been reported by SMALS et al. (1976). The crest time occurred during autumn. Despite differences related to method of data acquisition, geographic location, etc., these results are in good agreement with ours.

Table 1. Annual changes of circadian acrophases

Variable Pl = plasma Ur = urine	Annual 24 H mean M ± 1 SE (units)	Circadian Amplitude A (1) Pooled times series A in % of M (95% confidence limits)	 Acrophase Θ (2) Θ in h.min	Annual change of circadian acrophase Θ (3) Early location month: Θ in h.min (95% confidence limits)	 Late location
Pl FSH	7.63± 0.27 (m.U./ml)	No detection (4)		-	-
Pl LH	8.91± 0.29 (m.U./ml	4.9 (1.5-6.4)	03.02 (00.07-05.57)	No change (5)	
Pl prolactin	12.1 ± 1.6 (ng/ml)	28.9 (24.8-33.0)	04.44 (04.11-05.17)	No change (6)	
Pl thyroxin	8.45± 0.46 (µg/100 ml)	18.9 (11.3-26.5)	17.42 (16.00-19.24)	March: 14.21 (12.50-15.52)	September: 18.45 (17.45-19.45)
Pl cortisol	12.2 ± 6.8 (µg/100 ml)	7.9 (3.7-12.1)	09.01 (10.23-07.38)	September: 07.50 (06.46-08.54)	February: 10.18 (09.05-11.31)
Pl renin activity	3.45± 1.4 (ng/ml/h)	7.8 (2.6-13.0)	19.28 (17.07-21.49)	November: 17.01 (14.31-19.31)	March: 22.50 (18.10-03.50)
Pl testosterone	759 ±26 (ng/100 ml)	13 (7 -19)	11.10 (09.07-13.14)	May: 08.19 (04.53-11.45)	November: 14.14 (10.24-19.04)
Ur 17-OHCS	5.24± 0.3 (mg/24 h)	39 (28.9-49.1)	12.30 (09.13-15.47)	No change (7)	
Ur aldosterone	8.4 ± 2.7 (µg/24 h)	69.8 (29.4-110.2)	11.55 (10.07-13.43)	January: 11.07 (09.37-12.38)	June: 14.43 (12.42-16.46)
Ur potassium	51.9 ± 2.5 (mEQ/24 h)	55.5 (38.2-72.8)	13.44 (13.01-14.27)	December: 12.24 (11.44-13.04)	May: 15.47 (13.55-17.39)
Sexual activity	0.71+ 0.09 (no.of coitus+ mastur.)	26.6 (5.3-47.9)	03.30 (23.55-07.05)	No change (7)	

The annual phase relationship between plasma testosterone and sexual activity may reflect a causal relationship, as is the case in various vertebrate species (cf. BENOIT and ASSENMACHER, 1970; PENGELLEY, 1974), including nonhuman primates (CONAWAY and SADE, 1967; GORDON et al., 1976; VINCENT, 1969; PENG et al., 1973).

This does not mean that the circannual rhythm of plasma testosterone is the sole variable, but only one of the variables that may play a role in the circannual rhythm of sexual activity. Among others, plasma FSH and LH must be considered even if a difference of about 6 months occurs between Θ's reflecting pituitary and gonadal activity. A similar time difference between annual crests of these plasma hormones was observed in the Mallard drake by ASSENMACHER (1974).

One of the hypotheses to explain this fact is the existence of an annual cycle in gonadal sensitivity to gonadotropic hormones. Such a change has been demonstrated in the male Mallard among other animal species. Moreover, ASSENMACHER has shown the role played by the circannual rhythm of the thyroid activity in this phenomenon. The second hypothesis, which does not exclude the first, takes into consideration chronopharmacologic phenomena (REINBERG and HALBERG, 1971; REINBERG, 1976). The effectiveness of an agent (including hornomes) varies as a function of the timing of its administration (or of its circadian crest time in plasma concentration). The circadian Θ of plasma testosterone exhibits a 6-h shift between May and November (Table 1). Therefore, a circannual change in the effect(s) of this hormone on target organs can be related to a circannual change in its circadian crest time.

Let us add that in puberal girls, a circannual change of menarche has been observed (cf., reviews in REINBERG, 1970; ZACHARIAS et al., 1976) with a crest in late fall-early winter and a trough in spring for the northern hemisphere.

The question must be raised whether or not these annual rhythms are endogenous or have an endogenous component. A coherent body of knowledge emerges from other animal experiments: endogenous circannual rhythms (e.g., in gonadal activity and reproductive functions) are not induced by environmental information, but can be entrained by annual changes of external factors such as day length (FARNER, 1959; PENGELLEY, 1974), at least in certain species. If the extension from animals to man is acceptable, our species should have certain properties of short-day (or long-night) animals, with reference to reproductive functions. Pertinent for the discussion is a remark by CONAWAY and SADE (1965): "... it may well be that all primates including the human should be regarded as basically seasonal breeders."

(1) A is expressed in percent of the annual 24 h mean. (2) Θ (crest time) is given in hours and minutes. Θ reference: local midnight. (3) month: corresponding timing of Θ in the 24 h scale. The annual change of Θ is given only when statistically significant (F test). (4) FSH circadian rhythm was detected neither in any monthly time series nor in pooled data. (5) LH circadian rhythm was not detected in January, February, March and May. No change in validated Θ's. (6) Circadian ryhthm in prolactin were detected in each of the documented month, without annual change of Θ. (7) Circadian rhythms were detected. No annual change in circadian Θ locations.

Circannual Changes in the Feeding Behavior

Such changes have been validated for children under experimental conditions allowing the study of their spontaneous behavior (free choice in quality and quantity of food, etc.). DEBRY et al. (1975) demonstrated in healthy 4-year olds in Nancy (France) statistically significant circannual rhythms in the intake of lipids (crest in spring), carbohydrates (crest in summer) and resulting calories (crest in summer). No annual changes in protein intake were detected. Circannual changes in spontaneous food intake of North American infants (SARGENT, 1954), have a pattern associated with a circannual change in weight gain (crest, late summer-early fall). Soldiers in training camps, urban families and mill workers consumed significantly more colories in fall-winter than in spring-summer (SARGENT, 1954). According to SARGENT, the implicit mechanism is metabolic in nature, and seasonal variations would be governed by the nutritional demands and requirements of the tissues with annual changes in day length serving as the appropriate informative stimulus.

These annual changes in feeding behavior (more specifically carbohydrate intake) could be related - at least partially - to circannual changes of the plasma insulin response to glucose ingestion. Standardized glucose tolerance tests (GTT) were performed as a function of time (month) over two years, to document these changes in healthy young men living in Nancy (MÉJEAN et al., 1977).

The maximum level in the blood glucose curve shows a circannual rhythm with an acrophase Θ (annual crest time) = 29 September (± 56 days with 95% confidence limits) and an amplitude A (1/2 of the total variability) = 12.5% of the annual mean of the peak height 1.39 g/l. No statistically significant annual changes occur in the other GTT parameters.

Circannual rhythms of three parameters of the concentration/time curve of plasma insulin are validated. The maximum level of plasma insulin has its Θ = 27 October (± 58 days) associated with A = 19.7% of the annual mean (107.2 μu/ml). The span of time to reach the peak has its Θ = 5 May (± 52 days) associated with A = 18.2% of the annual mean (55.5 min). The area under the curve has a Θ = 16 August (± 23 days).

In other words, the plasma insulin response is both the most rapid and the strongest in fall. Such findings confirm those of CAMPBELL et al. (1975).

Circannual Changes in Incidence of Diseases

The analyses of death records in a Parisian hospital (1962-1967), in France as a whole (1962-1967) (REINBERG et al., 1973); in Minnesota (1941-1967), and other parts of the United States (SMOLENSKY et al., 1972) lead to similar results. Annual Θ's of deaths resulting from cerebral vascular lesions, heart diseases, as well as infections diseases (e.g., pneumonia and influenza) occur during winter months. In 48 states of the USA, Θ's of death due to pneumonia and influenza stand between the end of December and the end of February. If the risk of mortality for these lung diseases is higher in winter months, it is not necessarily because the weather is bad, but rather because the human organism is then more susceptible to this type of infection than at any other time. Annual changes in endocrine activities could play a role in the occurrence of annual changes in the resistance of the human organism resistance to potentially noxious factors. More precisely, there is a striking coincidence in time between annual Θ's of adrenal activity and the high risk of certain lung infections and cardiovascular diseases. With reference to the latter, it may be added that not only annual Θ's in aldosterone and plasma renin activity might be involved, but also annuals Θ's in adrenalin and noradrenalin which occur in May, (April to June) as demonstrated by DESCOVITCH et al. (1974) in Milan, Italy.

The effect (if any) of circannual rhythms in the adrenal activity on the incidence of diseases could involve circannual changes in immunologic processes. Analyses of blood samples gathered every other month (on a circadian basis) from healthy young Parisians (6 man and 3 women) validated the following circannual rhythms: blood leukocytes (annual Θ = December; from October to January); IgA (Θ = November; from September to January); IgM (Θ = September; from August to September) IgG (Θ = July; from early July to late August) (REINBERG et al., 1977).

We fully realize that, especially in this third part, we are dealing with a set of hypotheses. However, these hypotheses can be tested in the future as were hypotheses (formulated 12 years ago) concerning circadian rhythms in pathologic phenomena of patients suffering from allergic asthma (MCGOVERN et al., 1977). Component physiologic rhythms (including those of hormonal secretion) involved in these pathologic phenomena have been investigated.

Acknowledgments. We thank Drs. G. DEBRY, L. MÉJEAN (University of Nancy), and E. SCHULLER (Laboratoire d'Immunologie du Système Nerveux. Hôpital Sâlpétrière, Paris) for their permission to use data only published in abstract form when this paper was written.

References

AHUJA, M.M.S., SHARMA, N.J.: Adrenocortical function in relation to seasonal variations in normal indians. Indian J. Med. 59, 1893-1905 (1971)

ASSENMACHER, I.: External and internal components of the mechanism controlling reproductive cycles in drakes. In: Circannual Clocks. Pengelley, E.T. (ed.). New York: Academic Press, 1974, pp. 197-248

BATCHELET, E., HILLMAN, D., SMOLENSKY, M., HALBERG, F.: Angular-linear correlation coefficient for rhythmometry and circannually chang human birth rates at different geographic latitudes. Int. J. Chronobiol. 1, 183-202 (1973)

BENOIT, J., ASSENMACHER, I. (eds.): La photorégulation de la reproduction chez les oiseaux et les mammifères. (Colloques Int. CNRS. Montpellier 1967). CNRS 172 Paris (1970)

CAMPBELL, I.T., JARRETT, R.J., RUTLAND, P., STIMMER, L.: The plasma insulin and growth hormone response to oral glucose: diurnal and seasonal observations in the antactic. Diabetologia 11, 147-150 (1975)

CONAWAY, C.H., SADE, D.S.: The seasonal spermatogenetic cycle in free ranging rhesus monkeys. Folia Primat. 3, 1-12 (1965)

COPINSCHI, G., LECLERCQ, R., GOLSTEIN, J., ROBYN, C., DESIR, D., DE LAET, M.H., VIRASORO, E., VANHAELST, L., L'HERMITE, M., VAN CAUTER: Seasonal modifications of circadian and ultradian variations of ACTH, cortisol, β-MSH, hPrl and TSH in normal human. Chronobiologia 2, 106 (1977)

DEBRY, G., BLEYER, R., REINBERG, A.: Circadian, circannual and other rhythms in spontaneous nutrient and caloric intake of healthy four-year olds. Diabète et Métabolisme 1, 91-99 (1975)

DESCOVITCH, G.C., MONTALBETTI, N., KUHL, J.F.W., RIMONDO, S., HALBERG, F.: Age and catecholamine rhythms. Chronobiologia 1, 163-171 (1974)

FARNER, D.S.: Control of annual gonadal cycles in birds. In: Photoperiodism. Withrow, R.B. (ed.). Pb 55 AAAS. Washington D.S., 1959, pp. 717-750
GASTON, S., MENAKER, M.: Photoperiodic control of hamster testis. Science 158, 925-928 (1967)
GORDON, T.P., ROSE, R.M., BERNSTEIN, I.S.: Seasonal rhythm in plasma testosterone levels in the rhesus monkey. Hormones and Behavior 7, 229-243 (1971)
HALBERG, F., JOHNSON, E.A., NELSON, W., RUNGE, W., SOTHERN, R.: Autorhythmometry - procedures for physiologic self-measurements and their analysis. Physiology Teacher 1, 1 (1972)
HAMBURGER, C.: Six years' daily 17-ketosteroid determination on one subject; seasonal variations and independence of volume of urine. Acta Endocrinol. 17, 116-127 (1954)
HAUS, E., HALBERG, F.: Circannual rhythm in level and timing of serum corticosterone in standardized inbred mature C-mice. Environ. Res. 3, 81-106 (1970)
LAGOGUEY, M., CESSELIN, F., TOUITOU, Y., LAGOGUEY, A., GHATA, J., REINBERG, A.: Aspect endocrinien de la structure temporelle circannuelle de 5 parisiens jeunes, adultes et sains. Ann. Endocrinol. (Paris) 37, 459-460 (1976)
LAGOGUEY, M., REINBERG, A.: Circannual rhythms in plasma LH, FSH and testosterone and in the sexual activity of healthy young Parisian males. J. Physiol. 257, 19-20
LAGOGUEY, M., REINBERG, A., CESSELIN, F., ANTREASSIAN, J., DELASSALLE, A., LAGOGUEY, A.: Circannual and circadian rhythms in plasma cortisol, renin activity, thyroxine and in urinary aldosterone of five healthy young Parisian males. Chronobiologia 4, 126 (1977)
MCGOVERN, J., SMOLENSKY, M., REINBERG, A.: Chronobiology, Allergy and Immunology. Springfield, ill.: Charles Thomas, 1977
MEJEAN, L., REINBERG, A., GAY, G., DEBRY, G.: Circannual changes of the plasma insuline response to glucose tolerance test of healthy young males. Proc. Int. Union. Physiol. Sci. Paris, July 1977, Vol. XIII, p. 498 (1977)
MICHAEL, R.P., ZUMPE, D.: Environmental and endocrine factors influencing annual changes in sexual potency in primates. Psychoneuroendocrinology 1, 303-313 (1976)
PENG, M.T., LAI, Y.L., YANG, C.S., CHIANG, H.S., NEW, A.E., CHANG, C.P.: Reproductive parameters of the Taiwan monkey. Primates 14, 201-213 (1973)
PENGELLEY, E.T. (ed.): Circannual Clocks. (140th AAAS meeting San Francisco, 1974). New York: Academic Press, 1974
REINBERG, A.: Eclairement et cycle mensuel de la femme. In: La photorégulation chez les Oiseaux et les Mammifères. Colloque Int. CNRS (Montpellier, Juillet 1967). Benoit, J., Assenmacher, I. (eds.). Paris: CNRS, 1970, pp. 529-546
REINBERG, A.: Aspects of circannual rhythms in man. In: Circannual Clocks. Pengelley, E.T. (ed.). New York: Academic Press, 1974, pp. 423-505
REINBERG, A.: Advances in human chronopharmacology. Chronobiologia 3, 151-166 (1976)
REINBERG, A., GERVAIS, P., HALBERG, F., GAULTIER, M., ROYNETTE, N., ABULKER, C., DUPONT, J.: Rhythmes circadiens et circannuels de mortalité des adultes dans un hôpital parisien et en France. Nouvelle Presse Médicale 2, 289-294 (1973)
REINBERG, A., HALBERG, F.: Circadian chronopharmacology. Ann. Rev. Pharmacol. 11, 455-492 (1971)
REINBERG, A., LAGOGUEY, M.: Circadian and circannual rhythms in the sexual activity and in plasma hormones (FSH, LH, testosterone, etc.) of five healthy young parisian males. Arch. Sexual Behavior 7, 13-30 (1978)
REINBERG, A., LAGOGUEY, M., CHAUFFOURNIER, J.M., CESSELIN, F.: Circannual and circadian rhythms in plasma testosterone in five healthy young parisian males. Acta Endocrinol. 80, 732-743 (1975)
REINBERG, A., SCHULLER, E., DELASNERIE, N., CLENCH, J., HELARY, M.: Rythmes circadiens et circannuels des leucocytes, protéines totales. IgA, IgM, IgG d'adultes jeunes et sains. Nouvelle Presse Médicale 6, 3819-3823 (1977)
REINBERG, A., SMOLENSKY, M.H.: Circatrigintan secondary rhythms related to hormonal changes in the menstrual cycle: general considerations. in: Ferin, M., Halberg, F., Richart, R.M., Vande Wiele, R.L. (eds.). Biorhythms and Human Reproduction. New York: Wiley, 1974, pp. 241-258
SARGENT, F. (II): Season and the metabolism of fat and carbohydrate: a study of vestigial physiology. Meteorological Monographs 2 (3), 68-80 (1954)

SIMPSON, H., BOHLEN, J.: Latitude and the human circadian system. In: Biological Aspects of Circadian Rhythms. Mills, J.N. (ed.). London-New York: Plenum Press, 1973, pp. 85-120

SMALS, A.G.H., KLOPPENBORG, P.W.C., BENRAAD, TH.J.: Circannual cycle in plasma testosterone levels in man. J. Clin. Endocrinol. Metab. 42, 979-982 (1976)

SMOLENSKY, M., HALBERG, F., SARGENT, F. (II): Chronobiology of the life sequence. In: Advances in Climatic Physiology. Itoh, S., Ogata, K., Yoshimura, H. (eds.). Tokyo: Igaku Shoin Ltd, 1972, pp. 281-318

UDRY, J.R., MORRIS, N.M.: Seasonality of coitus and seasonality of birth. Demography 4, 673-680 (1967)

VINCENT, F.: Contribution à l'étude des prosimiens africains. Le Galago de Demidoff. Thèse D.S. Paris 1969. CNRS A.O. 3575.

WATANABE, G.I.: Seasonal variation of adrenal cortex activity. Arch. Environm. Hlth. 9, 192-200 (1964)

WEITZMAN, E.D.: Temporal patterns of neuro-endocrine secretion in man: relationship to the 24-hour sleep waking cycle. In: Aschoff, J., Ceresa, F., Halberg, F. (eds.). Chronobiological Aspects of Endocrinology. Stuttgart-New York: F.K. Schattauer, 1974, pp. 169-184

ZACHARIAS, L., RAND, W.M., WURTMAN, R.J.: A prospective study of sexual development and growth in American girl: the statistics of menarche. Obstetric & Gynecol. Survey. 31, 325-337 (1976)

Chapter II. Diurnal Endocrine Rhythms and Environment

1. Endocrine Concomitants of the Sleep-Wake Rhythm in Man

H.-J. QUABBE

The 24-h pattern of the concentration of growth hormone (GH) in human plasma reveals a close relation between secretory episodes of the hormone and the sleep-wake cycle. Since this discovery, the relation of other pituitary hormones and some hormones of peripheral glands to the sleep-wake rhythm has been studied and interesting patterns have been found.

Definitions and Technical Aspects. Acceptance of a functional relationship between the secretion of a hormone and the sleep-wake rhythm requires the demonstration of a difference of its total secretion and/or its secretory pattern (number, duration, magnitude of secretory episodes, etc.) between the states of wakefulness and sleep. This sleep-wake difference must be immediately entrained to any change of the sleep-wake pattern, e.g., a sleep-wake reversal. In contrast, a circadian rhythm dependent on an endogenous clock requires at least several days in order to be entrained to such a shift. Of course, a link between the secretion of a hormone and the sleep-wake cycle does not preclude the additional existence of a true endogenous circadian rhythm in the secretory pattern of this hormone.

From a technical aspect, studies of the relation between the sleep-wake rhythm and hormone secretion must assure that the frequency of blood sampling is adequate to (1) detect rapid changes in the plasma concentration of the hormone due to episodic secretion and a short half-time in plasma, and (2) to cope with rapid changes of sleep stages, if the possible influence of different sleep stages [slow-wave sleep (SWS), rapid eye-movement sleep (REM)] is to be investigated. For most hormones it is necessary to sample at least every 15-20 min throughout the entire 24-h day. Less frequent blood sampling is bound to lead to serious misinterpretations due to missing of secretory episodes, or to difficulties in relating the onset or termination of a secretory episode to a change in sleep stage.

Growth Hormone. In man, GH is secreted episodically and with a clear relation to the sleep-wake rhythm. Its plasma concentration is low during most of the day. A secretory episode occurs regularly in relation to the first SWS phase and smaller secretory bursts may be seen during subsequent SWS phases (QUABBE et al., 1966; TAKAHASHI et al., 1968; HONDA et al., 1969; SASSIN et al., 1969b; QUABBE et al., 1971). It has been shown that these nocturnal secretory episodes depend on the occurrence of sleep, more precisely, of SWS. A change in the sleep-wake rhythm is immediately accompanied by a concomitant change of the GH secretory pattern. SWS deprivation causes diminution or disappearance of the nocturnal GH secretion, but selective deprivation of REM sleep has no effect (SASSIN et al., 1969a; HONDA et al., 1969). However, while nocturnal GH secretion does not occur before the appearance of SWS activity, the EEG pattern of SWS may be present for as much as 60 min before GH secretion begins and during later SWS phases there is often no GH secretion. These and other observations indicate that SWS and nocturnal releases GH are both linked to a common determinator, but are not causally related to each other.

During daytime as well, bursts of GH secretion bear a relation to the state of arousal. They occur preferentially during morning and afternoon naps, i.e., during the rest phases of the so-called "basic rest-activity cycle" (PARKER and ROSSMAN, 1974). In the newborn this relationship of GH secretion to the sleep-wake rhythm develops when a concentration of sleep during the night and a stable non-REM/REM cycle are established. During old age, GH secretion during sleep seems to diminish. However, the link to SWS is preserved. Comparisons of this "endogenous program" of GH secretion with the influence of food intake, short- and long-term metabolic state of the body, etc. have revealed a remarkable stability of its secretory pattern, which makes it likely that the CNS program is of prime importance, and that metabolic factors merely play a modulating role (reviewed by QUABBE, 1977).

Prolactin. While small secretory episodes of prolactin (PRL) occur throughout the day, these become more frequent and more important during the night. In consequence, the overall nocturnal plasma concentration of PRL is higher than during the day. This increase is dependent on sleep, as demonstrated by sleep-delay studies. In contrast to the nocturnal GH pattern, the PRL concentration tends to be highest towards the end of the sleep period. During the day, PRL secretion increases during naps, and thus shows a relation to the 24-h basic rest-activity cycle (SASSIN et al., 1972; PARKER et al., 1973). A detailed analysis shows that PRL nadires often correspond to the REM phases, and peaks occur during non-REM phases (PARKER et al., 1974). As in the case of GH, this relation may represent only a superficial aspect of the sleep-PRL link. A decrease from the higher PRL concentrations during non-REM phases is already evident before the onset of the succeeding REM phase. Thus PRL secretion is apparently only triggered or facilitated, but not sustained, by non-REM sleep.

LH/FSH - Oestrogens/Testosterone. In adult female subjects, the plasma concentration of luteinizing hormone (LH) decreases during the first hours after sleep onset (KAPEN et al., 1973). A sleep-reversal study demonstrates entrainment of the LH nadir to the reversed sleep pattern. A "3-h day" (2 h waking and 1 h sleep) has been used to test whether the hormonal relationship with sleep persists despite a massive distortion of the normal sleep pattern. During such a 3-h sleep-wake schedule the LH plasma concentration was lower during the 1-h sleep periods than during the 2-h wake periods (KAPEN et al., 1976). Thus, in adult women, LH secretion seems to be inhibited by sleep, especially during the early part of sleep when SWS predominates. No relation to sleep stages has been found.

In adult men, no correlation of LH secretion to the sleep-wake rhythm or to sleep stages has been found. However, testosterone secretion increases during sleep and shows a relation to the sleep-stage cycle, with peaks occurring mostly in conjunction with REM sleep (EVANS et al., 1971). This may reflect an influence of the nocturnal PRL rise on testosterone secretion.

An interesting change in the secretion of gonadotropins and gonadal steroids occurs in puberty. In prepubertal children, there is no circadian or sleep-related pattern of LH secretion. With the onset of puberty, however, in both girls and boys, LH is secreted in larger amounts during sleep than during wakefulness. During later stages of puberty, the day-time LH concentrations also increase until the higher overall 24-h adult levels are attained. During puberty the LH secretory episodes usually begin during non-REM periods and end during REM periods (BOYAR et al., 1972). The association of this nocturnal increase in LH to sleep during puberty was demonstrated by sleep-delay experiments (KAPEN et al., 1974). An additional influence of an endogeneous circadian rhythm on the pubertal LH secretion becomes apparent in the sleep-reversal study, since the LH secretion during the nocturnal waking period did not decrease to the normal day-time waking levels. The increase of the nocturnal LH secretion is related to puberty and not to age as such, since the secretory pattern in patients with precocious puberty corresponds to their stage of puberty and not to their chronologic age (BOYAR et al., 1973).

The episodic secretion of follicle-stimulating hormone (FSH) during puberty is also higher during sleep than during waking in many children, but the difference is not as great as that of LH (BOYAR et al., 1973a). Episodic secretion of testosterone in boys shows a similar sleep-related increase during puberty and a link between the testosterone episodes and those of LH, both of which are not seen in adult men (BOYAR et al., 1974; JUDD et al., 1974). Estradiol secretion in pubertal girls, in contrast, is highest during the day (early afternoon). Since no sleep-delay studies have yet been done with determination of the estradiol concentration in plasma, it remains open at the present time whether this afternoon estradiol peak is due to an endogenous circadian rhythm or is dependent on the nocturnal increase in LH and FSH (BOYAR et al., 1976).

<u>TSH - Thyroid Hormones.</u> The 24-h pattern of thyroid-stimulating hormone (TSH) secretion suggests influences of both an endogenous circadian rhythm and a modulating influence of the sleep-wake rhythm. Nocturnal plasma concentrations of TSH are higher than those during daytime. However, the maximum of episodic TSH secretion occurs already in the late evening hours before sleep onset, and sleep seems to exert an inhibitory effect. Thus, during a sleep-reversal experiment, the late evening increase of TSH secretion persisted, and secretion was enhanced when the subjects were kept awake during the night. However, TSH secretion was low during the second nocturnal wake period. While this suggested to the authors a suppression of the TSH secretion by the elevated concentrations of the first nocturnal wake period (delayed negative feedback), further studies seem to be necessary to clarify this point (PARKER et al., 1976). Interestingly, the evening surge of TSH is not associated with a similar change of plasma thyroxin or triiodothyronine concentrations (AZUKIZAWA et al., 1976).

<u>ACTH - Cortisol.</u> The 24-h episodic secretion of ACTH/cortisol is associated primarily with time of day rather than with the sleep-wake rhythm. However, it is not entirely independent of the latter. When subjects live a "3-h day", the original circadian pattern of cortisol secretion is essentially preserved, but there is a clear entrainment of the cortisol secretory episodes to the hours of the waking periods (WEITZMAN et al., 1974). This suggests a modulating influence of the sleep-wake rhythm on ACTH/cortisol secretion. However, entrainment to other factors may also play a role in such a severely distorted sleep-wake pattern.

Thus, both the sleep-wake rhythm and an endogenous circadian rhythm are important determiners of the 24-h pattern of pituitary and pituitary-dependent hormones. For some (GH, PRL, LH during puberty) the link to the sleep-wake cycle is predominant. For others (ACTH/cortisol, TSH) an endogenous circadian rhythm is subjected to a modulating influence of the sleep-wake rhythm. The result is a characteristic pattern of secretion for each of the hormones, and a complicated temporal relationship among the plasma concentrations of individual hormones. Figure 1 summarizes the 24-h secretory patterns of some of the hormones that have been discussed.

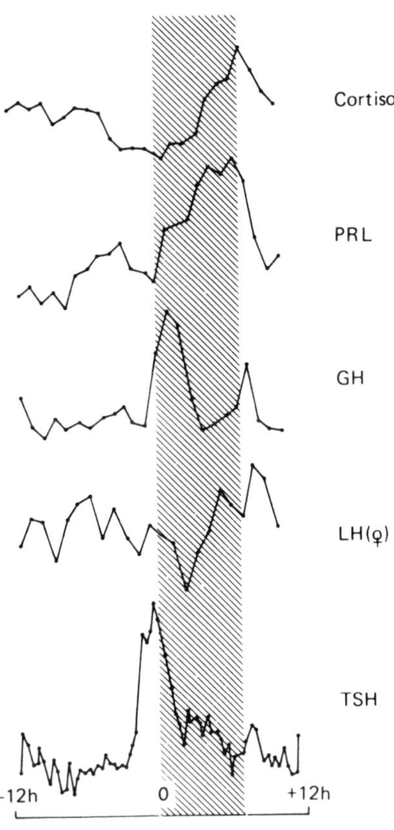

Fig. 1. Synoptic presentation of the 24-h plasma concentration of several hormones (expressed as percent of the 24-h mean. For cortisol the absolute plasma concentrations are given). Each hormone has its own characteristic temporal pattern and a different relation to the sleep-wake cycle. Data (some slightly modified) were taken from: SASSIN et al. (1972); KAPEN et al. (1973); WEITZMAN et al. (1974); PARKER et al. (1976). Shaded area: sleep time. O, indicates sleep-onset

Episodic secretion, link to the sleep-wake rhythm, and presence of endogenous circadian cycles all suggest a strong influence of the CNS on the temporal pattern of hormone secretion. The existence of this CNS program challenges to a certain degree the classical concept of hormone secretory regulation by a smoothly acting negative feedback through the peripheral hormone concentration.

Supporting evidence for a certain independence of pituitary hormone secretion from peripheral feedback has come from studies on certain patients. WU et al. (1976) described an 18-year old patient with XY gonadal agenesis, in whom the plasma concentration of LH and FSH was elevated to the castrate range, compatible with the absence of feedback from gonadal steroids. However, both LH and FSH were secreted episodically, and the LH concentration during sleep was significantly higher than during waking, indicating that the patient had entered "puberty." The CNS program of hormone secretion had apparently progressed to the late pubertal stage of the LH/FSH secretory program in the absence of gonads. Similar findings have been reported in patients with gonadal dysgenesis and after pharmacologic blockade of the testosterone/estrogen feedback in normal subjects (BOYAR et al., 1973b; NAFTOLIN et al., 1973). Likewise, in patients with Addison's disease, who produce no cortisol, the circadian pattern of episodic ACTH secretion is preserved, but the secretory program takes place at a higher set-point (KRIEGER and GEWIRTZ, 1974).

These results are compatible with, and support the concept that the temporal pattern of pituitary hormone secretion is due to a CNS program and relatively independent of peripheral feedback actions. However, the set-point at which this program is executed is apparently determined by a feedback action of the peripheral hormone concentration and also by metabolic factors for some hormones (e.g., glucose, free fatty acids, amino acids in the case of GH).

The physiologic significance of the relationship between pituitary hormone secretion and the sleep-wake rhythm is largely unknown. It can be speculated that it may serve a coordination of hormone action with other functions of the body that are entrained to the sleep-wake rhythm. For example, if sleep has a restorative function, the early nocturnal GH secretory peak may help to direct metabolism towards synthetic processes. A possible role of the GH peak for the development of subsequent sleep has also been discussed.

The application of the "frequent-sampling" hormone profile studies to patients with psychogenic and psychiatric diseases has revealed interesting changes of the temporal organization of hormone secretion in some cases. Two examples will be discussed.

Anorexia nervosa is a disease, usually of young females, in which severe, self-inflicted weight loss, due to relentless dieting, is associated with amenorrhea. The 24-h LH secretion in adult patients with this disease reverts to the pubertal or even prepubertal pattern, i.e., with either low day-time LH plasma concentration with an increase during sleep (pubertal pattern) or even low prepubertal LH concentrations during the entire 24-h day. Remission of the psychologic disturbance is accompanied by an improvement towards a more adult LH secretory pattern. A comparable abnormality of LH secretion is not seen in patients with amenorrhea due to nonpsychologic causes. It is possible that weight loss itself may play a role in the LH secretory abnormality, but there is evidence that a hypothalamic dysregulation is also involved, since amenorrhea is often present at the start or even before weight loss occurs (KATZ et al., 1976). Thus, in anorexia nervosa, the psychological disturbance manifests itself partly via a derangement of hypothalamic function: abnormal eating behavior leads to weight loss, and reversal of the 24-h gonadotropin secretion to the pubertal or prepubertal pattern leads to amenorrhea.

In children with psychosocial dwarfism, "environmental deprivation" ("noxious family influences") is associated with retarded growth. Sleep is poor. Endocrinologic investigations have revealed an impaired GH response to a number of stimulatory tests and - studied in one child - absence of sleep-related GH release. Improvement of the psychologic condition led to a recurrence of GH secretion during sleep. Impairment of GH secretion is most probably the cause of retardation of growth, since GH release normalizes during remissions and periods of poor growth correlate well with those of poor sleep (BROWN, 1976). While the significance of imparied GH release during (unphysiologic) stimulatory tests is uncertain, sleep-related GH secretion is a physiologic event and its absence in a disorder associated with poor growth may therefore be of more significance. Thus, in this disease, a psychosocial derangement manifests itself partly through an impairment of hypothalamic regulation of GH secretion and its link to sleep. The detailed mechanisms that lead in one psychologic disease to a derangement of LH secretion and in another to that of GH secretion are unknown.

A discussion of the possible neuroanatomic and neurochemical basis for the generation of episodic, circadian and sleep-linked secretion of hormones is beyond the scope of this review. There is evidence that episodic secretion of at least some hormones is generated within the medial basal hypothalamus (MBH) since it persists in animals with complete MBH deafferentation (WILLOUGHBY et al., 1977). The suprachiasmatic nucleus has been shown to be important for the entrainment of some circadian rhythms (sleep-wake, REM/non-REM, locomotor activity, estrous cyclicity, corticosterone; COINDET et al., 1975; IBUKA and KAWAMURA, 1975; STETSON and WATSON-WHITMYRE, 1976). Which structures are responsible for the link between sleep and pituitary hormone secretion remains to be investigated. It is known, however, that the hypothalamus receives direct and indirect afferents from many parts of the limbic system, and from other CNS areas that are involved in sleep regulation, including the pontine reticular formation. Recently, the demonstration of bidirectional hypothalamic neurons has opened the possibility that hypothalamic hormones may be released at the same time into the pituitary portal vessels and, as neurotransmitters, in extrahypothalamic CNS structures (RENAUD and MARTIN, 1975). The existence of such neurons may help to explain the close link between hypothalamic regulation of pituitary secretion and the state of CNS arousal.

Finally, it should be recognized that the existence of a CNS program for the temporal pattern of pituitary hormone secretion poses a problem for our understanding of the regulation of peripheral hormone action. How does the periphery cope with sudden, CNS-initiated changes of hormone concentration? Obviously, organ blood flow, cell receptor availability or intracellular mechanisms are all possible sites of regulation of hormone action. Different tissues could thus be differently responsive to a single short increase of the plasma hormone concentration. Humoral or nonhumoral feedback from different tissues could then individually influence the pituitary secretion, apparently unrelated to the overall plasma hormone concentration.

Acknowlegment. Original work of the author is supported by the Deutsche Forschungsgemeinschaft.

References

AZUKIZAWA, M., PEKARY, A.E., HERSHMAN, J.M., PARKER, D.C.: Plasma thyrotropin, thyroxine, and triiodothyronine relationships in man. J. Clin. Endocrinol. Metab. 43, 533-542 (1976)

BOYAR, R.M., FINKELSTEIN, J.W., DAVID, R., ROFFWARG, H., KAPEN, S., WEITZMAN, E.D., HELLMAN, L.: Twenty-four hour patterns of plasma luteinizing hormone and follicle stimulating hormone in sexual precocity. New Eng. J. Med. 289, 282-286 (1973a)

BOYAR, R., FINKELSTEIN, J., ROFFWARG, H., KAPEN, S., WEITZMAN, E., HELLMAN, L.: Synchronization of augmented luteinizing hormone secretion with sleep during puberty. New Eng. J. Med. 287, 582-586 (1972)

BOYAR, R.M., FINKELSTEIN, J.W., ROFFWARG, H., KAPEN, S., WEITZMAN, E.D., HELLMAN, L.: Twenty-four-hour luteinizing hormone and follicle-stimulating hormone secretory patterns in gonadal dysgenesis. J. Clin. Endocrinol. Metab. 37, 521-525 (1973b)

BOYAR, R.M., ROSENFELD, R.S., KAPEN, S., FINKELSTEIN, J.W., ROFFWARG, H.P., WEITZMAN, E.D., HELLMAN, L.: Human Puberty. Simultaneous augmented secretion of luteinizing hormone and testosterone during sleep. J. Clin. Invest. 54, 609-618 (1974)

BOYAR, R.M., WU, R.H.K., ROFFWARG, H., KAPEN, S., WEITZMAN, E.D., HELLMAN, L., FINKELSTEIN, J.W.: Human puberty: 24-hour estradiol patterns in pubertal girls. J. Clin. Endocrinol. Metab. 43, 1418-1421 (1976)

BROWN, G.M.: Endocrine aspects of psychosocial dwarfism. In: Hormones, Behavior and Psychopathology. Sachar, E.J. (ed.). New York: Raven Press, 1976, pp. 253-261

COINDET, J., CHOUVET, G., MOURET, J.: Effects of lesions of the suprachismatic nuclei on paradoxical sleep and slow wave sleep circadian rhythms in the rat. Neurosci. Lett. 1, 243-247 (1975)

EVANS, J.I., MACLEAN, A.W., ISMAIL, A.A.A., LOVE, D.: Concentrations of plasma testosterone in normal men during sleep. Nature (London) 229, 261-262 (1971)

HONDA, Y., TAKAHASHI, K., TAKAHASHI, S., AZUMI, K., IRIE, M., SAKUMA, M., TSUSHIMA, T., SHIZUME, K.: Growth hormone secretion during nocturnal sleep in normal subjects. J. Clin. Endocrinol. Metab. 29, 20-29 (1969)

IBUKA, N., KAWAMURA, H.: Loss of circadian rhythm in sleep-wakefulness cycle in the rat by suprachiasmatic nucleus lesions. Brain Res. 96, 76-81 (1975)

JUDD, H.L., PARKER, D.C., SILER, T.M., YEN, S.S.C.: The nocturnal rise of plasma testosterone in pubertal boys. J. Clin. Endocrinol. Metab. 38, 710-713 (1974)

KAPEN, S., BOYAR, R.M., FINKELSTEIN, J.W., HELLMAN, L., WEITZMAN, E.D.: Effect of sleep-wake cycle reversal on luteinizing hormone secretory pattern in puberty. J. Clin. Endocrinol. Metab. 39, 293-299 (1974)

KAPEN, S., BOYAR, R., HELLMAN, L., WEITZMAN, E.D.: The relationship of luteinizing hormone secretion to sleep in women during the early follicular phase: effects of sleep reversal and a prolonged three-hour sleep-wake schedule. J. Clin. Endocrinol. Metab. 42, 1031-1040 (1976)

KAPEN, S., BOYAR, R., PERLOW, M., HELLMAN, L., WEITZMAN, E.D.: Luteinizing hormone: changes in secretory pattern during sleep in adult women. Life Sci. 13, 693-701 (1973)

KATZ, J.L., BOYAR, R.M., WEINER, H., GORZYNSKI, G., ROFFWARG, H., HELLMAN, L.: Toward an elucidation of the psychoendocrinology of anorexia nervosa. In: Hormones, Behavior and psychopathology. Sachar, E.J. (ed.). New York: Raven Press, 1976, pp. 263-283

KRIEGER, D.T., GEWIRTZ, G.P.: The nature of the circadian periodicity and suppressibility of immunoreactive ACTH levels in Addison's disease. J. Clin. Endocrinol. Metab. 39, 46-52 (1974)

NAFTOLIN, F., JUDD, H.L., YEN, S.S.C.: Pulsatile patterns of gonadotropins and testosterone in man: the effects of clomiphene with and without testosterone. J. Clin. Endocrinol. Metab. 36, 285-288 (1973)

PARKER, D.C., PEKARY, A.E., HERSHMAN, J.M.: Effect of normal and reversed sleep-wake cycles upon nyctohemeral rhythmicity of plasma thyrotropin: evidence suggestive of an inhibitory influence in sleep. J. Clin. Endocrinol. Metab. 43, 318-329 (1976)

PARKER, D.C., ROSSMAN, L.G.: Sleep-wake cycle and human growth hormone, prolactin, and luteinizing hormone. In: Advances in Human Growth Hormone Research. Raiti, S. (ed.). DHEW Publ. No (NIH) 74-612, 1974, pp. 294-312

PARKER, D.C., ROSSMAN, L.G., VANDERLAAN, E.F.: Sleep-related, nyctohemeral and briefly episodic variation in human plasma prolactin concentrations. J. Clin. Endocrinol. Metab. 36, 1119-1124 (1973)

PARKER, D.C., ROSSMAN, L.G., VANDERLAAN, E.F.: Relation of sleep-entrained human prolactin release to REM-NonREM cycles. J. Clin. Endocrinol. Metab. 38, 646-651 (1974)

QUABBE, H.-J.: Chronobiology of growth hormone secretion. Chronobiologia 4, 217-246 (1977)

QUABBE, H.-J., HELGE, H., KUBICKI, S.: Nocturnal growth hormone secretion: correlation with sleeping EEG in adults and pattern in children and adolescents with non-pituitary dwarfism, overgrowth and with obesity. Acta Endocrinol. (Kbh.) 67, 767-783 (1971)

QUABBE, H.-J., SCHILLING, E., HELGE, H.: Pattern of growth hormone secretion during a 24-hour fast in normal adults. J. Clin. Endocrinol. Metab. 26, 1173-1177 (1966)

RENAUD, L.P., MARTIN, J.B.: Electrophysiological studies of connections of hypothalamic ventromedial nucleus neurons in the rat: evidence for a role in neuroendocrine regulation. Brain Res. 93, 145-151 (1975)

SASSIN, J.F., FRANTZ, A.G., WEITZMAN, E.D., KAPEN, S.: Human prolactin: 24-hour pattern with increased release during sleep. Science 177, 1205-1207 (1972)

SASSIN, J.F., PARKER, D.C., JOHNSON, L.C., ROSSMAN, L.G., MACE, J.W., GOTLIN, R.W.: Effects of slow wave sleep deprivation on human growth hormone release in sleep: preliminary study. Life Sci. 8, 1299-1307 (1969a)

SASSIN, J.F., PARKER, D.C., MACE, J.W., GOTLIN, R.W., JOHNSON, L.C., ROSSMAN, L.G.: Human growth hormone release: relation to slow-wave sleep and sleep-waking cycles. Science 165, 513-515 (1969b)

STETSON, M.H., WATSON-WHITMYRE, M.: Nucleus suprachiasmaticus: the biological clock in the hamster? Science 191, 197-199 (1976)

TAKAHASHI, Y., KIPNIS, D.M., DAUGHADAY, W.H.: Growth hormone secretion during sleep. J. Clin. Invest. 47, 2079-2090 (1968)

WEITZMAN, E.D., NOGEIRE, C., PERLOW, M., FUKUSHIMA, D., SASSIN, J., MCGREGOR, P., GALLAGHER, T.F., HELLMAN, L.: Effects of a prolonged 3-hour sleep-wake cycle on sleep stages, plasma cortisol, growth hormone and body temperature in man. J. Clin. Endocrinol. Metab. 38, 1018-1030 (1974)

WILLOUGHBY, J.O., TERRY, L.C., BRAZEAU, P., MARTIN, J.B.: Pulsatile growth hormone, prolactin, and thyrotropin secretion in rats with hypothalamic deafferentation. Brain Res. 127, 137-152 (1977)

WU, R.H., BOYAR, R.M., KNIGHT, R., HELLMAN, L., FINKELSTEIN, J.W.: Endocrine studies in a phenotypic girl with XY gonadal agenesis. J. Clin. Endocrinol. Metab. 43, 506-511 (1976)

2. Effect of Sex Hormones on the Circadian Rhythm of Slow-Wave and Paradoxical Sleep in Female Rats

M. KAWAKAMI, S. YAMAOKA, and M. MATSUSHIMA

In an earlier communication we (KAWAKAMI and SAWYER, 1959) have suggested the possible implication of sex hormones in the induction of EEG after-reaction. We wish to demonstrate here an example of the prominent influence of sex hormones on sleep biorhythm.

Adult albino rats were maintained under a controlled light-dark schedule (05.00-19.00 light, 19.00-05.00 dark), and were chronically implanted with electrodes for recording cortical EEG and dorsal neck EMG. Each recording was made successively for 8 to 10 days. The EEG pattern was divided into three stages, i.e., alertness (A), slow wave sleep (SWS), and paradoxical sleep (PS). The sum of the duration of each SWS or PS was expressed in seconds per 2-h interval. The results were as follows:

1. In the rat with regular 4- or 5-day vaginal cycle, SWS peaks were observed each day during 06.00-08.00 and 12.00-14.00 (morning SWS peak and afternoon SWS peak). PS peak was observed during 12.00-14.00, and a smaller one during 22.00-24.00 (night PS peak) was also observed each day except on proestrus (Fig. 1).

2. One month after ovariectomy, the circadian SWS rhythm was similar to that of the intact rat. Maxima in SWS were also observed during 06.00-08.00 and 12.00-14.00. However, the appearance of PS in the day time was decreased, and that in the night time was increased as compared with the intact female rat. PS maxima were observed twice, one in the day time (12.00-14.00 or 14.00-16.00) the other in the night time (22.00-24.00 or 00.00-02.00). The nocturnal maximum was more evident than that observed in the intact rat (Fig. 1).

3. Estradiol benzoate (20 µg) dissolved in sesame oil subcutaneously was administered to six ovariectomized rats. The amplitude of the nocturnal PS maximum was lower than that before the administration, and was maintained at low level even after the second administration of estradiol (20 µg). However, the amount of PS during day time was slightly increased (Fig. 2).

4. In the ovariectomized rat with bilateral septal lesions, the circadian rhythms in SWS and PS were maintained as in the intact ovariectomized rat. However, the first administration of estradiol failed to lower the night PS peak, and decreased the amount of PS during day time (Fig. 2).

5. The intact male rat showed circadian rhythms in SWS and PS with the maximum in SWS between 10.00-12.00, and that for the PS peak between 14.00-16.00 (Fig. 3).

6. The rat with constant estrus induced by neonatal administration of testosterone propionate (50 µg) showed a single maximum SWS at 10.00-12.00 resembling the pattern of SWS distribution in the male rat. Distribution of PS showed maxima during 02.00-04.00 and again during 14.00-16.00. The maximal appearance of SWS and PS in the afternoon were separated by four hour (Fig. 3).

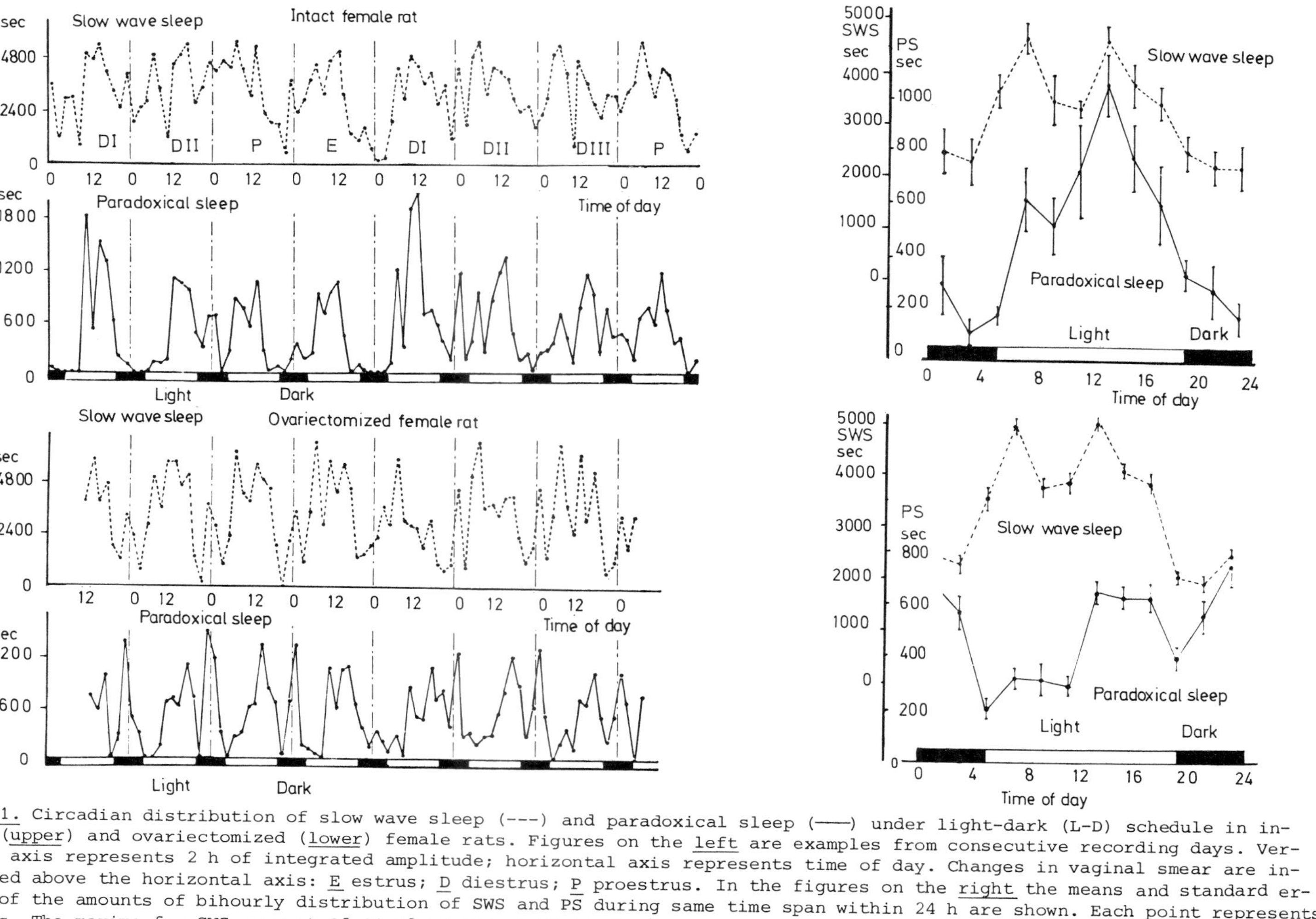

Fig. 1. Circadian distribution of slow wave sleep (---) and paradoxical sleep (——) under light-dark (L-D) schedule in intact (upper) and ovariectomized (lower) female rats. Figures on the left are examples from consecutive recording days. Vertical axis represents 2 h of integrated amplitude; horizontal axis represents time of day. Changes in vaginal smear are indicated above the horizontal axis: E estrus; D diestrus; P proestrus. In the figures on the right the means and standard errors of the amounts of bihourly distribution of SWS and PS during same time span within 24 h are shown. Each point represents 6 rats. The maxima for SWS were at 06.00-08.00 and 12.00-14.00 both in intact and ovariectomized female rats. In intact female rats, maximum PS was observed during 12.00-14.00 with a lower maximum during 22.00-24.00 (night PS peak) except on proestrus. In ovariectomized female rats, PS decreased in day time and increased at night with two maxima. Note the increase in the night PS peak

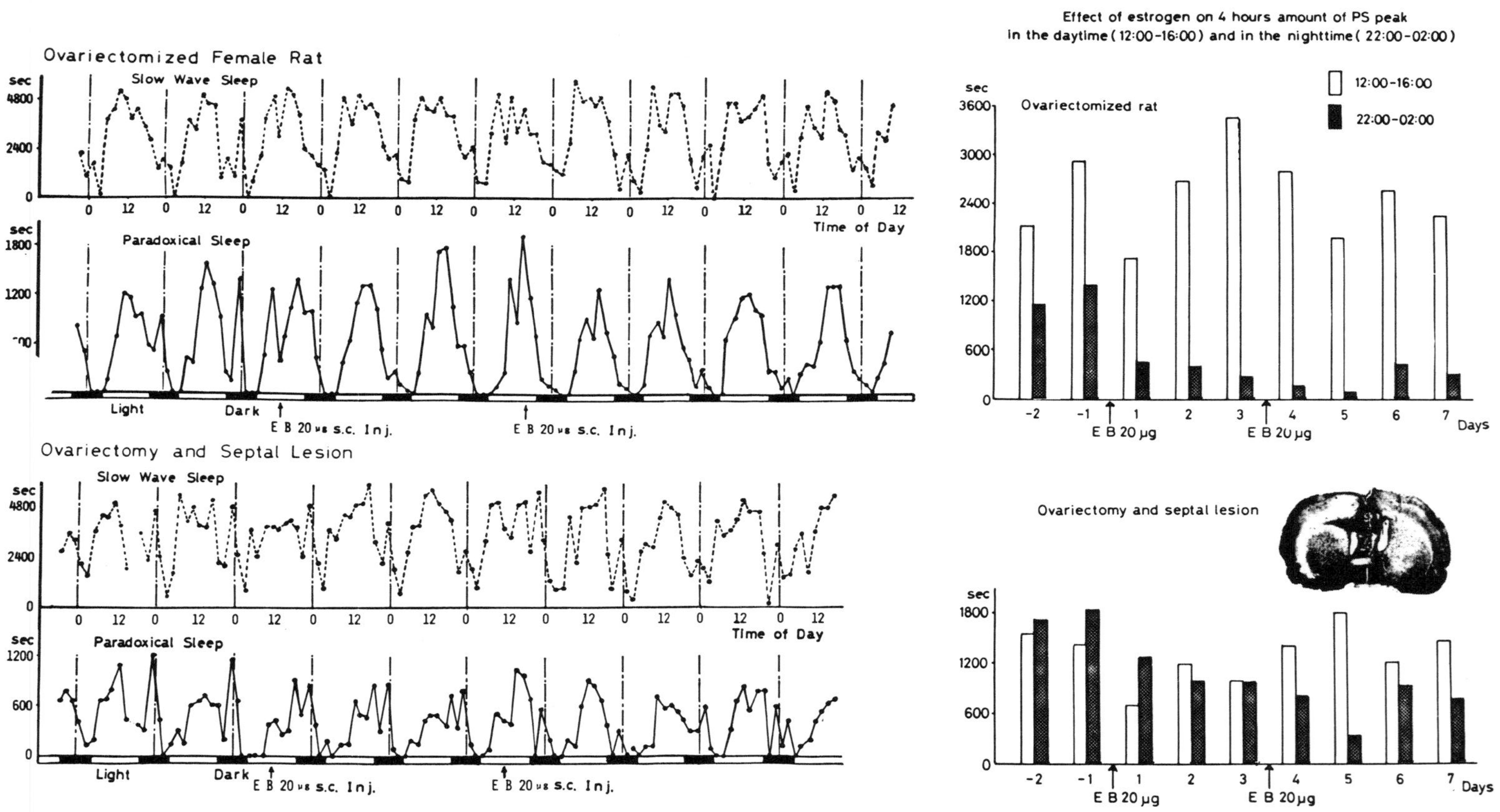

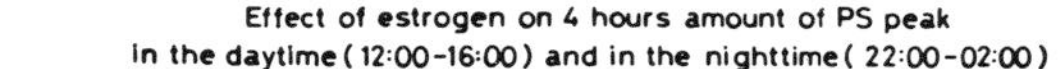

Fig. 2. Effects of estrogen on the bihourly distribution of SWS and PS through 24 h in an ovariectomized rat and in an ovariectomized, septal-lesioned rat. Administration of 20 μg estradiol benzoate (EB) occurred on the third day of EEG recordings and again 72 h later. Figures on right show 4 h of maximum PS in day time (12.00-16.00) and at night (22.00-02.00) of each day. In an ovariectomized rat (upper), nocturnal PS maxima decreased markedly and day time appearance of PS was slightly increased after EB administration. In an ovariectomized, septal-lesioned rat (lower), circadian rhythms in SWS and PS were changed after 20 μg EB and the night PS peak did not decrease so remarkably

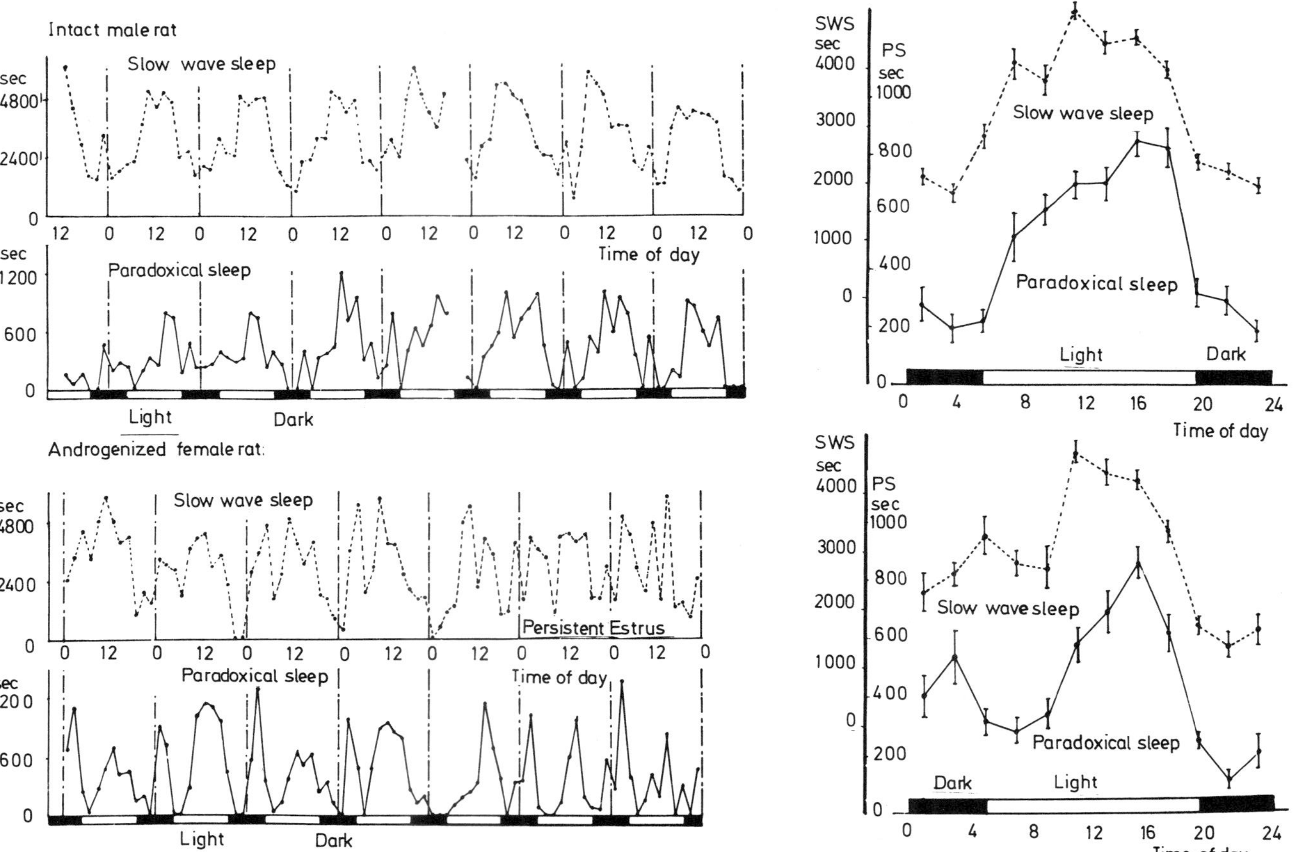

Fig. 3. Circadian rhythms of SWS and PS under L-D schedule in intact males and androgenized females. In an intact male rat (upper left), bihourly distribution of SWS and PS shows a single maximum - 10.00-12.00 in SWS and 14.00-16.00 in PS. In an androgenized female rat (lower left), single maximum in SWS during 10.00-12.00, and two in PS during 02.00-04.00 and 14.00-16.00. Figures on the right show the means and standard errors of the bihourly distribution of SWS and PS during same time span within 24 h. Each point represents six rats

Our previous data (HAGINO and YAMAOKA, 1974) have already demonstrated the decrease in SWS and PS in proestrus as COLVIN et al. (1968) had reported earlier, and our present data also confirm these findings. In the ovariectomized rat, the pattern of the circadian rhythm in SWS was the same as in the intact rat, but two maxima in PS were observed. The nocturnal increase in PS in the ovariectomized rat may be due partly to the lack of the feedback action of the sex hormone, since it decreased after the administration of estrogen. The important role of estrogen in the modification of the pattern of circadian rhythm of PS was suggested.

Previous studies (YAMAOKA, unpublished) demonstrated that neither septal lesions nor lesions in the roof of MPO alter the estrous cycle. The circadian rhyhtm in SWS also remained unchanged, but the nocturnal maximum in PS increased, except in proestrus. Failure of estrogen to decrease nocturnal PS in rats with ovariectomy and chronic septal lesion, as observed in the present experiment, may suggest that the action of estrogen to decrease nocturnal PS is mediated by the septal complex.

Conclusion

1. The low nocturnal appearance in PS in the rat at proestrus, and in the ovariectomized rat after the administration of estrogen may indicate an inhibitory feedback action of estrogen on the mechanism inducing PS. One of the estrogen feedback sites seems to be in the septum.

2. Neonatal exposure to androgen may modify the mechanism that controls the rhythms of SWS and PS.

References

COLVIN, G.B., WHITMOYER, D.I., LISK, R.D., WALTER, D.O., SAWYER, C.H.: Changes in sleep-wakefulness in female rats during circadian and estrous cycle. Brain Res. 7, 173-181 (1968)

HAGINO, N., YAMAOKA, S.: Role of biorhythm of sleep and wakefulness in the periodicity of gonadotropin secretion in the baboon (non-human primate). In: Biological Rhythms in Neuroendocrine Activity. Kawakami, M. (ed.). Tokyo: Igaku Shoin Ltd., 1974, pp. 326-337

KAWAKAMI, M., SAWYER, C.H.: Induction of behavioral and electroencephalographic changes in the rabbit by hormone administration or brain stimulation. Endocrinology 65, 631-643 (1959)

YAMAOKA, S.: Participation of limbic-hypothalamic structures in circadian rhythm of SWS and PS in the rat. (in preparation)

3. Role of Brain Monoamines in the Regulation of the Circadian Variations of Activity of some Neuroendocrine Axes

U. SCAPAGNINI, I. GERENDAI, G. CLEMENTI, L. FIORE, B. MARCHETTI, and A. PRATO

Brain Monoamines and Endocrine Circadian Rhythms. The main aim of this chapter is to give a general overview of the role of monoamines (MA) in the regulation of the circadian changes in secretion of three neuroendocrine axes. The axes that we have considered are the hypothamalo-hypophysial-adrenal-Axis (HHAA), the hypothalamo-hypophysial-thyroidal-Axis (HHTA) and the hypothalamo-hypophysial-prolactin-Axis (HHPRLA).

Two main strategies are generally used in experiments attempting to establish relationship between MA and hypothalamic hormones: (1)measurement of the effects on endocrine function of varying the functional activity of brain monoaminergic systems by administration of MA and/or their precursors, by neuropharmacologic treatment or by neurosurgical procedures; and (2) study of the effect on MA metabolism in the brain of natural or induced changes in endocrine activity. We will attempt to review some of the evidence obtained using mainly the first approach, focusing our attention on the serotoninergic, norepinephrinergic and dopaminergic neurons.

Brain MA in the Control of Circadian Activity of HHAA. Brain norepinephrine (NE) seems to be involved mainly with neuronal mechanisms that mediate the tonic inhibition of ACTH secretion (SCAPAGNINI, 1974). Decreasing central adrenergic tone by the synthesis inhibitor α-MpT (SCAPAGNINI et al., 1970) or by the specific neurotoxic agent for catecholaminergic endings, 6-OHDA (SCAPAGNINI and PREZIOSI, 1977), induces in rats an increase of plasma corticosterone (B) and ACTH that reaches stress levels at any time of the day clearly indepentent of the phase of the circadian cycle.

Unlike CA's, serotoninergic neurotransmission does not seem to be involved predominantly in acute response to stress but, instead, in the circadian periodicity of adrenal cortex secretion. A diurnal fluctuation of serotonin (5-HT) has been demonstrated in the whole brain, as well as in specific brain areas of several mammalian species (see MULLER et al., 1977); a positive correlation between 5-HT content in the limbic system and plasma B rhythm (characterized by a peak at 20.00) was found in the rat, suggesting that 5-HT may play a role in the regulation of diurnal fluctuation of ACTH secretion (SCAPAGNINI et al., 1971; SIMON and GEORGE, 1975). However the existence of a simple correlation between brain MA and plasma hormone levels does not demonstrate a causal relationship.

Experiments in which central 5-HT activity was modified by surgical or pharmacologic means provide more direct information concerning the role of 5-HT in the ACTH diurnal rhythm. Para-Chloro-Phenyl-Alanine (pCPA), the 5-HT synthesis blocker, eliminated the diurnal fluctuation of plasma corticosteroids in birds, rats and cats (see MULLER et al., 1977). In rats treated with the soluble form of pCPA-methylester (pCPA m.e.) the abolition of the rhythm was difficult to observe (ROTSZEJN et al., 1977). However, in comparable experiments it was demonstrated that the insoluble form of pCPA (300 mg/kg) given 48 h earlier or pCPA m.e.

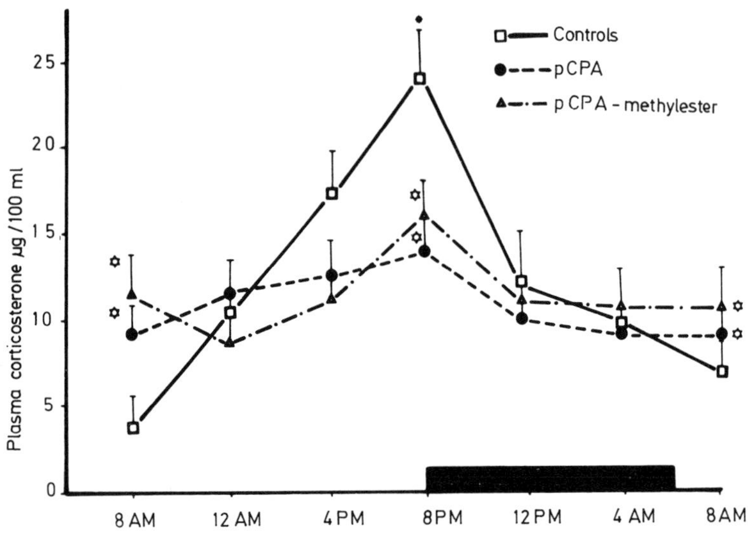

Fig. 1. Effect on plasma corticosterone circadian rhythm of a pretreatment with insoluble pCPA (300 mg/kg/ip) and soluble pCPA (methylester) given respectively 48 or 24 h before each point. Controls received solvent at the same time. Each point represents the mean ± S.E. of 10 to 12 animals. * $p < 0.01$ if compared to the 08.00 (8 a.m.), 12.00 (12 a.m.), 24.00 (12 p.m.), 04.00 (4 a.m.)

Table 1. Action on plasma corticosterone levels (B) at 08.00 and 20.00 after pretreatment with soluble pCPA (300 mg/kg/ip) given 48 or 72 h before cacrifice + pCPA methylester (m.e.; 50 mg/kg/ip) given 24 h before killing

Treatment	Plasma B 100 µg/100 ml	
	08.00	20.00
Saline 72 h + Saline 24 h	6.50 ± 1.8	23.50 ± 3.0
pCPA 48 h + Saline 24 h	13.50 ± 2.5[a]	16.00 ± 1.8[a]
pCPA 72 h + Saline 24 h	7.20 ± 2.0	24.00 ± 2.5
pCPA 72 h + pCPA m.e. 24 h	15.20 ± 2.3	15.00 ± 2.3[a]
Saline 72 h + pCPA m.e. 24 h	5.50 ± 2.0	24.00 ± 2.5

[a] $p < 0.01$ if compared to the control values at the corresponding time.

(200 mg/kg) given 24 h earlier resulted in constant plasma B levels throughout the day, that were higher than normal in the morning, but lower than normal in the evening (Fig. 1).

Interestingly, 48-72 h after injection of pCPA, in spite of the continual depletion of brain 5-HT levels, a normal diurnal rhythmicity of plasma B was restored (VERNIKOS-DANELLIS et al., 1973). These data can be explained by the reappearance, after pCPA administration, of a small functional 5-HT pool produced as a consequence of the induction of tryptophan-hydroxylase (Tr-H) activity due to feed-back stimulation (see MULLER et al., 1977). In fact in rats pretreated 72 h earlier with insoluble pCPA (300 mg/kg), an injection of pCPA m.e. at a dose (50 mg/kg), which is unable to modify the HHAA activity in control rats, abolishes the diurnal rhythmicity of plasma B (Table 1).

Intraventricular injection of the neurotoxic tryptamine derivative 5,6-dihydroxytryptamine (5,6-DHT) produces a blunting of B circadian rhythm detectable 5 but not 21 days after treatment (Fig. 2). In preliminary experiments using the serotonin agonist Quipazine there is a suggestion of supersensitivity of 5-HT receptors 3 weeks after 5,6-DHT.

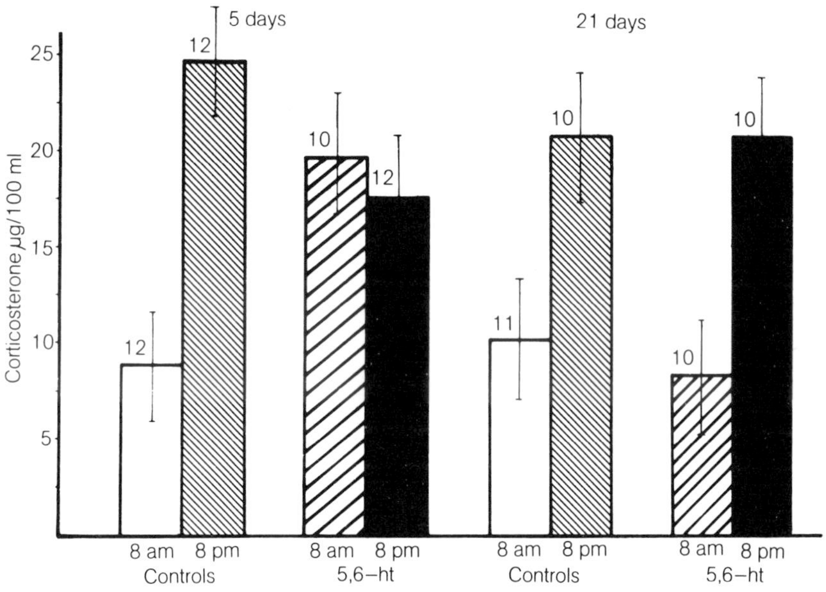

Fig. 2. Effect of an injection into the lateral ventricle of the brain of 5,6-DHT (50 µg/An) on the plasma B level at 08.00 (8 a.m.) and 20.00 (8 p.m.) 5 and 21 days later. Controls received solvent at the same time. In brackets the number of animals. * $p < 0.01$ if compared to the control values at the corresponding time

The above findings are in keeping with the observations made by FUXE et al. (1973) after 5,6-DHT-induced degeneration of the 5-HT mesencephalic-hypothalamic pathways.

Further support for the view that 5-HT pathways play a modulating role in the phasic regulation of ACTH secretion was suggested by the observation that in rats lesions of 5-H-containing cell bodies in the raphe nuclei abolished the circadian rhythm of plasma B. However, the specific location of the lesions seems to be of critical importance since in more recent studies smaller lesions of the raphe nucleus were ineffective in contrast with the above experiments (BALESTRERY and MOBERG, 1976; ROTSZTEJN et al., 1977); it is possible that the reason for the discrepancy is due to the fact that most of the fibers coming from the medial raphe nucleus (m.r.n.) reach the hypothalamus directly whereas those leaving the dorsal raphe nucleus reach the limbic system. Lesions including both nuclei can produce effects different from lesions specifically destroying m.r.n. or d.r.n.

Microsurgical procedures isolating the hypothalamus by complete (c.c.) or frontal deafferentation decreased hypothalamic 5-HT (see MULLER et al., 1977) and blocked the diurnal ACTH cycle (HALÁSZ, 1969). Additional evidence that the mechanism(s) for the normal circadian fluctuation of B secretion is located in the limbic area, and is probably serotoninergic in nature, is provided by the observation that section of the fornix (MOBERG et al., 1971; LENGVÀRI and HALÁSZ, 1973) or septal lesions (HARRINGTON et al., 1973) also resulted in disappearance of usual circadian rhythms with intermediate (fornix) or high (septum) B levels. However three weeks after transection of the fornix, a significant diurnal variation reappeared (LENGVÀRI and HALÁSZ, 1973). Preliminary results suggest that in animals submitted to so-called roof cut (disconnections of all the afferents to the hypothalamus from the dorsal brain areas), the fornix cut produces a cessation of the circadian rhythm of plasma B also for three weeks.

<u>Brain MA in the Control of Circadian Activity of HHTA.</u> In vivo and in vitro experiments using mcroiontophoretic, pharmacologic and surgical approaches support the notion of central MA participation in the regulation of TRH-TSH secretion. The findings obtained in these experiments suggest that the acute, cold-induced release of TRH is under two different MA control systems, with a positive NE and a negative 5-HT component (see MULLER et al., 1977). The evidence concerning the involvement of the MA in the circadian regulation of plasma TSH secre-

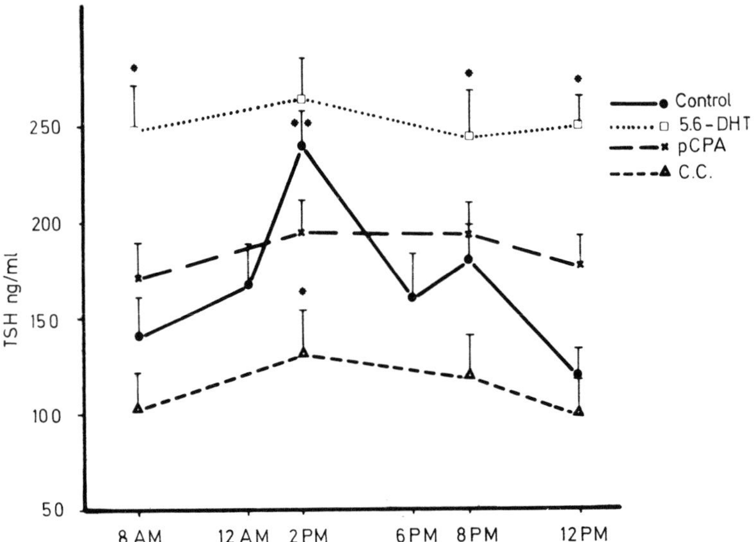

Fig. 3. Effect of hypothalamic deafferentation (c.c.), 5,6-DHT (50 µg/An 5 days earlier), pCPA (300 mg/kg/ip 48 h earlier) on the circadian rhythm of plasma TSH of rats adapted for one week at 30° C. Each point represents the mean ± S.E. of 10 to 14 animals. * $p < 0.01$ if compared to the other points of the control curve

tion is more limited (JORDAN et al., 1976). In our experiments, male rats adapted for one week to 30°C showed a circadian pattern of plasma TSH level characterized by a peak at 14.00. Complete deafferentation of the hypothalamus (c.c.), pCPA 48 h earlier (300 mg/kg) and 5,6-DHT 5 days earlier (50 µg/An into III Ventricle) all abolished the diurnal fluctuation of plasma TSH. However, while c.c. decreases the levels at all times explored, pCPA produces constant intermediate and 5,6-DHT constant high levels of plasma TSH throughout the day (Fig. 3). In 5,6-HDT pretreated rats, a hyperrespose to the 5-HT agonist quipazine was observed, suggesting supersensitivity of 5-HT receptors.

Brain MA in the Control of Circadian Rhythm of HHPRLA. Among the anterior pituitary hormones, PRL is unique in that its secretion in mammals is tonically inhibited by the CNA. The existence of a PRL-inhibiting factor (PIF) has been proved; however, the nature of PIF is still unclear. Anatomic, biochemic and pharmacologic experiments strongly suggest that hypothalamic MA plays a strategic role in the regulation of the secretion of PRL. Conclusions derived from a large number of in vivo and in vitro experiments are that dopamine (DA) directly at the pituitary level (or indirectly through PIF stimulation) is responsible for a tonic inhibition of PRL secretion that can occasionally be overcome by acute (stress) or cyclic events (see MULLER et al., 1977).

Two surges of plasma PRL, one during the day and one at night occur in the male rat (DUNN et al., 1972) or pseudopregnant female (MCLEAN and NIKITOVICH-WINER, 1975). A preliminary report in 1975 (MULLOY and MOBERG) showed that pCPA and destruction of midbrain raphe nuclei caused

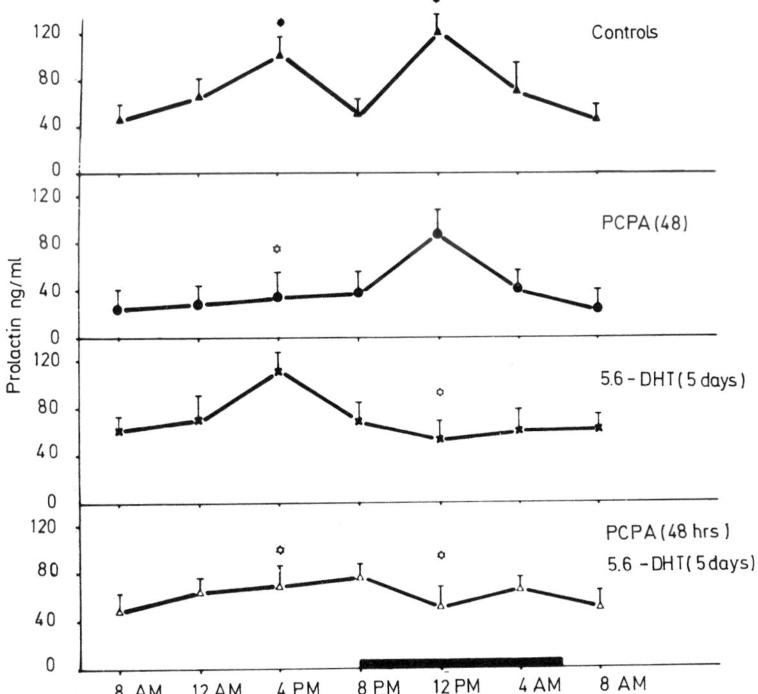

Fig. 4. Effect of pCPA (300 mg/kg/ip 48 h before killing). 5,6-DHT (50 µg/An/iv 5 days before killing) and of pCPA + 5,6-DHT on the circadian rhythm of plasma PRL. Each point represents the mean ± S.E. of 9 to 14 animals. *, $p < 0.01$ if compated to the 08.00 (8 AM) and 20.00 (8 PM) values. **, $p < 0.01$ if compared to the values of the controls at the corresponding time

coincident decreasing of 5-HT in the forebrain and in plasma PRL levels. In our experiments pCPA (300 mg/kg/ip) abolished 48 h later only the afternoon peak (16.00) but not the nocturnal (24.00) peak of plasma PRL. Conversely, the intraventricular injection of 5,6-DHT (50 µg/AN) causes after five days the disappearance of the nocturnal but not the afternoon peak (all the diurnal points exhibit a general tendency to an increase). Combined treatments with pCPA (300 mg/kg/48 h earlier) plus 5,6-DHT (50 µg/An 5 days earlier) completely abolishes circadian variation of PRL at low level (Fig. 4). It is tempting to speculate, on the basis of these results, that the two circadian peaks are, at least in part, regulated by the variation of activity of two separate serotoninergic systems acting independently. Recently the presence of a small intrahypothalamic 5-HT system, similar to the tuberoinfundibular dopaminergic (TIDA) one, has been postulated (BEAUDET and DESCARRIES, 1976). In fact after the surgical isolation of the medio-basal hypothalamus (MBH), NE concentration falls completely within the island, while DA is relatively unaffected, and 5-HT is decreased by about 50% (WEINER et al., 1972; PALKOVITS, 1977). In animals with c.c. of MBH, the circadian rhythm does not disappear, but the shape of the curve is totally modofied: instead of the two peaks at 16.00 and 24.00, only one peak is present at 20.00. We, therefore, suggest that the MA imputs (NE and/or 5-HT) responsible for the biphasic circadian variation of PRL from areas located outside the MBH reach the TIDA (and/or the intrahypothalamic 5-HT) system producing the typical rhythm of PRL release. When extrahypothalamic afferents are disconnected, an autonomous free-running rhythm characterized by a single peak appears.

In conclusion, from the above results the critical importance of the central monoaminergic system(s) in the regulation of the circadian variation of activity of HHAA, HHTA and HHPRLA appears to be clearly demonstrated.

References

BALESTRERY, F.G., MOBERG, G.P.: Effect of midbrain raphe nuclei lesions of the circadian rhythm of plasma corticosterone in the rat. Brain Res. 118, 503-508 (1976)

BEAUDET, A., DESCARRIES, L.: A serotonin-containing nerve cell groups in rat hypothalamus. Neurosci. Abstr. 11, 479 (1976)

DUNN, J.D., ARIMURA, A., SCHEVING, L.E.: Effect of stress on circadian periodicity in serum LH and prolactin cincentration. Endocrinology 90, 29-34 (1972)

FÜXE, K., HOKFELT, T., JOHNSSON, G, LEVINE, S., LIDBRINK, P., LOFSTROM, A.: In: Brain-Pituitary-Adrenal Interrelationships. Brodish, A., Redgate, E.S. (eds.). Basel: S. Karger, 1973, pp. 239-263

JORDAN, D., PONSIN, G., MORNEX, R.: Serotoninergic stimulation of thyrotropic function in the rat. Proc. 5th Int. Congr. Endocrinol. Hamburg 1976

HALÁSZ, B.: The endocrine effects of isolation of the hypothalamus from the rest of the brain. In: Frontiers in Neuroendocrinology. Ganong, W.F., Martini, L. (eds.). Oxford: University Press, 1969, pp. 307-342

HARRINGTON, R.J., SCAPAGNINI, U., MOBERG, G.P.: Diurnal plasma B after raphe and septal lesions. J. Anim. Sci. 37, 313 (1973)

LENGVÁRI, I., HALÁSZ, B.: Evidence for diurnal fluctuation in plasma corticosterone levels after fornix transection in the rat. Neuroendocrinology 11, 191-196 (1973)

MCLEAN, B.K., NIKITOVICH-WINER, M.B.: Cholinergic control of the nocturnal prolactin surge in the pseudopregnant rat. Endocrinology 17, 763-770 (1975)

MOBERG, G.P., SCAPAGNINI, U., DE GROOT, J., GANONG, W.F.: Effect of sectioning the fornix on diurnal fluctuation in plasma corticosterone levels in the rat. Neuroendocrinology 7, 11-15 (1971)

MÜLLER, E., NISTICÒ, G., SCAPAGNINI, U.: In: Neurotransmitters and Anterior Pituitary Function. New York: Academic Press, 1977, pp. 220-323

MULLOY, MOBERG, G.P.: Diurnal prolactin rhythm and brain serotonin

PALKOVITZ, M.: Transmitter of the suprainfundibular system. In: Nonstriatal Dopaminergic Neurons. Costa, D., Gessa, G.L. (eds.). New York: Raven Press, 1977, pp. 71-78

ROTSZTEJN, W.H., BEAUDET, A., ROBERGE, A.G., LALONDE, J., FORTIER, C.: Role of brain serotonin in the circadian rhythm of corticosterone secretion and the corticotropic response to adrenalectomy in the rat. Neuroendocrinology 23, 126-140 (1977)

SCAPAGNINI, U.: Pharmabological studies of brain control over ACTH secretion. In: The Neurosciences. Schmitt, F.O., Worden, F.G. (eds.). 3rd Study Program. Cambridge: MIT Press, 1974, pp. 565-569

SCAPAGNINI, U., MOBERG, G.P., VAN LOON, G.R., DE GROOT, J., GANONG, W.F.: Relation of brain 5-hydroxytriptamine content to the diurnal variation in plasma corticosterone in the rat. Neuroendocrinology 7, 90-96 (1971)

SCAPAGNINI, U., PREZIOSI, P.: Role of brain norepinophrine and serotonin in the tonic and phasic regulation of HHAA. Archs. Int. Pharmacodyn. Ther. Supp. 196, 205-208 (1972)

SCAPAGNINI, U., PREZIOSI, P.: The Endocrine Function of the Human Adrenal Cortex. Int. Symp. Florence, October 1977, Acta

SCAPAGNINI, U., VAN LOON, G.R., MOBERG, G.P., GANONG, W.F.: Effect of α-Methyl-p-Tyrosine on the circadian variation of plasma corticosterone in rats. Eur. J. Pharmacol. 11, 266-268 (1970)

SIMON, M.L., GEORGE, R.: Diurnal variations in plasma corticosterone and growth hormone as correlated with regional variations in norepinephrine, dopamine and serotonin content in rat brain. Neuroendocrinology 17, 125-138 (1975)

VERNIKOS-DANELLIS, J., BERGER, P., BARCHAS, J.D.: Brain serotonin and pituitary-adrenal function. Progr. Brain Res. 39, 301-308 (1973)

WEINER, R.J., SHRYNE, J.E., GORSKY, R.A., SAWYER, C.H.: Changes in the catecholamine content of the rat hypothalamus following deafferentation. Endocrinology 90, 867 (1972)

4. Diurnal Rhythms and the Seasonal Reproductive Cycle in Birds

F. TUREK

The seasonal reproductive cycle in the vast majority of temperate-zone birds is under the temporal control of the seasonal change in day length (for review see: FARNER, 1975). Since ROWAN (1925) first discovered that the length of the day was a primary environmental signal regulating the seasonal reproductive cycle in birds, a great deal of attention has been directed toward answering the question; how do birds measure the length of the day? The present working hypothesis of most of those who study avian photoperiodism as well as photoperiodism in other species, is that measurement of day length somehow involves endogenous circadian rhythmicity. Although BÜNNING suggested as early as 1936 that endogenous diurnal rhythms may be involved, it was not until 1963 that W.M. HAMNER reported experimental evidence to support this hypothesis in birds. HAMNER utilized what is still today one of the most powerful methods for testing the involvement of circadian rhythmicity in the measurement of day length in photoperiodic responses, "resonance light cycles" (NANDA and K.C. HAMNER, 1958). Resonance light cycles consist of a photophase of fixed duration with scotophases of varying duration so that the period (T) of the cycle is systematically changed. (A typical series of resonance light cycles is depicted on the left side of Fig. 1). Positive results from resonance experiments (i.e., photoperiodic induction rises and falls as a function of T) demonstrate that neither the duration of light nor the duration of dark in the cycle is the determining factor in inducing a photoperiodic response. Instead, such results indicate that the measurement of time in photoperiodic responses involves an endogenous rhythm with a period of about 24 h. Through the use of resonance light cycles, this role of circadian rhythmicity has been implicated in a number of different photoperiodic species during the initiation and maintenance of gonadal activity, as well as during the maintenance of the gonadal refractory condition (HAMNER, 1963; FOLLETT and SHARP, 1969; TUREK, 1972, 1974).

Although a number of studies indicate that a daily biologic clock is somehow involved in time measurement in photoperiodic responses, neither the mechanism for such time-measuring capabilities nor the location of such a clock is known. The twofold objective of the present paper is (1) to examine some of the experimental evidence that supports the two major hypotheses that have been advanced to explain the role of diurnal rhythms in time measurement in photoperiodic responses, and (2) to discuss the available information on the anatomic location for the biologic clock involved in photoperiodic phenomena.

External Vs Internal Coincidence

There are two, although not necessarily mutually exclusive, hypotheses that have been formulated to describe the possible role of a diurnal rhythm(s) in measuring the length of the day in birds as well as other organisms. PITTENDRIGH (1972) has termed these two hypotheses the "external coincidence" and "internal coincidence" models. The external

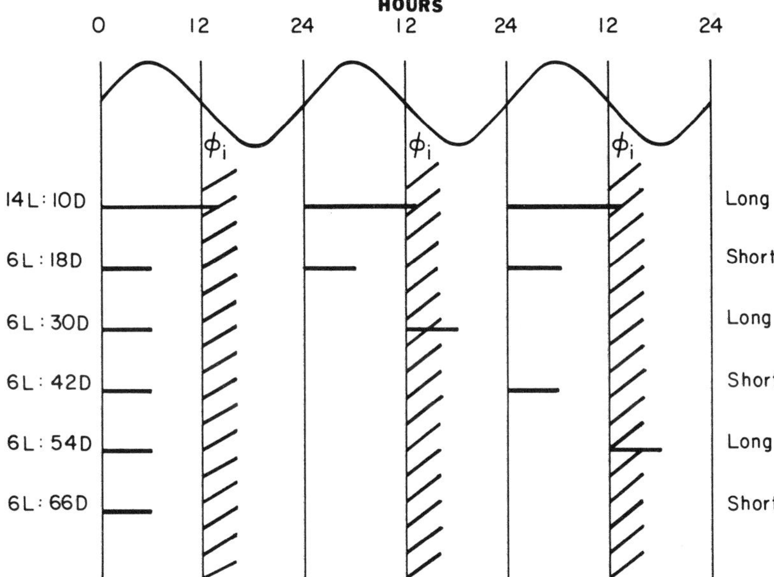

Fig. 1. Diagrammatical representation of an external coincidence model and the way in which this model is used to explain the response of birds to resonance light cycles. The light portion of the cycles is represented by the horizontal bars and whether or not the environmental light cycle will be interpreted as a long or short day is shown on the right. The model predicts that there is a circadian rhythm of sensitivity to light, drawn as a sine wave at the top, which is entrained by the environmental light cycle. When light is coincident with the photoinducible phase of the sensitivity rhythm ($\emptyset_i$: crosshatched bars), drawn arbitrarily between 12 and 16 h after the onset of light, the animal will interpret the light cycle as being a long day. In birds exposed to resonance light cycles consisting of a main 6-h light period, the cycle will be interpreted as a short day when the cycle is 24, 48 or 72 h in duration, but will be interpreted as a long day when the cycle is 36 or 60 h in length

coincidence model predicts that photoperiodic induction occurs when light is coincident (or not coincident) in time with a certain phase (termed the photosensitive or photoinducible phase) of a daily biologic rhythm of sensitivity to light. A diagrammatic representation of this model is shown in Figure 1. An important feature of this model is that light has a dual function: first, it serves to entrain a biologic rhythm which is presumed to be an endogenous free-running circadian rhythm, and second, light induces a particular response when it is coincident with a particular phase of the rhythm that it is entraining.

The internal coincidence model predicts that photoperiodic induction occurs when two or more diurnal rhythms are in a particular phase relationship with respect to one another. In this model light serves only as an entraining agent and does not play an active role in inducing a photoperiodic response. As the length of the day changes, different phase relationships will inevitably be established between various circadian rhythms and only under certain durations of the environmental photophase will the phase relationship between the internal oscillators be such that photoperiodic induction will occur (DANILEVSKY et al., 1970; PITTENDRIGH, 1972).

Experiments that might permit complete exclusion or prove the involvement of either internal or external coincidence in the physiology of photoperiodic induction have not been carried out in birds, although the results from a number of studies appear to favor one model or the other. The next two sections will examine the main experimental evidence that supports each of the two models.

Experimental Support for External Coincidence. Some form of the external coincidence model is usually evoked by most avian biologists to explain the measurement of day length in photoperiodic birds. This is probably due to its earlier formulation in the literature, and because it appears to be the simplest hypothesis that can explain the photoperiodic response of birds subjected to resonance and night-interruption experiments. In most night-interruption experiments carried out in birds, it is found that if the night of an otherwise short day is interrupted by a short pulse of light (e.g., 1 h), photoperiodic induction will occur (e.g., LOFTS et al., 1970). Positive results from both night-interruption and resonance experiments have usually been interpreted to indicate that photoperiodic induction depends upon the coincidence of light with a particular phase of a diurnal rhythm in the bird. While the results from such studies are easy to conceptualize in terms of an external coincidence model, they do not conclusively rule out the possibility of internal coincidence. Although detailed models have never been constructed for birds, the light in resonance and night-interruption light cycles may be altering the phase relationship of internal oscillators such that photoperiodic induction can occur.

Experimental support for some form of the external coincidence model being involved in the measurement of day length in photoperiodic birds is found in studies utilizing low-intensity light to separate the photic-mediated gonadal response from the entrainment response. In one such study carried out in house sparrows (*Passer domesticus*), MENAKER and ESKIN (1967) observed that when a 75-min period of bright white light (light intensity ≈ 500 lux) is superimposed late during the dim light portion of a nonphotoperiodic inductive 14 DL (dim light): 10 D cycle (DL ≈ 0.1 lux green light) which will entrain the circadian rhythm of activity, testis weight is maintained. In contrast, if the period of white light does not occur, or if it falls early in the dim light portion of the cycle, testis weight is not maintained. These results are readily interpretible in terms of the external coincidence model since only when the 75-min pulse of white light is given late in the dim light portion of the cycle is it expected to be coincident with the photoinducible phase of the rhythm of sensitivity that is being entrained by the green light cycle. To explain these results in terms of internal coincidence, it is necessary to postulate that even though the dim green light is not maintaining the proper phase relationship between internal oscillators, it is somehow affecting the oscillators so that the phase relationship necessary for photoperiodic induction is established when the pulse of bright light falls late in the dim light phase of the cycle. While this may be theoretically possible, it would involve a number of as yet unsubstantiated assumptions about the interaction of bright and dim light in the entrainment of biological rhythms.

Experimental Support for Internal Coincidence. The discussion of the role of diurnal rhythms in measurement of day length in photoperiodic birds usually involves some form of the external coincidence model. However, MEIER and his colleagues (MEIER and MACGREGOR, 1972; MEIER and DUSSEAU, 1973) have suggested that the internal phase relationship between diurnal hormone rhythms may play an important role in photoperiodic phenomena. MEIER and DUSSEAU (1973) have suggested that injections of corticosterone, with prolactin in a photosensitive position, entrain a daily rhythm of a photoinducible phase. This hypothesis for photoperiodic induction involves elements of both the internal and external coincidence models. While the experiments of MEIER and his colleagues demonstrate that the testicular response can be altered by various temporal injection patterns of prolactin and corticosterone, these changes are often minor, i.e., 2-3 fold difference in testis weight, compared with photic-induced changes in testicular weight of 50-100 fold (MEIER and MACGREGOR, 1972; MEIER and DUSSEAU, 1973; FARNER and LEWIS, 1973). Further studies, and a more rigidly defined hypothesis concerning the mechanism by which internal hormonal phase relationships can entrain a diurnal rhythm of sensitivity to light are necessary before it can be determined if the temporal relationship between the diurnal rhythms of corticosterone and prolactin play a major role in photoperiodic induction in birds.

Studies on birds transferred from a photostimulatory light cycle into either short days or constant darkness suggest that some features of the internal coincidence model may be involved in photoperiodic time measurement. In one such study Slate-Colored Juncos (*Junco hyemalis*) were exposed to a photoinductive light schedule (16L 8D) for 8 days, and then transferred to either constant darkness (DD) or a nonstimulatory (9L 15D) light cycle (WOLFSON, 1966). After 19 days under these conditions, the birds exposed to DD had enlarged testes (mean testis weight = 117.9 mg, N = 4), while the birds exposed to short days had fully regressed testes (mean testis weight = 7.9 mg, N = 7).

Because the studies with juncos involved only a few birds, and the testicular condition of the birds prior to transfer to 16L 8D was not known, I have attempted to confirm WOLFSON'S results using White-Crowned Sparrows (*Zonotrichia leucophrys*). The results with White-Crowned Sparrows have never been as dramatic as those for juncos, however, they do suggest that the testicular response of sparrows transferred from long days into DD may be different than in birds transferred from long days into short days (TUREK, 1973). In one study, testicular development was induced in White-Crowned Sparrows by maintaining them on 18L 6D for 25 days before transfer to either DD or 8L 16D (Fig. 2). A third group of birds remained on 18L 6D. The testes of birds in DD were significantly larger ($p < 0.05$) than the testes of birds transferred to short days 10, 20, 30 and 40 days after transfer from 18L 6D, indicating that testicular regression occurs sooner in birds maintained on short days than in DD. Testicular regression in both groups of birds preceded spontaneous testicular regression that eventually occurred in the birds maintained on 18L 6D throughout the study. FARNER and his colleagues (FARNER et al., 1977) have also observed that testicular regression is more conspicuous in photostimulated house sparrows transferred into short days than in birds transferred into DD.

The observation that testicular regression does not occur equally in DD and in short days is difficult to explain in terms of a simple external coincidence model. This model predicts that testicular regression should occur at the same rate when birds are transferred into either DD or short days, since in either case light will not be coincident with the photoinducible phase. However, if exposure to short days actively inhibits testicular development in some undetermined manner, while testicular regression in DD is just a passive response to the absence of photostimulation, then these results would be compatible with a modified external coincidence model.

The slower rate of testicular regression in birds transferred into DD is readily interpretable in terms of the internal coincidence model. The diurnal oscillators involved in photoperiodic induction are pre-

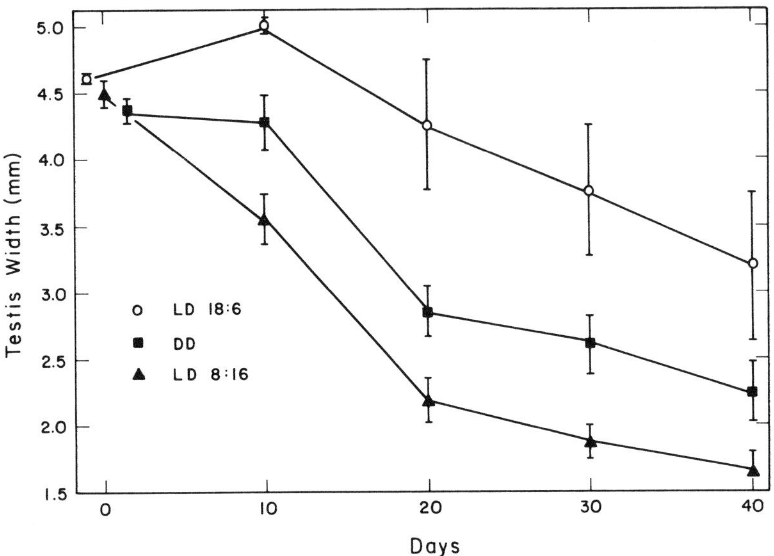

Fig. 2. Testis width (± S.E.) of White-Crowned Sparrows that were maintained on a photostimulatory 18L 6D light cycle for 25 days (Day 0). Birds were then transferred to either constant darkness (DD), 8L 16D, or remained on 18L 6D. The birds were laparatomized at 10-day intervals and the width of the left testis was determined

dicted to be in a particular phase relationship that supports gonadal activity when the birds are exposed to long days. The phase relationship established between the internal oscillators upon transfer from long to short days does not stimulate gonadal development, and therefore gonadal regression occurs. If upon exposure to DD the long-day phase relationship between internal oscillators is maintained for a longer period of time than when birds are transferred to short days, it would be expected that gonadal regression would be slower in birds exposed to DD as opposed to short days. Additional studies examining gonadal activity in photostimulated birds transferred into DD or short days are necessary in order to determine if the results from this type of experiment do indeed support the internal coincidence model.

Conclusions: External or Internal Coincidence? It has not been possible to determine whether the role of diurnal rhythms in the measurement of day length in photoperiodic responses involves internal and/or external coincidence. While certain experiments seem to support one model or the other, no definitive experiments that rigorously test either model have been carried out. The observation that there is experimental evidence to support either model may indicate that time measurement involves aspects of both internal and external coincidence, or as FARNER (1975) has pointed out, there may be multiple origins of the evolution of mechanisms for measurement of day length in birds, and therefore one hypothesis will not fit for all species. At least part of the difficulty in trying to obtain experimental evidence that conclusively disproves either internal or external coincidence is that both models are so loosely formulated that they can be modified quite easily to fit new experimental observations. More information about the physiology of the photoperiodic response is necessary before it will be possible to define more clearly the role of diurnal rhythms in the measurement of day length in photoperiodic birds.

Location of the Biologic Clock Involved in Photoperiodic Time Measurement

At the present time there is no experimental evidence to even suggest a possible location of a biologic clock that may be responsible for the generation of a diurnal rhythm(s) involved in the measurement of day length in avian photoperiodic systems. This is not surprising in view of the fact that it has proved very difficult to locate a self-sustained endogenous oscillator controlling any biologic rhythm. Indeed, the only organ or tissue that has been implicated in the generation of circadian rhythmicity in birds is the pineal gland. Although the precise role of the avian pineal organ within the circadian system is not known, it has been suggested that it may act as a self-sustained oscillator driving measurable circadian rhythms, or as a coupling device between such an oscillator and other components of the system (ZIMMERMAN and MENAKER, 1975). These hypotheses are principally based on the observation that pinealectomy can abolish the free-running circadian rhythm of locomotor activity, body temperature and migratory restlessness in sparrows (GASTON and MENAKER, 1968; BINKLEY et al., 1971; MCMILLAN, 1972), and the transplantation of a pineal gland to the anterior chamber of the eye can restore rhythmicity in a pinealectomized arrhythmic bird (ZIMMERMAN and MENAKER, 1975). Furthermore, the pineal product melatonin, when administered via intraperitoneally placed silastic capsules can either shorten the free-running period of activity or induce continuous activity in house sparrows (TUREK et al., 1976). Since the pineal gland is involved in the generation

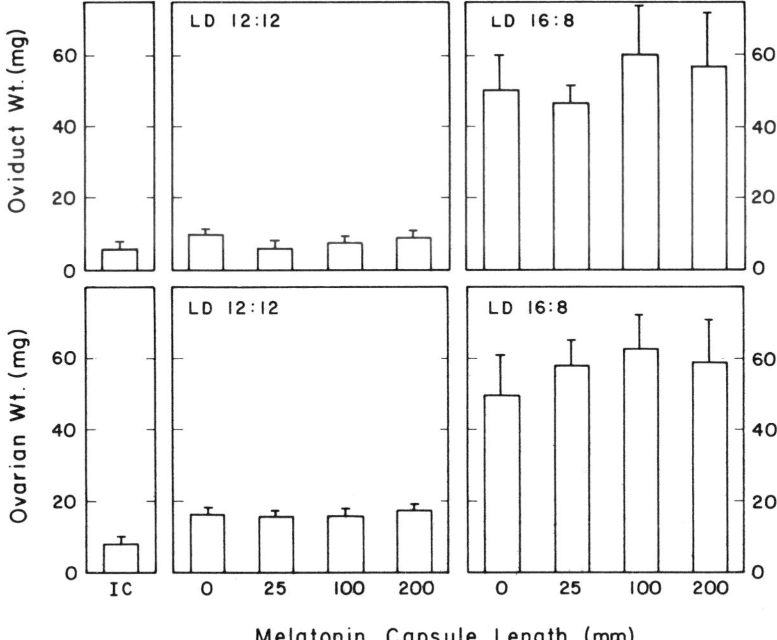

Fig. 3. Ovarian and oviduct weight (± S.E.) in White-throated Sparrows that received implants of either empty (O) or melatonin-filled capsules of various sizes, and were maintained under either a 12L 12D light cycle, or a photostimulatory 16L 8D light cycle for 50 days. Values for initial control animals are shown in the left hand panel. Melatonin-filled capsules had no effect on the development of either the ovaries or the oviducts in birds maintained under either light cycle. (TUREK and WOLFSON, 1978)

of at least three different diurnal rhythms, it might be expected also to be involved in the control of the diurnal rhythm(s) involved in measurement of day length. However, while pinealectomy and treatment with melatonin have profound effects on measurable circadian rhythms, they have very little, if any, effect upon photoperiodically controlled gonadal development (OISHI and LAUBER, 1974; MENAKER and OKSCHE, 1974; Fig. 3).

The absence of an observable effect of pinealectomy or treatment with melatonin on the avian photosexual response indicates that the avian pineal gland is not involved in photoperiodic phenomena. However, a critical reevaluation of the data suggests that previous experimental results may not have excluded a possible role for the pineal gland in photoperiodic induction because the design of these experiments was inadequate. Previous attempts to find a role for the pineal gland in photoperiodic phenomena have usually involved the maintenance of birds on normal light:dark cycles (e.g., 8L 16D or 16L 8D). The use of 24-h light dark cycles may have masked the normal role of the pineal gland: in the measurement of day length just as these cycles can mask the role of the pineal gland in the regulation of circadian locomotor activity. The importance of the lighting conditions in experiments on the role of the pineal gland in regulating the rhythm of activity is demonstrated by the observation that pinealectomy profoundly effects the free-running rhythm of activity in sparrows housed in constant darkness, but has little effect upon the ability of the birds to entrain to normal light-dark cycles (GASTON and MENAKER, 1968; BINGLEY et al., 1971). One interpretation of these results is that the pineal gland is a self-sustained endogenous oscillator that drives a second, damped oscillator which, in turn, directly controls locomotor activity (GASTON and MENAKER, 1968). An important feature of this hypothesis is that the damped oscillator, in the absence of the pineal gland, can be driven directly by a light cycle. If the diurnal rhythm(s) involved in measurement of

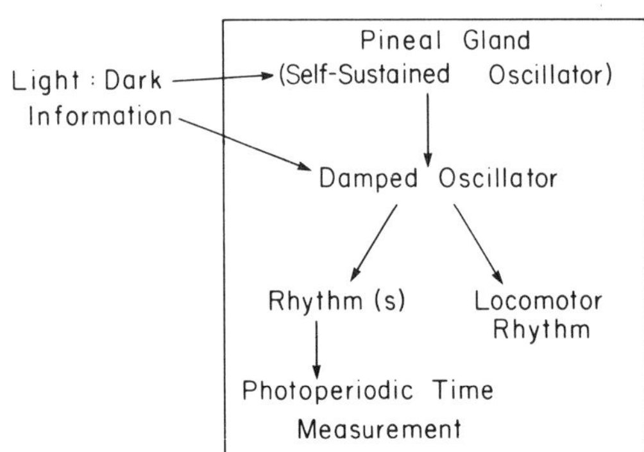

Fig. 4. Diagram of a hypothetical scheme of involvement of the pineal gland in the control of a diurnal rhythm(s) involved in measurement of day length. In an intact bird an endogenous self-sustained oscillator located within the pineal gland is entrained by the light:dark cycle. This oscillator in turn drives a damped oscillator(s) that regulates directly the rhythm(s) involved in the measurement of day length as well as other diurnal rhythms such as locomotor activity. In the absence of the pineal gland, the damped oscillator can be entrained directly by the light cycle, and under normal light cycles the pattern of entrainment is similar to that observed in intact birds. Therefore, pinealectomy will alter neither the photoperiodic response, not the activity rhythm in birds exposed to normal light-dark cycles, even though in the intact bird the pineal gland is involved in the control of the rhythms ultimately responsible for regulating locomotor activity and photoperiodic induction

day length has a similar relationship to the pineal gland and a second damped oscillator, then an effect of pinealectomy on a photoperiodic response may not be observed in birds exposed to normal light cycles. A diagrammatical representation of this hypothesis is shown in Figure 4. According to this model, the rhythm(s) involved in photoperiodic time measurement may normally be under the control of the pineal gland, but in the absence of the pineal gland, the rhythm can be entrained by the light cycle. If this hypothesis is correct, then in order to determine if the pineal gland is involved in avian photoperiodism, it may be nesessary to examine the photoperiodic response during exposure to unusual light cycles that require an intact pineal gland for normal entrainment to occur.

Acknowledgments. Unpublished experiments reported here were supported by NSF Grant PCM 76-09955 and NIH Grant HD-09885.

References

BINKLEY, S., KLUTH, E., MENAKER, M.: Pineal function in sparrows: Circadian rhythms and body temperature. Science 174, 311-314 (1971)

BÜNNING, E.: Die endogene Tagesrhythmik als Grundlage der photoperiodischen Reaktion. Ber. Deut. Bot. Ges. 54, 590-607 (1936)

DANILEVSKY, A.S., GORYSHIN, N.I., TYSHCHENKO, V.P.: Biological rhythms in terrestrial arthropods. Ann. Rev. Entomology 15, 201-214 (1970)

FARNER, D.S.: Photoperiodic controls in the secretion of gonadotropins in birds. Am. Zool. 15 (suppl. 1), 117-135 (1975)

FARNER, D.S., DONHAM, R.S., LEWIS, R.A., MATTOCKS, P.W., DARDEN, T.R., SMITH, J.P.: The circadian component in the photoperiodic component of the House Sparrow, *Passer domesticus*. Physiol. Zool. 50, 247-268 (1977)

FARNER, D.S., LEWIS, R.A.: Field and experimental studies of the annual cycles of white-crowned sparrows. J. Reprod. Fert. Suppl. 19, 35-50 (1973)

FOLLETT, B.K., SHARP, P.J.: Circadian rhythmicity in photoperiodically induced gonadotropin release and gonadal growth in the quail. Nature (London) 223, 968-971 (1969)

GASTON, S., MENAKER, M.: Pineal function: The biological clock in the sparrow? Science 160, 1125-1127 (1968)

HAMNER, W.M.: Diurnal rhythm and photoperiodism in testicular recrudescence of the house finch. Science 142, 1294-1295 (1963)

LOFTS, B., FOLLETT, B.K., MURTON, R.K.: Temporal changes in the pituitary-gonadal axis. Mem. Soc. Endocrinol. 18, 545-575 (1970)

MEIER, A.H., DUSSEAU, J.W.: Daily entrainment of the photoinducible phases for photostimulation of the reproductive system in the sparrows *Zonotrichia albicollis* and *Passer domesticus*. Biol. Reprod. 8, 400-410 (1973)

MEIER, A.H., MACGREGOR, R.: Temporal organization in avian reproduction. Am. Zool. 12, 257-271 (1972)

MENAKER, M., ESKIN, A.: Circadian clock in photoperiodic time measurement: A test of the Bünning hypothesis. Science 157, 1182-1185 (1967)

MENAKER, M., OKSCHE, A.: The avian pineal organ. In: Avian Biology. New York: Academic Press, 1974, pp. 79-118

MCMILLAN, J.P.: Pinealectomy abolishes the circadian rhythm of migratory restlessness. J. Comp. Physiol. 79, 105-112 (1972)

NANDA, K.R., HAMNER, K.C.: Studies on the nature of the endogenous rhythm affecting photoperiodic responses of Biloxi soybean. Bot. Gaz. 120, 14-25 (1958)

OISHI, T., LAUBER, J.K.: Pituitary-pineal-endocrine relationships in Japanese quail. Endocrinology 94, 1731-1734 (1974)

PITTENDRIGH, C.S.: Circadian surfaces and the diversity of possible roles of circadian organization in photoperiodic induction. Proc. Natl. Acad. Sci. USA 69, 2734-2737 (1972)

ROWAN, W.: Relation of light to bird migration and development changes. Nature (London) 115, 494-495 (1925)
TUREK, F.W.: Circadian involvement in termination of the refractory period in two sparrows. Science 178, 1112-1113 (1972)
TUREK, F.W.: Photoperiodic phenomena in white-crowned and golden-crowned sparrows (Genus Zonotrichia), Dissertation 1973
TUREK, F.W.: Circadian rhythmicity and the initiation of gonadal growth in sparrows. J. Comp. Physiol. 92, 59-64 (1974)
TUREK, F.W., MCMILLAN, J.P., MENAKER, M.: Melatonin: Effects on the circadian locomotor rhythm of sparrows. Science 194, 1441-1443 (1976)
TUREK, F.W., WOLFSON, A.: Lack of an effect of melatonin treatment via silastic capsules on photic-induced gonadal growth and the photorefractory condition in white-throated sparrows. Gen. Comp. Endocrinol., in press (1978)
WOLFSON, A.: Environmental and neuroendocrine regulation of annual gonadal cycles and migratory behavior in birds. Rec. Progr. Horm. Res. 12, 177-244 (1966)
ZIMMERMAN, N.H., MENAKER, M.: Neural connections of sparrow pineal: Role in circadian control of activity. Science 190, 477-479 (1975)

5. Central Neural Control of Endocrine Rhythms in the Rat

S. P. KALRA and P. S. KALRA

The organization of neuroendocrine systems in relation to time in the "spontaneously" ovulating laboratory rat was disclosed in 1953 by EVERETT and SAWYER. However, the complex nature of the relationships was not appreciated until accurate measurements of hormones became feasible with the advent of radioimmunoassays. During the past few years we have concerned ourselves with the characterization of the temporal organization of pituitary and gondadal hormones in the blood, and the nature of the central control exercised by the hypothalamus on the secretion of these two endocrine glands in the rat (KALRA and KALRA, 1974a, b, 1977, 1977a). In this paper, we will first summarize our studies on the circadian periodicity in the circulating gonadal hormones in male and female rats and present evidence that the daily pattern of progesterone secretion, that does not appear to affect gonadotropin release, may regulate the gonadal steroid secretion. Further experimental evidence will show that rhythmic oscillations in the secretions of the hypothalamo-hypophysio-adrenal axis exercise a profound modulating influence on testicular secretion. In the second section of this paper we deal with the daily periodicities in the hypothalamic content of luteinizing hormone-releasing hormone (LH-RH) in male and female rats.

Temporal Variations in Gonadal Steroids and Gonadotropins during the Estrous Cycle

Several laboratories have described the temporal relationship among the hormonal events of the estrous cycle (KALRA and KALRA, 1974a, 1974b, 1977; BUTCHER et al., 1974; SMITH et al., 1975). The important feature of our studies was the demonstration of a reciprocal relationship between the serum concentrations of estradiol and progesterone in the presence of basal levels of LH (Fig. 1). During the cycle, serum progesterone levels displayed a daily rhythm; the lowest values recorded around noon were invariably succeeded by relatively higher rates of secretion that resulted in peak concentrations during the first half of the dark period. These intervals of augmented secretion of progesterone were followed by a marked decrease in serum levels of estradiol. Exogenous administration of ovulation-inhibiting doses of progesterone at different times during the cycle caused a rapid and relatively prolonged suppression in estradiol (Fig. 2) but serum levels of LH were unaltered. This indicates that progesterone may suppress serum estradiol by direct inhibition of production of estrogen. These findings have important implications with respect to the central regulation of ovulation and the estrous cycle. The neuroendocrine events involved in the ovulatory surge of gonadotropins and in ovulation are estrogen-dependent (EVERETT, 1964; KALRA, 1975). It seems likely that progesterone, by serving as an internal regulator of estrogen secretion, plays a key role in determining the precise time of coupling of the estrogen-dependent neural (hypothalamic) and endocrine (hypophysial)

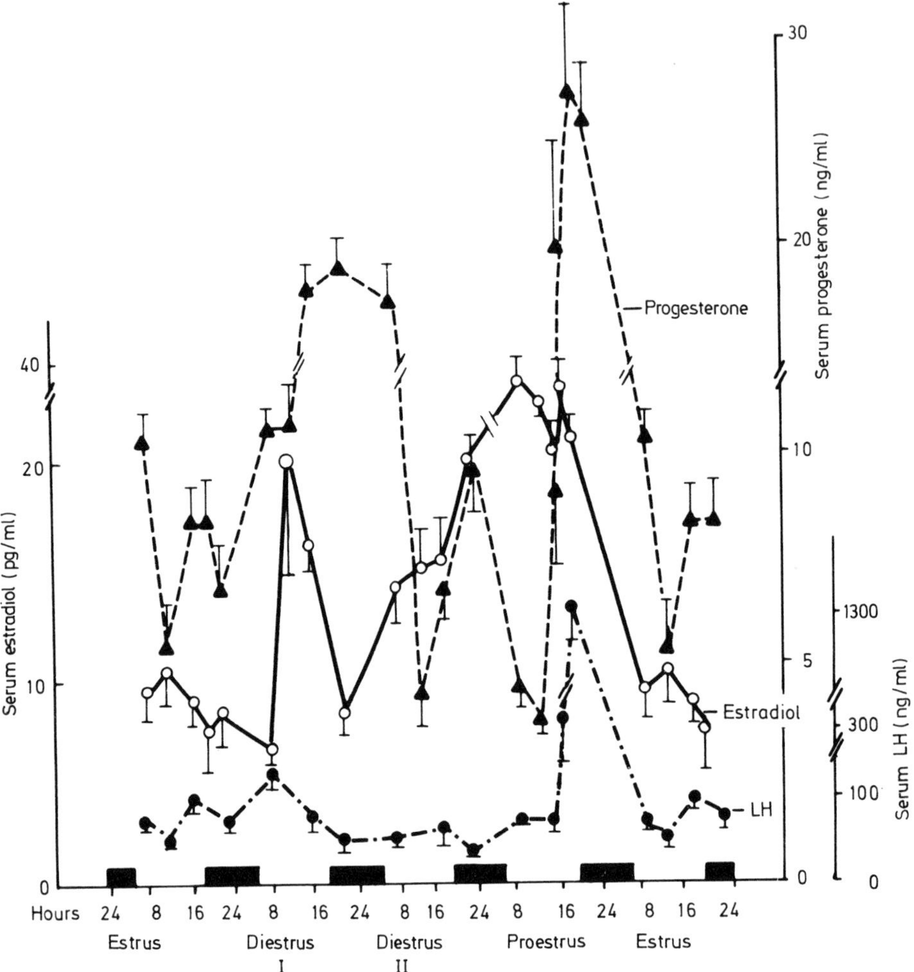

Fig. 1. Serum levels of LH, estradiol and progesterone in the rat. Each point represents the mean and one SEM for 10-21 rats killed at various times during the 4-day estrous cycle. (From KALRA and KALRA, 1974b)

events with the central "trigger clock"; the latter ultimately signals the preovulatory discharge of gonadotropins.

Temporal Variations in Serum Levels of Gonadal Steroids in Male Rats

As in females, serum levels of progesterone also displayed a circadian pattern in male rats (Fig. 3), the levels being lowest between 05.00-11.00 h and highest between 16.00-22.00 h. In addition, the serum androgens, testosterone and dihydrotestosterone, fluctuated rhythmically in these rats (Fig. 3). The rhythms of serum progesterone and androgens appeared to be inversely related; increments in serum androgens were found when the progesterone level decreased, and similarly de-

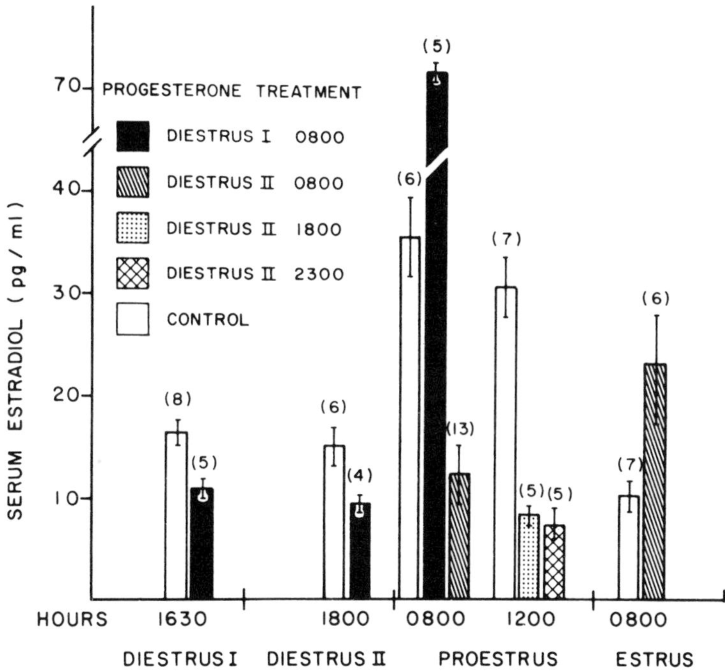

Fig. 2. Effects of exogenous progesterone (4 mg/rat) on serum estradiol in intact cyclic rats. Progesterone was administered at the times indicated by shading of bars and the animals were sacrificed at the times indicated on the abscissa. Numbers in parentheses represent the number of rats. Progesterone treatment at 08.00 h of diestrus I resulted in a significant reduction of estradiol levels at 16.30 h of diestrus I and at 18.00 h of diestrus II; however, estradiol levels were elevated at 08.00 h of proestrus. Similarly, administration of progesterone during diestrus II resulted in reduced estradiol levels on proestrus and higher values at 08.00 h of estrus (48 h after progesterone treatment on 08.00 h of diestrus II). (From KALRA and KALRA, 1974b)

crements in serum androgens occurred during the interval of high serum concentrations of progesterone. These findings in male rats are consistent with the postulate elaborated above that the circadian pattern of progesterone secretion may modulate gonadal secretion.

Further studies were designed to identify the source of serum progesterone and to attempt to define more precisely the role of adrenals in the circadian pattern of secretion of testicular androgens.

Effects of Adrenalectomy on Daily Patterns of Serum Progesterone and Testosterone

Analysis of the circadian pattern of serum testosterone and progesterone two weeks after adrenalectomy presented an interesting picture (Fig. 4). A typical AM-to-PM increase in serum progesterone was still descernible in the adrenalectomized rats, thereby indicating that the testes may secrete progesterone rhythmically. On the other hand, adrenalectomy abolished the rhythm in serum testosterone without adverse

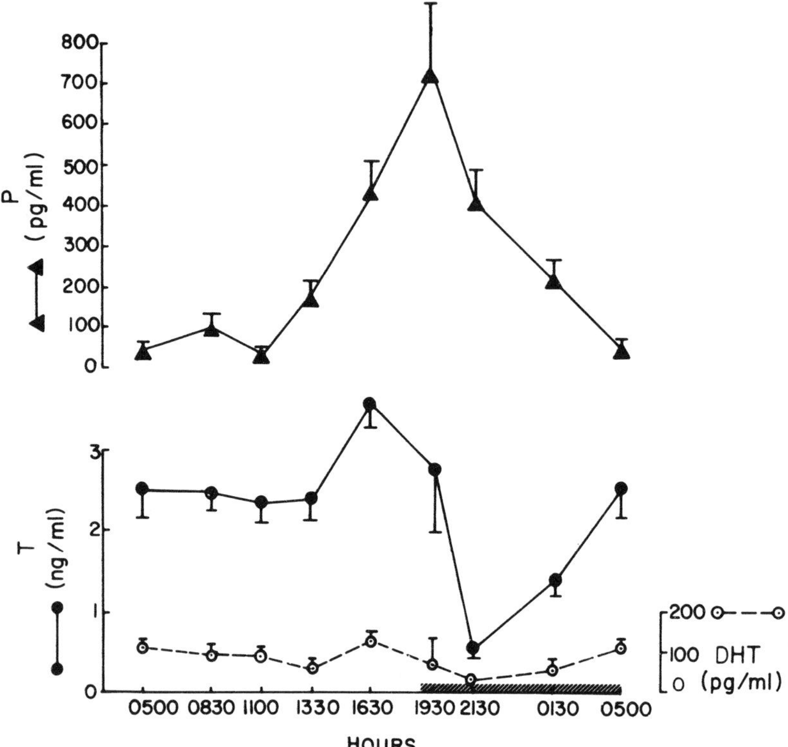

Fig. 3. Serum levels of progesterone (P), testosterone (T) and dihydrotestosterone (DHT) in male rats killed at the times designated on the abscissa. The levels represent the mean and one SEM for 5-6 rats at each point. (From KALRA and KALRA, 1974a)

effect on serum LH. Since serum testosterone levels in castrate rats are undetectable, our observations strongly support the hypothesis that adrenal secretion may be responsible for the apparent circadian variations in serum levels of testosterone (KALRA and KALRA, 1977a). These studies suggest that the adrenal product(s) is secreted rhythmically and may stimulate the diurnal hypersecretion of testosterone; the nature of this product(s) is under investigation.

Effects of Anterior-Hypothalamic Deafferentation on Serum Testosterone and Progesterone Rhythms

The temporal organization of the various components of the adrenal-glucocorticoid system has been extensively studied. The hormonal variables in the hypothalamo-hypophysio-adrenal axis have been shown to possess a 24-h periodicity (YATES, 1974). Based on the evidence from investigations involving lesions and deafferentations, the neural links between the preoptic-anterior hypothalamic area (POA-AHA) and the medial basal hypothalamus (MBH) represent the common final neural pathway in the central regulation of adrenal-glucocorticoid periodicities (CRITCHLOW et al., 1963; HALASZ, 1969). In view of our observation of a close relationship between adrenal secretion and production of tes-

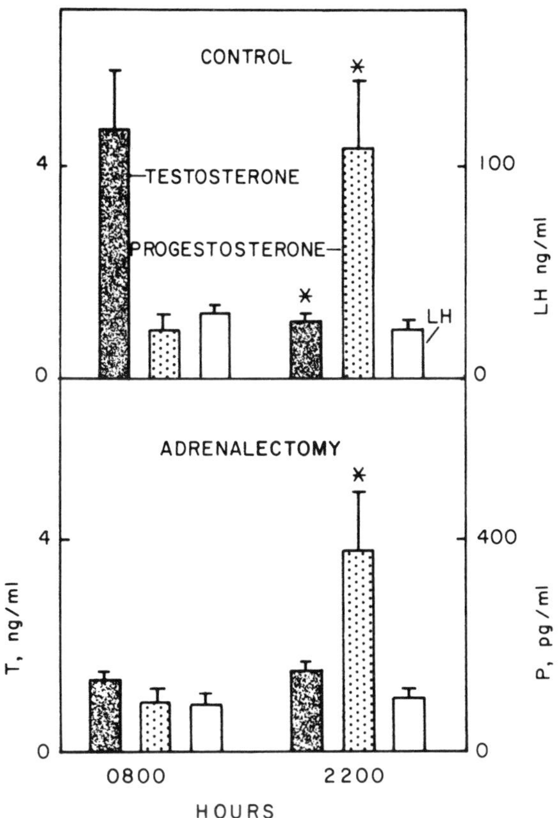

Fig. 4. Serum levels of LH, testosterone and progesterone at 08.00 h and 22.00 h in sham-operated control male rats (upper panel) and 2 weeks after bilateral adrenalectomy (lower panel). Levels are mean and one SEM for 6-14 rats per group. (* $p <$ 0.05 in comparison with the respective 08.00-h levels)

tosterone by the testes, the effects of severing the neural links between the POA-AHA and the MBH (by Halász-type knife) on the rhythms of serum testosterone and progesterone were investigated. In deafferented rats, the typical AM-to-PM decrements in serum levels of testosterone were attenuated, resulting in extinction of the daily pattern (Fig. 5). The nocturnal hypersecretion of progesterone was also suppressed by deafferentation. Furthermore, we have found, in agreement with other investigators (HALÁSZ, 1969), that the reproductive system and gonadotropin release were normal in these deafferented rats (KALRA and KALRA, 1977a). One can, therefore, assume that the disruption of circadian oscillations of the hypothalamo-pituitary-adrenal axis in the deafferented rats was responsible for the marked alterations in the daily pattern of serum levels of testosterone.

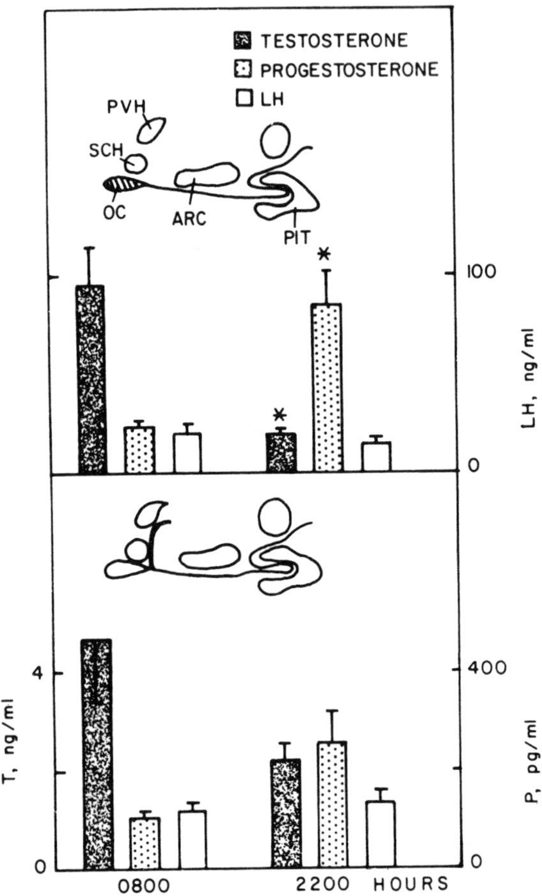

Fig. 5. Serum levels of LH, testosterone and progesterone at 08.00 and 22.00 h in male rats. The animals were killed 33 days after either anterior hypothalamic deafferentation (lower) or sham operation (upper). The location of the knife-cut is shown by the thick black line in the diagrammatic inset of the hypothalamus. ARC, arcuate nucleus; OC, optic chaism; PIT, pituitary; PVH, paraventricular nucleus; SCH, suprachiasmatic nucleus). * $p < 0.05$ in comparison with 08.00-h values

Daily Periodicity in Hypothalamic LH-RH Activity

It is well documented that secretion of the hypothalamic hormone, LH-RH, regulates pituitary release of LH which, in turn, controls the gonadal steroid-hormone secretion. LH-RH is widely distributed in the hypothalamus and in extra-hypothalamic regions. LH-RH-containing fiber systems are present in the broad band of neural tissue between anterior commissure and suprachiasmatic nucleus, and extend further back into the basal hypothalamus. These fiber systems terminate in the organum vasculosum of stria terminalis, and in the median eminence (BARRY et al., 1973; NAIK, 1975). Our experiments involving anterior hypothalamic deafferentation indicated that 80% of LH-RH normally found in the MBH of male and female rats is derived from that synthesized in the rostral regions including the preoptic area, while the remaining amount in the

MBH is probably produced in the arcuate nucleus (KALRA, 1976a; KALRA et al., 1977). More recent histofluorescent studies have indeed visualized LH-RH-containing perikarya scattered in the preoptic area and in the arcuate nucleus (NAIK, 1975).

The preoptic brain has been implicated in the regulation of the cyclic discharge of LH in female rats. Recently, we have found that in intact cyclic rats, LH-RH content in the preoptic region changes significantly through the 24-h period (Fig. 6). The amounts of LH-RH are generally

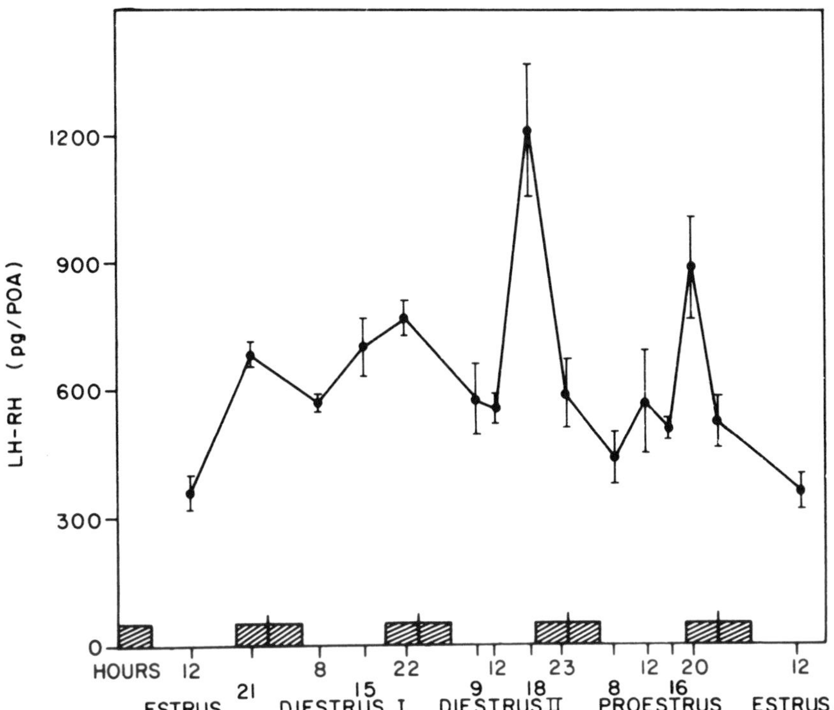

Fig. 6. Daily fluctuation in LH-RH in the preoptic area (POA). Each point represents the mean ± SE of values for 5 rats killed at the times designated on the abscissa. Hatched horizontal bars designate the period of darkness between 19.00-05.00 h. (From KALRA, 1976)

higher during the first half of the dark period than during the day (KALRA, 1976). Similar circadian periodicity in the LH-RH content of POA was not observed in male rats. On the contrary, the levels of LH-RH in serum and in the MBH in males fluctuated rhythmically, although these rhythms were unrelated to the serum gonadotropin levels (KALRA and KALRA, 1977a). At present it is uncertain whether the hypothalamic LH-RH rhythms are endogenously controlled within the neurons that synthesize this hormone, or by other neural inputs from the central pacemaker (suprachiasmatic nuclei?), which may itself take cues from external environmental factors.

Summary and Conclusion

The foregoing brief discussion of our recent findings is presented in Figure 7. Several environmental parameters (light, temperature, food, etc.) have been shown to be capable of producing marked disturbances

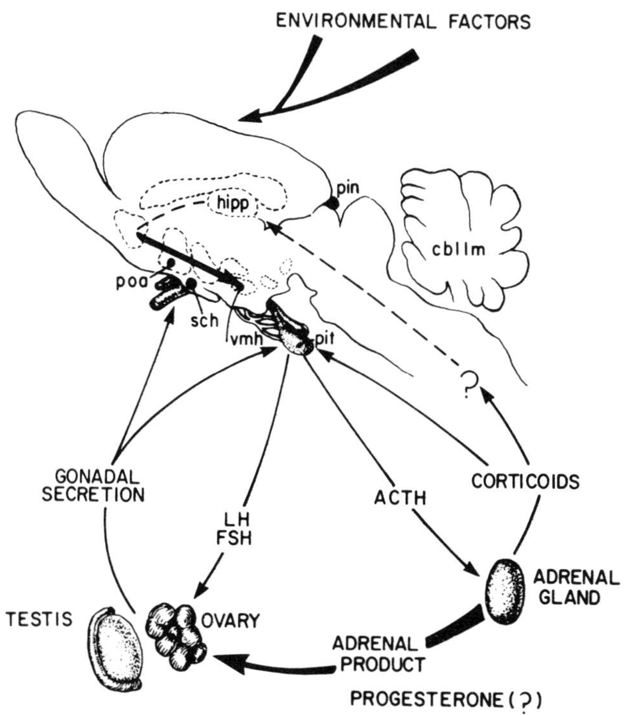

Fig. 7. Our current view of the apparent coupling between the hypothalamo-hypophysio-adrenal and hypothalamo-hypophysio-gonadal axis. Circadian oscillations in adrenal secretion are regulated by the feedback action of corticoids on the pituitary and central nervous system, although the efferent pathways of this feedback loop within the brain have not yet been fully determined (dashed line). Participation of the limbic system (hippocampus) in the adrenal-corticoid secretion has been suggested. The neural links between the preoptic-anterior hypothalamic area (POA-AHA) and the medial basal hypothalamus (MBH) are essential in the circadian oscillations in secretion of adrenal corticoids (thick line). Our experiments show that disruption of the hypothalamo-hypophysio-adrenal axis at two levels, (1) transection of these neural links between POA-AHA and MBH, or (2) ablation of adrenal glands, abolish the rhythm in secretion of gonadal steroid. This has led us to hypothesize that adrenal product(s) (progesterone?) are essential in maintaining the 24-h periodicity in secretion of gonadal steroid hormones. (ACTH, Adrenocorticotropic hormone; Cbllm, cerebellum; FSH, follicle stimulating hormone; hipp, hippocampus; LH, luteinizing hormone; pin, pineal; pit, pituitary; poa, preoptic area; sch, suprachiasmatic nucleus; vmh, ventromedial nucleus)

in the hypothalamo-hypophysio-gonadal and hypothalamo-hypophysio-adrenal systems. The experiments discussed here indicate that various hormonal components in the hypothalamo-hypophysio-gonadal axis have circadian patterns and that gonadal steroid secretion is closely linked with the hypothalamo-hypophysio-adrenal system. Though the precise mechanism of adrenal modulation of gonadal steroid secretion is unknown, evidence suggests that in female rats, adrenal progesterone could modify ovarian estrogen production. A most exciting finding is that the hypothalamic content of LH-RH shows temporal variations. In this respect, the study of the interaction of external (light) and internal environmental factors (gonadal steroid feed-back action, coupling with adrenal glucocorticoid system) in the organization of the hypothalamic LH-RH rhythms offers a fruitful area of investigation.

Acknowledgments. Supported by grants from NIH (HD 80634). Secretarial help of Lyn Thomas is gratefully acknowledged.

References

BARRY, J., DUBOIS, M.P., POULAIN, P.: LRF-producing cells of the mammalian hypothalamus. Z. Zellforsch. 146, 351-366 (1973)

BUTCHER, R.L., COLLINS, W.E., FUGO, N.W.: Plasma concentrations of LH, FSH, prolactin, progesterone and estradiol-17β throughout the 4-day estrous cycle of the rat. Endocrinology 94, 1704-1708 (1974)

CRITCHLOW, V., LIEBOLT, R.A., BARSELA, M., MOUNTCASTLE, W., LIPSCOMB, H.S.: Sex differences in resting pituitary-adrenal function in the rat. Am. J. Physiol. 205, 807-815 (1963)

EVERETT, J.W.: Central neural control of reproductive functions of the adenohypophysis. Physiol. Rev. 44, 373-431 (1964)

EVERETT, J.W., SAWYER, C.H.: A 24-hour periodicity in the "LH-release apparatus" of female rats, disclosed by barbiturate sedation. Endocrinology 47, 198-218 (1953)

HALÁSZ, B.: The endocrine effects of isolation of the hypothalamus from the rest of the brain. In: Frontiers in Neuroendocrinology. Ganong, W.F., Martini, L. (eds.). New York: Oxford University Press, 1969, pp. 307-342

KALRA, P.S., KALRA, S.P.: Temporal changes in the hypothalamic and serum luteinizing hormone-releasing hormone (LH-RH) levels and the circulating ovarian steroids during the rat estrous cycle. Acta Endocrinol. 85, 449-455 (1977)

KALRA, P.S., KALRA, S.P.: Circadian periodicities of serum androgens, progesterone, gonadotropins and LH-RH in male rats: the effects of hypothalamic deafferentation, castration or adrenalectomy. Endocrinology 101, 1821-1827 (1977a)

KALRA, S.P.: Observations on facilitation of the preovulatory rise of LH by estrogen. Endocrinology 96, 23-28 (1975)

KALRA, S.P.: Circadian rhythm in luteinizing hormone-releasing hormone (LH-RH) content of preoptic area during the rat estrous cycle. Brain Res. 104, 354-358 (1976)

KALRA, S.P.: Tissue levels of luteinizing hormone-releasing hormone in the preoptic area and hypothalamus, and serum concentrations of gonadotropins following anterior hypothalamic deafferentation and estrogen treatment of the female rat. Endocrinology 99, 101-107 (1976a)

KALRA, S.P., KALRA, P.S.: Effects of circulating estradiol during rat estrous cycle on LH release following electrochemical stimulation of preoptic brain or administration of synthetic LRF. Endocrinology 94, 845-851 (1974a)

KALRA, S.P., KALRA, P.S.: Temporal interrelationships among circulating levels of estradiol, progesterone and LH during the rat estrous cycle. Effects of exogenous progesterone. Endocrinology 95, 1711-1718 (1974b)

KALRA, S.P., KALRA, P.S., MITCHELL, E.O.: Differential response of luteinizing hormone releasing hormone in the basal hypothalamus and the preoptic area following anterior hypothalamic deafferentation and/or castration in male rats. Endocrinology 100, 201-204 (1977)

NAIK, D.V.: Immunoreactive LH-RH neurons in the hypothalamus identified by light and fluorescent microscopy. Cell and Tissue Res. 157, 423-436 (1975)

SMITH, M.S., FREEMAN, M.E., NEILL, J.D.: The control of progesterone secretion during estrous cycle and early pseudopregnancy in the rat: prolactin, gonadotropins and steroid levels associated with rescue of the corpus luteum of pseudopregnancy. Endocrinology 96, 219-226 (1975)

YATES, F.E.: Modeling periodicities in reproductive, adrenocortical and metabolic systems. In: Biorhythms and Human Reproduction. Ferin, M., Halberg, F., Richart, R.M., VandeWiele, R.L. (eds.). New York: Wiley, 1974, pp. 133-144

6. Circadian Pattern of Secretion of Hormones by the Anterior Pituitary Gland with Particular Reference to the Involvement of Serotonin in Their Rhythmic Regulation

C. KORDON, M. HERY, F. GOGAN, and W. H. ROTSZTEJN

The first clear-cut evidence of the existence of circadian endocrine rhythms in the rat was reported 30 years ago, when EVERETT and SAWYER (1950) demonstrated that the ovulatory surge of LH in the course of the estrous cycle could be blocked by anesthetics, but only at given periods of the nychtemera. Under these conditions, ovulation was postponed by 24 h and the procedure could be repeated on consecutive days, provided the anesthetics were always administered between 13.00 and 16.00.

Precise evaluations of the circadian patterns of FSH and LH secretion are not easy in intact cycling animals. In the course of the estrous cycle, several peripheral parameters also interfere with the release of gonadotropins, in particular marked changes in pituitary sensitivity occurring under the influence of steroid circulating levels. More recently, KARSCH et al. (1973a, b); LEGAN et al. (1975) and CHAZAL et al. (1974) described a preparation in which peripheral steroid concentrations can be rendered invariant. They were able to show that, in castrated females implanted with a solid source of estradiol, plasma estradiol and pituitary sensitivity to LHRH no longer fluctuated during the day. Under these conditions, a very marked increase in plasma levels of LH begins between 13.00 and 15.00, peaks between 17.00 and 19.00 and returns to basal levels around 21.00 (Fig. 1). This schedule seems to be valid for animals kept on a standard 14L 10D light schedule as well as for rats held on 12L 12D. In parallel, plasma prolactin shows a fluctuation pattern very closely related to that of LH; in contrast, plasma FSH, as well as the hypothalamic content of LHRH, show variations of a much smaller amplitude. In addition, rhythms of FSH secre-

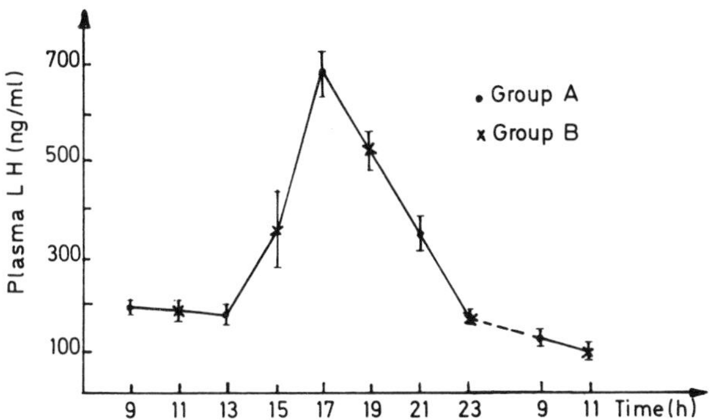

Fig. 1. Plasma levels of LH during the nychtemera in ovariectomized, estradiol-implanted castrated rats. Sequential blood sampling was performed under light ether anesthesia, alternately on two separate groups of animals; each was sampled every 4 h

tion and of hypothalamic content of LHRH have been found to be rather inconsistent; daily fluctuations of the latter hormones are hardly superimposable from one experiment to the other, and a seasonal component in their cyclic pattern cannot be excluded.

In castrated, estradiol-implanted female rats, the initial elevation in plasma levels of LH appears synchronously with those of ACTH, a finding that suggests that at least three hormones - LH, prolactin and ACTH - could be stimulated by a common trigger mechanism in the course of the estrous cycle.

Here, we first review some characteristics of the cyclic LH and ACTH patterns observed in castrated, estradiol-treated females, or in normal males, and then attempt to evaluate the role of central neurotransmitters and of discrete neuronal pathways in regulating this circadian rhythm.

Characteristics of the Cyclic LH Pattern

It is of interest to note that a cyclic pattern of LH secretion can only be obtained after castration and estradiol implantation in female, and not in male animals (Fig. 2). It has been proposed a long time ago

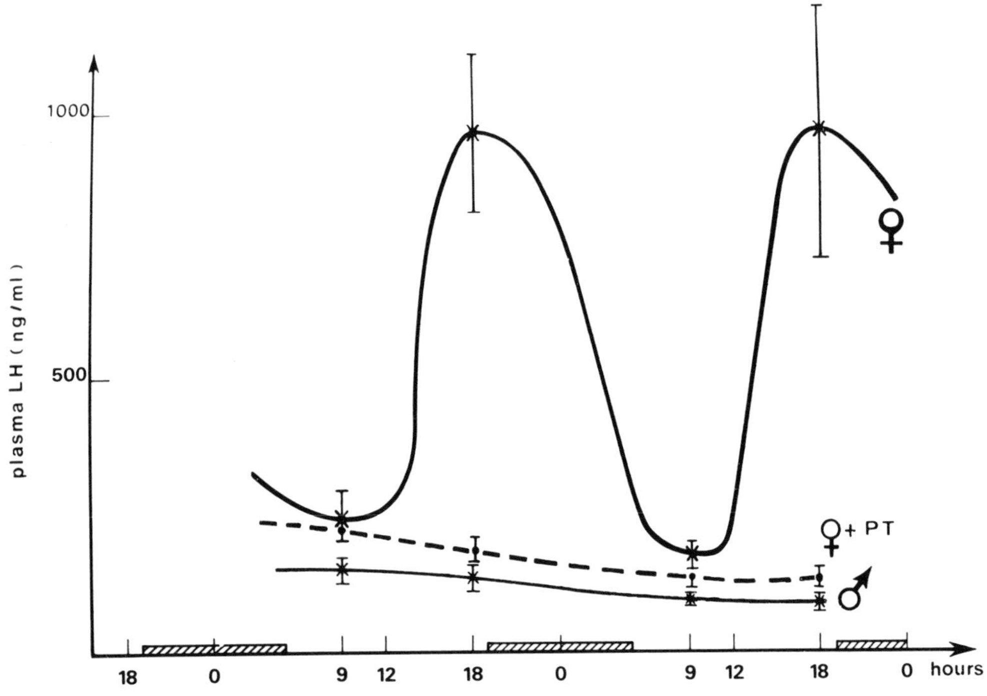

Fig. 2. Fluctuations of plasma LH in castrated females bearing estradiol implants (full line), in castrated males also implanted with estradiol (thin line) and in females kept under the same conditions, but treated within 5 days of birth with testosterone propionate (broken line)

(PFEIFFER, 1936) that neural structures able to control cyclicity of hormonal reproductive functions were sexually differentiated. The existence of a sexual dimorphism in the synaptic articulation of discrete afferents to the preoptic area was subsequently demonstrated by RAISMAN and FIELD (1973). This differentiation does not seem to depend upon the genetic sex of the animal, but upon its exposure to sex steriods during a critical period of ontogenetic development. The circadian pattern of LH secretion in castrated, estradiol-implanted animals also depends on this ontogenetic differentiation, since it is absent in normal males and in females injected with testosterone during the first 5 days of neonatal life (Table 1).

Table 1. The effect of exogenous estradiol on plasma levels of LH

	LH plasma levels (ng/ml)	
	Basal levels (09.00 h)	Maximal levels (18.00 h)
Control (1)	256 ± 13	745 ± 60
Male (2)	148 ± 20	130 ± 21
Androgenized female (3)	233 ± 26	190 ± 24

(1) castrated female rats implanted with estradiol.
(2) castrated male rats implanted with estradiol.
(3) androgenized female rats at birth and implanted with estradiol.

The sensitivity of the pituitary response to LHRH is strongly enhanced after estradiol implantation (CHAZAL et al., 1977). In particular, a massive increase of in vitro secretion of LH can be obtained when LHRH concentrations in the range of 10^{-10} M are added to the incubation medium; pituitaries from castrated animals exhibit a much smaller capacity to release LH under the same conditions. This sensitivity probably accounts for the very high amplitude of the LH daily fluctuations observed after estradiol implantation. In addition, a progressive decrease in pituitary sensitivity, which can be observed when implanted animals are tested after long periods of implantation, accounts for a parallel decrease in the amplitude of the LH cycle (Fig. 3 and 4).

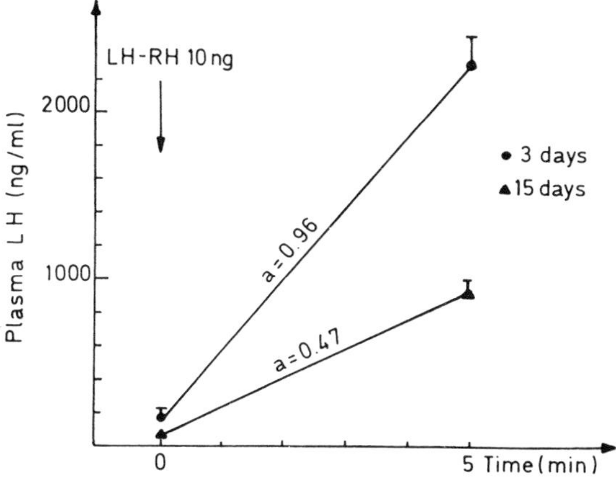

Fig. 3. Differential effectiveness of a single injection of LHRH (10 ng i.v.) on LH plasma levels in castrated females implated with estradiol for 3 days (dots) or for 15 days (triangles). Note the progressive decrease in pituitary sensitivity

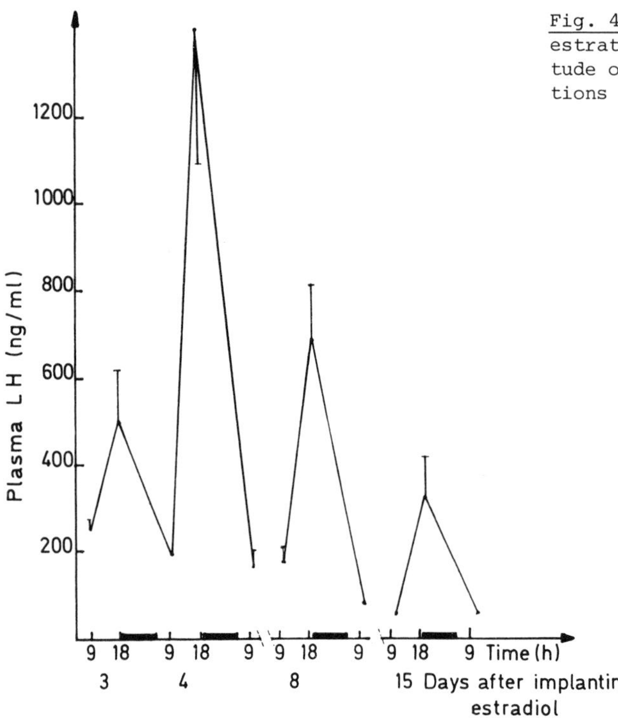

Fig. 4. Effect of the duration of estratiol implantation on the amplitude of the daily plasma LH fluctuations

In contrast to reports that indicated that adrenal steroids may interfere with the timing of the estrous cycle (BROWN-GRANT, 1971), the circadian LH secretion observed in estradiol-implanted animals is totally unaffected by adrenalectomy (CHAZAL et al., 1974; HERY et al., 1975a, b).

A markedly different pattern of LH-regulating mechanisms has been described in monkeys (KARSCH et al., 1973) in which the ovulatory release of LH may depend entirely upon a direct sensitization of the pituitary by estradiol, since a massive release of the hormone can be elicited by the steroid even after complete transection of all afferents to the hypothalamus from other parts of the brain (KREY et al., 1975). It must be stated, however, that all authors do not agree with this conclusion (NORMAN et al., 1976). At any rate, such species differences, as well as the different time course of LH release observed in rodents and in primates (during the estrous cycle, LH is only released in rodents during 2 to 4 h, whereas elevated LH plasma level can be maintained in primates for much longer periods), could be rationalized by postulating only differences in the relative importance of pituitary sensitization processes in both species. In primates, pituitary sensitization by estradiol would trigger LH release, provided a minimal basal amount of LHRH reaches the pituitary; no additional fluctuation in the flux of LHRH from the median eminence is required to result in hormonal stimulation. In contrast, in the rat, pituitary sensitivity never reaches a level at which basal concentrations of LHRH effectively release gonadotropins; this will only occur when an additional amount of LHRH is released from the median eminence, and it is this additional release that is submitted to a circadian periodicity.

Involvement of Serotonin (5-HT) in the Control of the Circadian Cycle of LH and ACTH

Brain serotonin has been shown to undergo wide circadian variations (HERY et al., 1972). In addition, an interference of this transmitter in a number of autonomous or endocrine rhythms has been postulated (JOUVET, 1969; BREISCH et al., 1976; POPOVA et al., 1972).

Inhibition of 5-HT biosynthesis by drugs such as p-chlorophenylalanine (pCPA) results in failure to ovulate in cyclic animals (HERY et al., 1975a). In castrated, estradiol-implanted females, circadian fluctuations in LH plasma levels are almost completely abolished 24 h after treatment with pCPA, and totally eradicated after 48 h (Fig. 5). Under

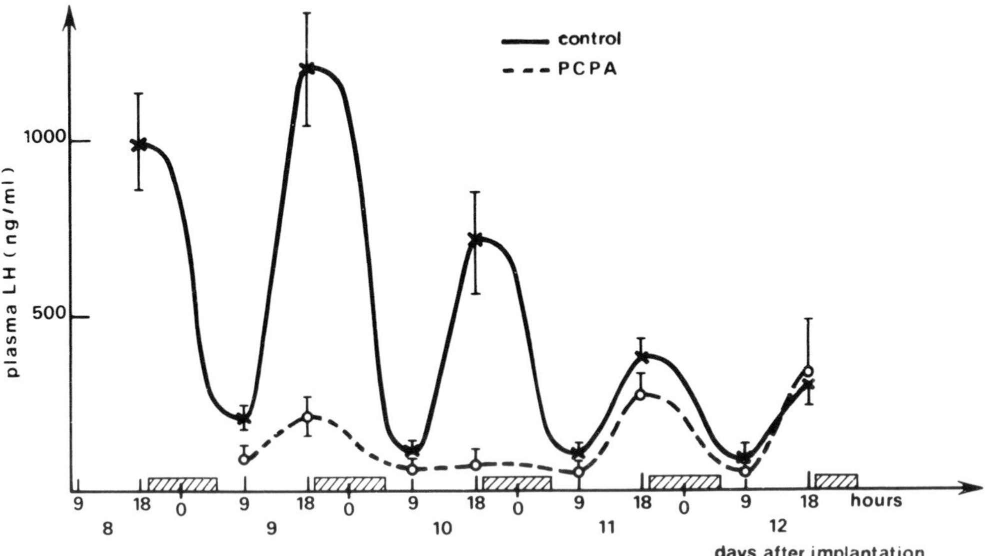

Fig. 5. Effect of inhibition of 5-HT synthesis on the amplitude of daily plasma LH fluctuations. Full line, control animals; broken line, pCPA-treated subjects

these conditions, restoration of endogenous levels of the transmitter by administration of the immediate precursor of the amine, 5-hydroxytryptophan (5-HTP) restores the capacity of the hypothalamo-hyophyseal unit to release LH at the expected time of the nychtemera, provided the precursor is administered between 0 and 4 h of the expected LH rise (HERY et al., 1976). This response can be obtained by systemic as well as by intraventricular administration of small doses of 5-HTP (HERY et al., 1976), and is not strictly related to the time of injection. Drugs that block the effects of serotonin at the level of post-synaptic receptors, such as methysergide or metergoline, also inhibit the cyclic release of LH (HERY et al., 1976), thus suggesting that these effects really involve a serotoninergic synaptic transmission and cannot be accounted for by nonspecific drug effects.

Only few data are available on circadian fluctuations of ACTH secretion, mainly because accurate evaluation of resting levels of plasma ACTH is still difficult (MATSUYAMA et al., 1972; COWAN, 1976). Therefore, most authors investigated modifications of the pituitary hormone secretion indirectly, be measuring plasma corticosterone levels.

Serotonin also seems to be involved in the circadian periodicity of secretion by the adrenal cortex. Correlations have been described between 5-HT fluctuations in various parts of the brain and the daily rhythm of plasma corticosterone (DIXIT and BUCKLEY, 1967; FRIEDMAN and WALKER, 1968; SCAPAGNINI et al., 1971; SIMON and GEORGE, 1975; TELEGDY et al., 1976), but it should be noted that the existence of such correlations does not necessarily imply a causal relationship. Systemic administration of pCPA elevates morning and lowers evening levels of plasma corticosterone (SCAPAGNINI et al., 1971; VERNIKOS-DANELLIS et al., 1973), but it seems that in most cases the amplitude of the circadian fluctuation of the steroid is decreased, and not entirely suppressed (VAN DELFT et al., 1973; TELEGDY et al., 1976; ROTSZTEJN et al., 1977). This may be due to the fact that, under certain conditions, corticosterone concentrations can continue to fluctuate even in the absence of variations in ACTH (DALLMAN et al., 1976).

Neuronal Pathways Involved in the Control of Cyclic Hormone Regulation

Since most 5-HT ascending projections originate in mesencephalic Raphé nuclei, it was of interest to attempt to localize 5-HT-containing neurons which may eventually be connected with the regulation of LH rhythms. Lesions of the medial Raphé, even when extending fairly rostrally to the site of the nucleus, did not deplete hypothalamic 5-HT by more than 50%; the extraneuronal metabolite 5-hydroxyindoleatic acid (5HIAA) was also not as massively blunted under these conditions as after synthesis inhibition of the amine. In contrast, large mesencephalic lesions involving both the medial and the dorsal Raphé, or transections of 5-HT-containing fibers in the mediopontine area, before they enter the medial forebrain bundle, depleted 5-HT and its metabolite to an extent comparable to that of pCPA administration. In parallel, the amplitude of the LH fluctuation was unaffected by the two first kinds of lesion, and was strongly inhibited by the two latter. However, even under conditions of maximal hypothalamic depletion of 5-HT and 5HIAA, the LH cycle was never completely abolished, but only inhibited by approximately 70% (Table 2) (HERY et al., 1977). Lesions

Table 2. Effects of Raphé lesions and mediopontine transections on daily variations of LH and on hypothalamic neurotransmitters concentrations

Experimental groups	Amplitude of LH rhythms (ng/ml)	Hypothalamic concentration (ng/g)		
		5HT	5HIAA	NA
Controls	771 ± 63	783 ± 15	937 ± 29	2281 ± 72
Medial + dorsal Raphé lesions	291 ± 80	137 ± 21	245 ± 57	2280 ± 60
Controls	557 ± 41	599 ± 40	1140 ± 38	2544 ± 101
Transections	141 ± 33	394 ± 32	477 ± 63	2242 ± 178

aimed at destroying the Raphé area were reported to abolish also diurnal corticosteroid variations, inducing either constant intermediate (SCAPAGNINI and PREZIOSI, 1972), or very high baseline levels of the hormone (TELEGDY et al., 1976); however, these lesions were not analyzed histologically, and may have affected also ascending noradrenergic fibers, known to inhibit corticosterone secretion (SCAPAGNINI and PREZIOSI, 1972). More selective destruction of the nucleus centralis superior or of the Raphé dorsalis, which reduce 5-HT concentrations in both hypothalamus and dorsal hippocampus without affecting norepinephrine levels, was shown to reduce the amplitude of plasma corticosterone fluctuations without totally suppressing the rhythm (ROTSZTEJN et al., 1977), as in the case of LH discussed above. This result was recently confirmed by BALESTRERY and MOBERG (1976), although these authors did not observe any modification of the amplitude of the steroid rhythm one week after Raphé lesions.

How can one explain that in spite of a similar depletion of hypothalamic stores of 5-HT and 5HIAA, complete transection of mesencephalic fibers ascending to the hypothalamus is not as effective as pharmacologic blockade of the synthesis of the transmitter to inhibit the rhythm of LH? Only speculative answers can be given as yet. The recent discovery of a serotoninergic neuron system, that appears to lie entirely within the hypothalamus (BEAUDET and DESCARRIES, 1976), could provide the basis of an explanatory hypothesis. The exact location of the terminals of these neurons is not yet known with precision. However, if they could be assumed to innervate hypothalamic structures involved in neuroendocrine control, one could understand why pharmacologic inhibition of the amine, that can be expected to affect all central serotoninergic neurons, is more effective than mesencephalic lesions or transections, that would spare any neuron system originating rostrally to the transection.

Whether one or two 5-HT-containing fiber systems are involved in the control of cyclic endocrine variations and the exact structure at which they exert their effect, has not been elucidated as yet. However, a number of data suggest that the suprachiasmatic nucleus, a structure very rich in 5-HT (FUXE, 1965; SAAVEDRA et al., 1974), and which exhibits a clear-cut circadian rhythm in its ability to take up serotonin (MEYER and QUAY, 1976), plays an important role in impulsing circadian patterns. Its destruction has been shown to disrupt the rhythm of sleep, locomotor activity, eating and drinking behavior, as well as that of a number of hormonal fluctuations (TALEISNIK and MCCANN, 1961; MOORE and EICHLER, 1972; SZAFARCZYK et al., 1977). It is therefore very tempting to speculate that fibers originating in the dorsal Raphé, and possibly intrahypothalamic serotoninergic fibers as well, could terminate in the suprachiasmatic nucleus and initiate there a rhythmic tuning of autonomous functions.

At any rate, a central clock seems involved in the control of several neuroendocrine rhythms. No particular structure can be considered as representing the clock itself; everything seems to indicate that various neuronal circuits each represent a part of the clock mechanism. The hypothesis that the function of the suprachiasmatic nucleus would be to integrate information originating in these separate clock parts does not seem unlikely in the light of our present knowledge.

References

BALESTRERY, F.G., MOBERG, G.P.: Effect of midbrain Raphe nuclei lesions on the circadian rhythm of plasma corticosterone in the rat. Brain Res. 118, 503-508 (1976)

BEAUDET, A., DESCARRIES, L.: A serotonin containing nerve cell group in rat hypothalamus. Neurosci. Abstract II 479, Congr. Soc. Neurosci. Toronto (1976)

BREISCH, S.T., ZEMLAM, F.P., HOEBEL, B.G.: Hyperphagia and obesity following serotonin depletion by intraventricular parablorophenylalanine. Science 192, 382-384 (1976)

BROWN-GRANT, G.: The role of steroid hormones in the control of gonadotropin secretion in adult female mammals. In: Steroid Hormones and Brain Function. Sawyer, C.H., Gorski, R. (eds.). Los Angeles: California Press, 1971, pp. 269-288

CHAZAL, G., FAUDON, M., GOGAN, F., HERY, M., KORDON, C., LAPLANTE, E.: Circadian rhythm of luteinizing hormone secretion in the ovariectomized rat implanted with estradiol. J. Endocrinol. 75, 251-269 (1977)

CHAZAL, G., FAUDON, M., GOGAN, F., HERY, M., LAPLANTE, E.: Mise en évidence d'un implant d'oestradiol. J. Physiol. 69, 190A (1974)

COWAN, J.S.: Loss of ACTH biological activity in plasma during extraction with a commercial radioimmunoassay kit. Can. J. Physiol. Pharmacol. 54, 160-176 (1976)

DALLMAN, M.F., SIEDENBURG, F., SHINASKO, J.: Parachlorophenylalanine (pCPA) treatment changes adrenal sensitivity to ACTH. Proc. 5th Int. Congr. Endocrinol. Hamburg, Abstract 423, p. 173 (1976)

DELFT, A.M.L. VAN, KAPLANSKI, J., SMELIK, P.G.: Circadian periodicity of pituitary-adrenal function after p-chlorophenylalanine administration in the rat. J. Endocrinol. 59, 465-474 (1973)

DIXIT, B.N., BUCKLEY, J.P.: Circadian changes in brain 5-hydroxytryptamine and plasma corticosterone in the rat. Life Sci. 6, 755-758 (1967)

EVERETT, J.W., SAWYER, C.H.: A 24-hour periodicity in the "LH-release apparatus" of female rats disclosed by barbiturate sedation. Endocrinology 47, 198-218 (1950)

FRIEDMAN, A.H., WALKER, C.A.: Circadian rhythms in rat midbrain and caudate nucleus biogenic amine levels. J. Physiol. 197, 77-85 (1968)

FUXE, K.: Evidence for the existence of monoamine neurons in the central nervous system. IV. Distribution of monoamine terminals in the central nervous system. Acta Physiol. Scand. 64, Suppl. 247, 37-85 (1965)

HERY, M., LAPLANTE, E., KORDON, C.: Role of pituitary sensitivity and adrenal secretion in the effect of serotonin depletion on luteinizing hormone regulation. J. Endocrinol. 67, 463-464 (1975a)

HERY, M., LAPLANTE, E., KORDON, C.: Participation of serotonin in the phasic release of LH. I: Evidence from pharmacological experiments. Endocrinology 99, 496-503 (1976)

HERY, M., LAPLANTE, E., KORDON, C.: Participation of serotonin in the phasic release of LH. II: Effects of lesions of serotonin-containing pathways in the CNS. Endocrinology (in press, 1978)

HERY, M., LAPLANTE, E., PATTOU, E., KORDON, C.: Interaction de la serotonine cérébrale avec la libération cyclique de LH chez la ratte. Ann. Endocrinol. 36, 123-130 (1975b)

HERY, F., ROUER, E., GLOWINSKI, J.: Daily variation of serotonin metabolism in the rat brain. Brain Res. 43, 445-465 (1972)

HOFFMAN, R.A., REITER, R.J.: Responses of some endocrine organs female hamsters to pinealectomy and light. Life Science 5, 1147-1151 (1966)

IBUKA, N., KAWAMURA, H.: Loss of circadian rhythm in sleep-wakefulness cycle in the rat by suprachiasmatic lesions. Brain Res. 96, 76-81 (1975)

JOUVET, M.: Biogenic amines and the states of sleep. Science 163, 32-41 (1969)

KARSCH, F.J., DIERSCHKE, D.J., WEICK, R.F., YAMAJI, T., HOTCHKISS, J., KNOBIL, E.: Positive and negative feed-back control by estrogen of luteinizing hormone secretion in the Rhesus monkey. Endocrinology 92, 799-804 (1973a)

KARSCH, F.J., WEICK, R.F., BUTLER, W.R., DIERSCHKE, D.J., KREY, L.C., WEISS, G., HOTCHKISS, J., YAMAJI, T., KNOBIL, E.: Induced LH surges in the Rhesus monkey: strength-duration characteristics of the estrogen stimulus. Endocrinology 92, 1740-1747 (1973b)

KREY, C.L., BUTLER, W.R., KNOBIL, E.: Surgical disconnection of the medial basal hypothalamus and pituitary function in the Rhesus monkey. I: Gonadotropin secretion. Endocrinology 96, 1073-1087 (1975)

LEGAN, S.J., ALLYN COON, E.G., KARSCH, F.J.: Role of estrogen as initiator of daily LH surges in the ovariectomized rat. Endocrinology 96, 5056 (1975)

MATSUYAMA, H., RUHMANN-WENNHOLD, A., JOHNSON, L.R., NELSON, D.H.: Disappearance of exogenous and endogenous ACTH from rat plasma measured by bioassay and radioimmunoassay. Metabolism 21, 30-35 (1972)

MEYER, D.C., QUAY, W.B.: Hypothalamic and suprachiasmatic uptake of serotonin in vitro: twenty four hour changes in male and proestrus female rats. Endocrinology 98, 1160-1165 (1976)

MOORE, R.Y., EICHLER, V.B.: Loss of circadian adrenal corticosterone rhythm following suprachiasmatic lesions in the rat. Brain Res. 42, 201-206 (1972)

NORMAN, R.L., RESKO, J.A., SPIES, H.G.: The anterior hypothalamus: how it affects gonadotropin secretion in the Rhesus monkey. Endocrinology 99, 59-71 (1976)

PFEIFFER, C.A.: Sexual differences of the hypophysis and their determination by the gonads. Am. J. Anat. 58, 195-225 (1936)

POPOVA, N.K., MASLOV, L.M., NAUMENKO, E.V.: Serotonin and the regulation of the pituitary-adrenal-system after deafferentation of the hypothalamus. Brain Res. 47, 61-67 (1972)

RAISMANN, G., FIELD, P.M.: Sexual dimorphism in the neuropil of the preoptic area of the rat and its dependence on neonatal androgen. Brain Res. 54, 1-29 (1973)

ROTSZTEJN, W.H., BEAUDET, A., ROBERGE, A.G., LALONDE, J., FORTIER, C.: Role of brain serotonin in the circadian rhythm of corticosterone secretion and the corticotropic response to adrenalectomy in the rat. Neuroendocrinology 23, 157-170 (1977)

SAAVEDRA, J.M., PALKOVITS, M., BROWNSTEIN, M., AXELROD, J.: Serotonin distribution in the nuclei of the rat hypothalamus and preoptic region. Brain Res. 77, 157-165 (1974)

SCAPAGNINI, U., MOBERG, G.P., VAN LOON, G.R., DE GROOT, J., GANONG, W.F.: Relation of brain 5-hydroxytryptamine content to the diurnal variation in plasma corticosterone in the rat. Neuroendocrinology 7, 90-96 (1971)

SCAPAGNINI, U., PREZIOSI, P.: Role of brain norepinephrine and serotonin in the tonic and phasic regulation of hypothalamic hypophyseal adrenal axis. Arch. Int. Pharmacodyn. Suppl. 196, 205-220 (1972)

SIMON, M.L., GEORGE, R.: Diurnal variations in plasma corticosterone and growth hormone as correlated with regional variations in norepinephrine, dopamine and serotonin content of rat brain. Neuroendocrinology 17, 125-138 (1975)

SREBRO, B., LORENS, A.S.: Behavioral effects of selective midbrain Raphé lesions in the rat. Brain Res. 89, 103 (1975)

STEPHAN, F.K., ZUCKER, I.: Circadian rhythms in drinking behavior and locomotor activity of rats are eliminated by hypothalamic lesions. Proc. Nat. Acad. Sci. USA 69, 1583-1586 (1972)

SZAFARCZYK, A., IXART, G., MALAVAL, F., NOUGUIER-SOULE, J., ASSENMACHER, I.: Short-term effects of stereotaxic destruction of the suprachiasmatic nucleus on the diurnal rhythms of plasma ACTH and corticosterone and locomotor activity in rats. Proc. Int. Union Physiol. Sci. (Paris) Vol. XIII, Abstract 2179, p. 733 (1977)

TALEISNIK, K.S., MCCANN, S.M.: Effects of hypothalamic lesions on the secretion and storage of hypophyseal luteinizing hormone. Endocrinology 68, 263-272 (1961)

TELEGDY, G., VERMES, I., LISSAK, K.: Correlation between the diurnal rhythm of brain serotonin and plasma corticosterone in rats. In: Cellular and Molecular Bases of Neuroendocrine Processes. Endröczi, E. (ed.). Budapest: Académiai Kiaido, 1976, pp. 451-459

VERNIKOS-DANELLIS, J., BERGER, P., BARCHAS, J.D.: Brain serotonin and pituitary-adrenal function. Prog. Brain Res. 39, 301-310 (1973)

7. Circadian Rhythms Within and Outside Their Ranges of Entrainment

J. Aschoff

Circadian rhythms can be entrained to various periods not too far from their own "natural period". The size of this "range of entrainment" depends mainly on two factors: the degree of persistance of the oscillation (KLOTTER, 1960) and the strength of the entraining Zeitgeber. The term "strength" as used here comprises the physical characteristics of the Zeitgeber, especially its "amplitude", as well as the responsiveness of the biologic system to the entraining signals (ASCHOFF, 1960). Within the range of entrainment, the phase-angle difference between the rhythm and the Zeitgeber changes in a predictable manner, with increasingly leading phases towards long periods, and lagging phases towards short periods. Ranges of entrainment differ among species, but may also be different for various functions within an organism. In the following paragraphs, several of these aspects are discussed from a comparative aspect.

Phase-Angle Differences within the Range of Entrainment

To test the entrainability of circadian rhythms to various periods, the period of the Zeitgeber should be changed in small steps, because with too large steps entrainment may be lost before the "true" limits of range of entrainment are reached ("Haltebereich" versus "Fangbereich"; WEVER, 1962). An example of such an experiment presented in Figure 1 includes four sections of a longer record of activity from a Lesser Redpoll (*Acanthis flammea cabaret*) kept in light-dark cycles (LD) of low amplitude (5:1 lux) with interposed twilights. For the first ten days the cycle consists of 12 h 7.5 min L and 12 h 7.5 min D (T = 24.25 h). There is continuous activity (black marks) throughout the light-time, but onset of activity occurs already about 3 h before dawn. With a further increase of the T from 24.25 to 24.75, this positive phase-angle difference between onset of activity and dawn becomes larger, and eventually onset of activity occurs shortly after dusk, when the period is 24.75. A shortening of T to values below 24 h (not shown here), resulted in changes of the phase-angle difference in the opposite direction. The insert in Figure 1 shows the dependence of phase on T for the full range of entrainment.

As a second example, Figure 2 presents data derived from the activity records of mice. Peaks of activity, as indicated by the three symbols, occur shortly after "light-off" in the 24-h day, and progressively later as T is shortened to 23, 22, and 21 h. Two animals escape from the Zeitgeber at T = 20 h, and the third at T = 19. (When exposed to periods longer than 24 h, one of the animals lost entrainment at T = 28, and the two others at T = 29.) The insert in Figure 2 demonstrates the change of phase for two animals within their full range of entrainment. Outside the range of entrainment, the Zeitgeber still has an influence on the circadian system: the two animals that lost entrainment at the 20-h day, lock on to the Zeitgeber temporarily and then drift away again after a few periods. As a consequence of this "relative coordination" (ASCHOFF and WEVER, 1962; ASCHOFF, 1965; WEVER, 1972)

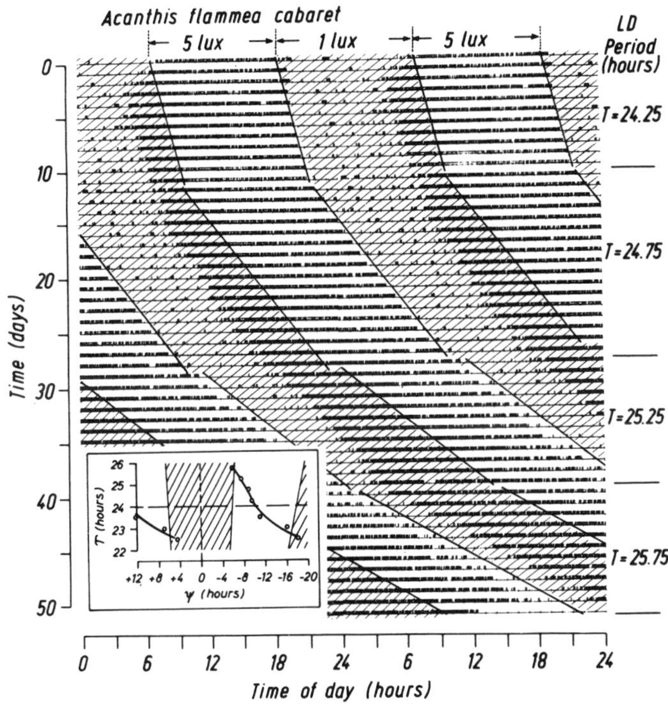

Fig. 1. Activity rhythm of a Lesser Redpoll (*Acanthis flammea cabaret*), entrained to light-dark cycles (5:1 lux) with periods (T) varying from 24.25 to 25.75 h. Original record duplicated along the abscissa. Oblique lines represent the mid-point of artificial 1-h twilights. Insert; mean phase-angle difference (Ψ) between midpoint of activity time (circles) and midpoint of dark-time at various Zeitgeber periods (T) for the full range of entrainment for three birds. (From ASCHOFF and POHL, 1978)

between rhythm and Zeitgeber, the mean period of the nonentrained rhythm is somewhat longer than it would be were it free-running without the influence of a Zeitgeber. A summary of these findings is given in Figure 3.

Within the range of entrainment, the changes of phase-angle difference between rhythm and Zeitgeber are similar for birds and for mice (cf. the inserts in Figs. 1 and 2). To compare data from different organisms, it is useful to express all phase-angles in angular degrees (instead of in h), with each Zeitgeber period corresponding to 360°. Such a procedure has been used to draw the "phase curves" shown in Figure 4, referring to the middle of dark-time as reference phase of the Zeitgeber (= zero degrees). The data from the Japanese Quail and from the rat are singled out by dashed lines because it is likely that in these experiments the extreme values of Zeitgeber period do not belong to the primary range of entrainment but to secondary ones, either at multiples or at submultiples of the circadian range (e.g., T = 13 in case of the quail, or T = 48 in case of the rat). Pecularities of these findings, that indicate partial entrainment, are discussed below. The protocols of the experiments on which the four solid lines are based suggest that the full ranges of entrainment had been exploited in these species. With an increase in range of entrainment, the slope of the phase curve decreases. The general validity of this rule has re-

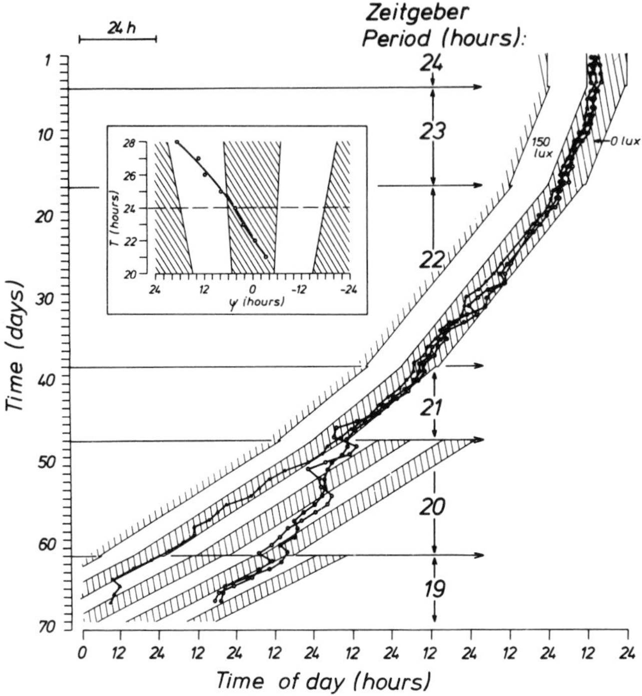

Fig. 2. Entrainment and loss of entrainment of the activity rhythms of three mice under the influence of light-dark cycles varying from 24 to 19 h. Points represent time of maximum motor activity. Insert, phase-angle difference (Ψ) between peak of activity (mean of two animals) and mid-point of dark-time at various Zeitgeber periods (T) for the full range of entrainment. (Data from TRIBUKAIT, 1956)

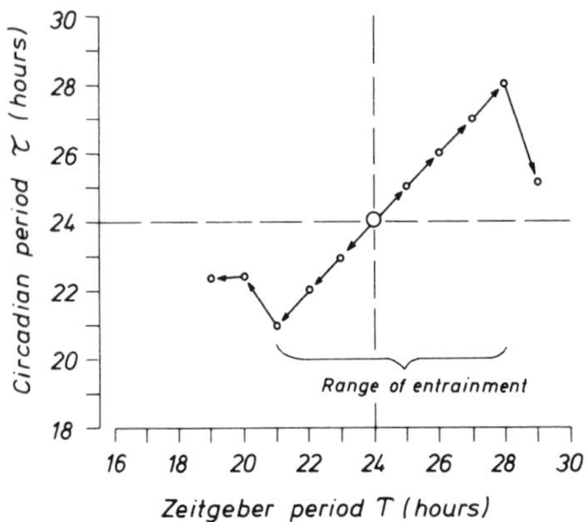

Fig. 3. Circadian period (τ) of the activity rhythm of mice (n = 2), drawn as a function of the period T of a light-dark cycle as Zeitgeber. (Data from TRIBUKAIT, 1956)

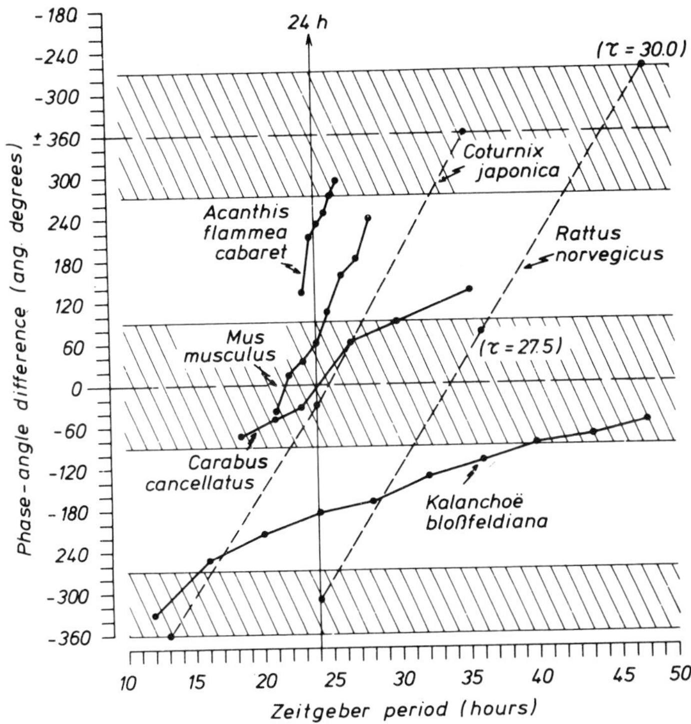

Fig. 4. Phase-angle difference between circadian rhythm and mid-point of dark-time, drawn as a function of Zeitgeber period. Shaded area, dark time. Rhythm measured and source: Activity for Acanthis (ASCHOFF and POHL, 1978), Mus (TRIBUKAIT, 1956) and Carabus (LAMPRECHT and WEBER, 1973). Leaf movement for Kalanchoe (BÜNSOW, 1953); Plasma corticosteroids for Cortunix (BOISSIN and ASSENMACHER, 1971) and Rattus (SZARFACZYK et al., 1974) (in parenthesis, second frequency component within that time series)

cently been discussed on the basis of data from 19 species (ASCHOFF and POHL, 1978). The 19 phase curves have been submitted to a simple regression analysis, and the regression coefficients have been found to be negatively correlated with the range of entrainment according to a hyperbolic function, indicating that within their full range of entrainment, most species change their phase-angle difference more or less by the same amount (Fig. 5).

The differences in ranges of entrainment as indicated in Figure 5 are representative in so far as, in general, larger ranges have been found in insects and plants than in mammals. This may be partly due to the fact that stronger Zeitgebers were applied to the lower organisms. A more detailed analysis, however, reveals that part of the difference must be explained by the effects of two other interfering factors: as compared to insects and plants, vertebrates are either less sensitive to the signals of the entraining light-dark cycles, or their oscillators have a higher degree of persistance (cf. the discussion in ASCHOFF and POHL, 1978).

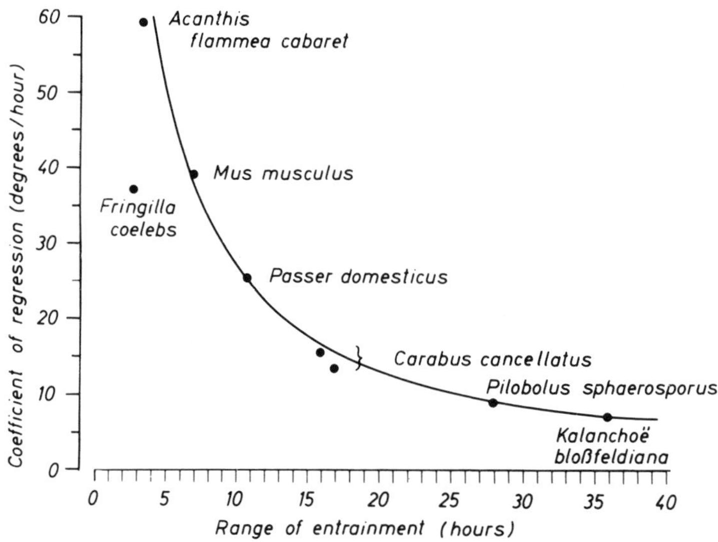

Fig. 5. Regression coefficients of phase curves (cf. Fig. 4), drawn as a function of range of entrainment. Hyperbola, Behavior of model oscillators that change their phase within their ranges of entrainment by 265°. Rhythm measured and source: Activity for *Acanthis* (ASCHOFF and POHL, 1978), *Fringilla* (WEVER, unpublished), *Mus* (TRIBUKAIT, 1956), *Passer* (ESKIN, 1971) and *Carabus* (LAMPRECHT and WEVER, 1973); Spore formation for *Pilobolus* (UEBELMESSER, 1954); Leaf movement for *Kalanchoe* (BÜNSOW, 1953)

Entrainment of Human Circadian Rhythms

Apart from observations in animals that demonstrate splitting of the activity rhythm into two components (for references cf. PITTENDRIGH and DAAN, 1976), it is mainly the phenomenon of spontaneous and forced "internal desynchronization", as observed in human subjects, that suggests a multioscillatory structure of the circadian system. As an introduction to this problem, a few facts about free-running circadian rhythms in man are presented. In complete isolation and without any time cue, about 66% of all subjects show free-running rhythms with periods close to 25 h (ASCHOFF and WEVER, 1976; WEVER, 1975a). Another 28% of the subjects lengthen their activity rhythms to periods of about 30 to 36 h. When this occurs, the rhythms of autonomic functions such as body temperature or urine excretion separate from the activity rhythm and continue to free-run with periods close to 25 h. This phenomenon is called *spontaneous internal desynchronization*. Since the different rhythmic functions can be considered to be controlled by separate oscillators which are usually coupled to each other, internal desynchronization represents a loss of coupling between previously entrained oscillators, and hence suggests smaller ranges of entrainment for rhythms of autonomic functions than for the activity rhythm (WEVER, 1975a).

Stronger support for the hypothesis that ranges of entrainment differ among various rhythmic functions comes from experiments in which attempts have been made to entrain human circadian rhythms to periods deviating from 24 h in an isolation unit (ASCHOFF et al., 1969; WEVER,

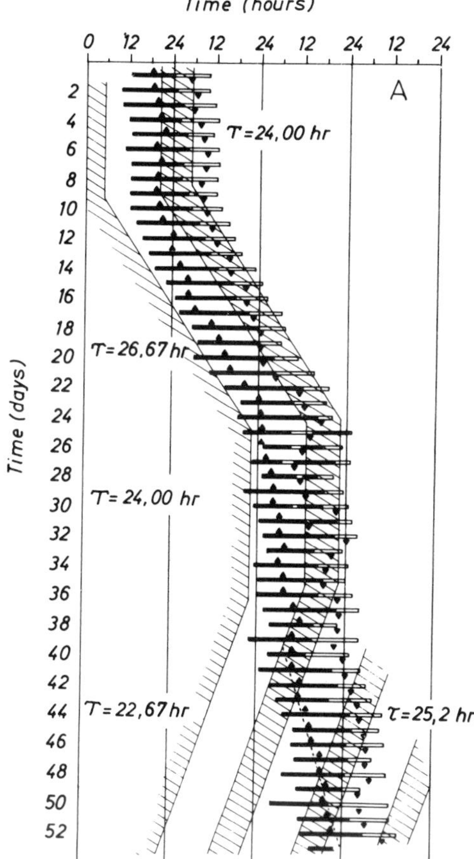

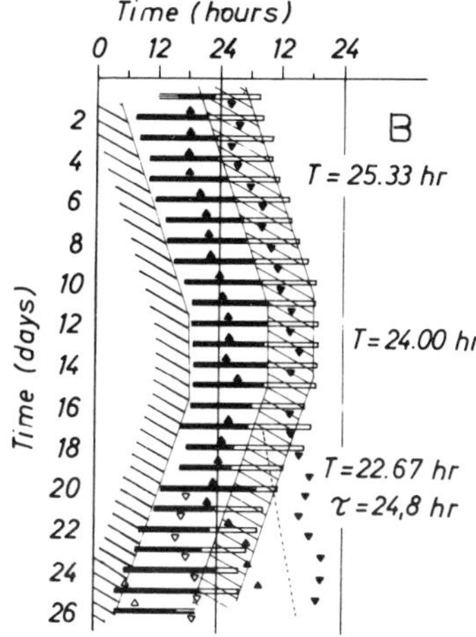

Fig. 6A, B. Circadian rhythms of isolated subjects under the influence of light-dark cycles with added gong signals. ("Weak" Zeitgeber: reading lamps available). Horizontal black and white bars, wakefulness and sleep. Triangles, maxima (above bars) and minima (below bars) for rectal temperature. Shaded area, darkness. T, Zeitgeber period; τ, circadian period. (Fig. 6A from ASCHOFF et al., 1969; Fig. 6B from WEVER, 1977)

1970). The main lights at the ceiling, which together with regular gong signals serve as the Zeitgeber, are controlled externally, while the subject can make use of small reading lamps as desired. As a consequence, the subject has his choice either to follow the Zeitgeber or to ignore it. Examples of entrainment to such a "weak" Zeitgeber as well as of failure of entrainment are given in Figure 6A and B. The following general features of entrainment are illustrated in Figure 6A: (1) In the 24-h day, the subject keeps a substantial negative phase-angle difference between awakening and light-on which becomes zero and even positive after T has been changed to 26.67 h; (2) The internal phase-angle difference between rectal temperature and the activity rhythm changes into the same direction; (3) When, after the change for 12 days to T = 24, T is shortened to 22.67 h, entrainment is lost, and the now free-running rhythm "crosses" through the Zeitgeber with a slight indication of relative coördination. The conclusion to be drawn is that, given this subject and the special type of a weak Zeitgeber, a period of 26.67 h is within, and a period of 22.67 h outside the range of entrainment for both the rhythms of activity and of rectal temperature. In contrast to this experiment in which the circadian system remained internally snychronized, the data reproduced in Figure 6B demonstrate a case of "forced" internal desynchronization. The rhythms of activity and of rectal temperature are both entrained to 25.33 and to 24.00 h, but in the 22.67-h day only the activity rhythm remains entrained, while the rhythm of rectal temperature starts to free-run with a mean period of 24.8 h.

Forced internal desynchronization, as examplified in Figure 6B, can be attained readily under conditions in which no reading lamps are available, i.e., conditions in which the subject has no alternative but to follow the Zeitgeber at least with his activity rhythm. Entrainment of a subject to such a "strong" Zeitgeber is shown in Figure 7.

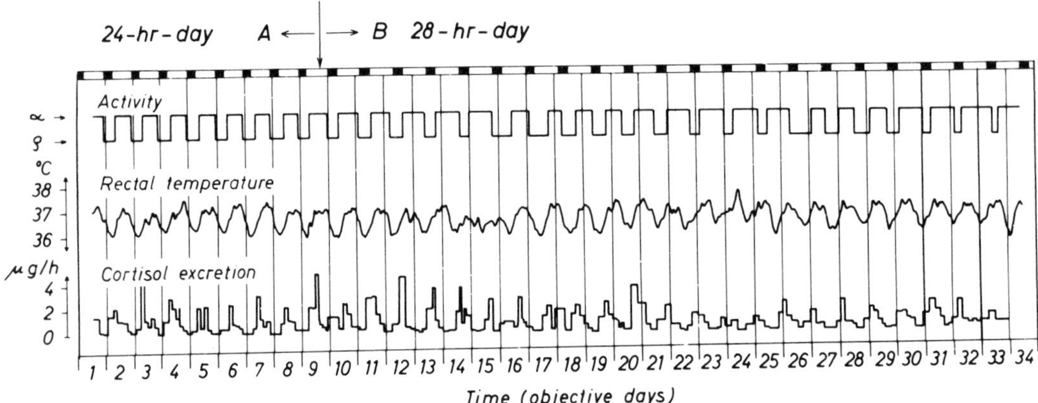

Fig. 7. Circadian rhythms of wakefulness (α) and sleep (ρ), rectal temperature and urinary cortisol excretion in an isolated subject exposed first to a 24-h day, thereafter to a 28-h day (light and dark indicated by white and black bars on top of the diagram; from WEVER, 1975b)

As expected, the activity rhythm follows the Zeitgeber in the 24-h day as well as in the 28-h day. Contrary to this, the rhythms of rectal temperature and of urinary cortisol excretion, while being entrained in the 24-h day, free run in the 28-h day with a common period of about 25 h. To demonstrate this more clearly, power spectra computed separately for the two parts of the experiment are presented in Figure 8. The time series obtained during exposure to a 28-h day (part B), shows a predominant peak for activity at the Zeitgeber period, while temperature and cortisol have their main peaks at a period of 24.8 h.

Intra-Individual Differences in the Entrainability of Rhythms

From the findings discussed in the foregoing paragraphs two conclusions can be drawn: (1) the circadian system consists of a multiplicity of oscillators that are usually coupled to each other, that change their phase-angle differences within the range of entrainment, and that may become uncoupled either spontaneously or under the influence of artificial Zeitgebers; (2) the experiments with forced internal desynchronization demonstrate large differences in the entrainability of various circadian rhythms within one organism.

In Table 1, results from experiments carried out in the isolation unit with "strong" Zeitgebers are listed under No. 1. In all four conditions (T = 20 h through T = 32 h) the activity rhythms of the subjects

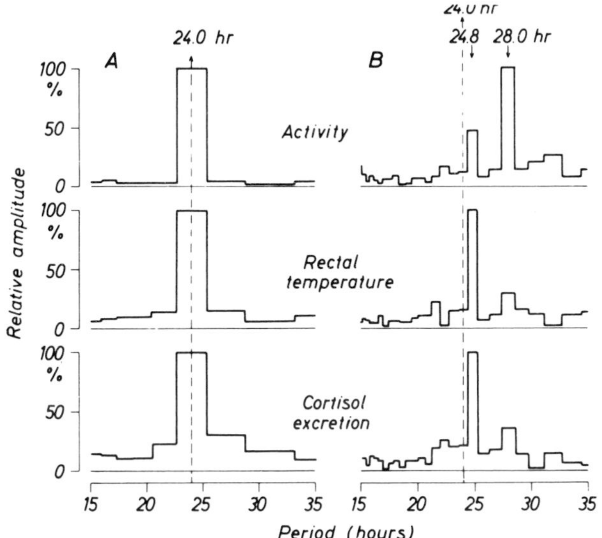

Fig. 8. Power spectra of three circadian rhythms measured in an isolated subject, exposed first to a 24-h day (A), thereafter to a 28-h day (B) (cf. Fig. 7; from WEVER, 1975b)

Table 1. Survey of experiments showing forced internal desynchronization

Species	T (hours)	Variable	τ (hours)	τ (hours)
1. Man (Isolation Unit)	20	Activity	20.0	(25.0)
		Body temp.	25.0	(20.0)
	28	Activity	28.0	(24.8)
		Body temp.	28.0	24.8
		Urine cortisol	24.8	(28.0)
	30	Activity	30.0	(24.9)
		Body temp.	24.8	(30.0)
	32	Activity	32.0	(24.8)
		Body temp.	24.8	
2. Man (Spitzbergen)	22	Activity	22	
		Urine potassium	22	24
3. Man (Spitzbergen)	21	Activity	21	
		Body temp.	21	
		Urine volume	21	(24)
		potassium	24	21
	27	Activity	27	
		Body temp.	27	
		Urine potassium	24	(27)
4. Man (Spitzbergen)	21	Activity	21	
		Urine 17-OHCS	24.2	
		potassium	24.3	
		sodium	24.0	
5. Rat	36	Activity	36.0	(26.0)
		Plasma corticost.	27.5	(36.0)
	48	Activity	48.0	(25.5)
		Plasma corticost.	30.0	(48.0)

T, Zeitgeber period. τ, circadian period; First figure, main component; Second figure, minor component in the period analysis (if not in parenthesis: both components of about equal weight). Sources: 1. WEVER (1977); 2. LEWIS and LOBBAN (1956); 3. LEWIS and LOBBAN (1957a, b); 4. SIMPSON et al. (1970); 5. SZAFACZYK et al. (1974).

were entrained to the Zeitgeber (main peak in the power spectrum corresponding with the period of the Zeitgeber), while the rhythms of autonomic functions were free-running with periods close to 25 h. Comparable results have been obtained from human subjects living in Spitzbergen on abnormal time schedules (LEWIS and LOBBAN, 1956, 1957a, 1957b; SIMPSON and LOBBAN, 1968; SIMPSON et al., 1970). While in the first two of these studies (Table 1, Nos. 2 and 3) it can still be questioned whether the about 24-h components observed in some variables represent free-running rhythms or entrainment to a still-present Zeitgeber (cf. the discussion to LOBBAN, 1960), the data of the third study as summarized under No. 4 strongly suggest that the rhythms of urinary constituents were free-running during the 21-h routine. In a recent study with 25 subjects living in an isolation unit on either 21- or 27-h days, MILLS and coworkers (1976) observed two frequency components in the rhythms of body temperature and urinary constituents (a 24-h component, and a component corresponding with the artificial day.)

There are, finally, data from experiments on rats (SZAFARCZYK et al., 1974) that suggest forced internal desynchronization (Table 1, No. 5; cf. also Fig. 4). As in the human data, two frequency components have been extracted from the time series of the two variables measured. The major component in the activity rhythm corresponds to the Zeitgeber period, while the analysis of plasma corticosteroids indicates free-running rhythms. This is not surprising in case of T = 36 h, but noteworthy for T = 48 h in which entrainment to the Zeitgeber in a 1:2 ratio could have been expected.

The observations of internal desynchronization, of differences in entrainability between variables, and of two frequency components in the times series of desynchronized rhythms can be incorporated into and even demand the hypothesis that the circadian system consists of more than one basic oscillator, and that the various overt rhythms are influenced by all oscillators, but to different extents. (For details cf. WEVER, 1975a.)

Conclusions

In physiology, a sequence of events is often viewed as a sequence of causes and effects. That such a point of view, fruitful as it may be in many cases, can lead to a misinterpretation of observations is clearly demonstrated by the facts reviewed in the three foregoing sections. The drastic changes in mutual phase-relationships between rhythmic function, and more so the phenomena of spontaneous and forced internal desynchronization contradict a simple cause-and-effect relationship (e.g., between activity and temperature, or hormone secretion), but point to a more complex system with some degree of independence among at least some variables. Under these aspects, it may be useful to reconsider, not the least in endocrinology, accepted doctrines on interactions within the organism as well as with the environment.

References

ASCHOFF, J.: Exogenous and endogenous components in circadian rhythms. Cold Spring Horbor Symp. Quant. Biol. 25, 11-28 (1960)

ASCHOFF, J.: Response curves in circadian periodicity. In: Circadian Clocks. Aschoff, J. (ed.). Amsterdam: North Holland, 1965, pp. 95-111

ASCHOFF, J., PÖPPEL, E., WEVER, R.: Circadiane Periodik des Menschen unter dem Einfluß von Licht-Dunkel-Wechseln unterschiedlicher Periode. Pflügers Arch. 306, 58-70 (1969)

ASCHOFF, J., POHL, H.: Phase-relations between a circadian rhythm and its zeitgeber within the range of entrainment. Naturwissenschaften 65, 80-84 (1978)

ASCHOFF, J., WEVER, R.: Biologische Rhythmen und Regelung. In: Probleme der zentralnervösen Regulation. Bad-Oeynhausener Gespräche V. Berlin-Göttingen-Heidelberg: Springer, 1962, pp. 1-15

ASCHOFF, J., WEVER, R.: Human circadian rhythms: A multi-oscillatory system. Federation Proc. 35, 2326-2332 (1976)

BOISSIN, J., ASSENMACHER, I.: Entrainment of the adrenal cortical rhythm and of the locomotor activity rhythm by ahemeral photoperiods in the quail. J. Interdiscipl. Cycle Res. 2, 437-443 (1971)

BÜNSOW, R.: Endogene Tagesrhythmik und Photoperiodismus bei Kalanchoe Blassfeldiana. Planta 42, 220-252 (1953)

ESKIN, A.: Some properties of the system controlling the circadian activity rhythm of sparrows. In: Biochronometry. Menaker, M. (ed.). Nat. Acad. Sci. USA 1971, 55-80

KLOTTER, K.: General properties of oscillating systems. Cold Spring Harbor Symp. Quant. Biol. 25, 185-187 (1960)

LAMPRECHT, G., WEBER, F.: Mitnahme, Frequenzmultiplikation und Maskierung der Laufaktivität von Carabus-Arten (Coleoptera) durch Lichtzyklen. J. Insect. Physiol. 19, 1579-1590 (1973)

LEWIS, P.R., LOBBAN, M.C.: Patterns of electrolyte excretion in human subjects during a prolonged period of life on a 22-hour day. J. Physiol. 133, 670-680 (1956)

LEWIS, P.R., LOBBAN, M.C.: The effects of prolonged periods of life on abnormal time routines upon excretory rhythms in human subjects. Quart. J. Exp. Physiol. 42, 356-370 (1957a)

LEWIS, P.R., LOBBAN, M.C.: Dissociation of diurnal rhythms in human subjects living on abnormal time routines. Quart. J. Exp. Physiol. 42, 371-386 (1957b)

LOBBAN, M.: The entrainment of circadian rhythms in man. Cold Spring Harbor Symp. Quant. Biol. 25, 325-332 (1960)

MILLS, J.N., MINORS, D.S.: Waterhouse: Urinary and temperature rhythms on days of abnormal length. J. Physiol. 257, 54-55P (1976)

PITTENDRIGH, C.S., DAAN, S.: A functional analysis of circadian pacemakers in nocturnal rodents. V. Pacemaker structure: a clock for all seasons. J. Comp. Physiol. 106, 333-355 (1976)

SIMPSON, H.W., LOBBAN, M.C.: Effect of a 21-hour day on the human circadian excretory rhythms of 17-hydroxycorticosteroids and electrolytes. Aerospace Med. 38, 1205-1213 (1968)

SIMPSON, H.W., LOBBAN, M.C., HALBERG, F.: Arctic chronobiology. Urinary near 24-hour rhythms in subjects living on a 21-hour routine in the arctic. Arctic Anthropology 7, 144-164 (1970)

SCAFARCZYK, A., NOUGUIER-SOULÉ, J., ASSENMACHER, I.: Diurnal locomotor and plasma corticosterone rhythms in rats living on photoperiodically lengthened 'days'. Int. J. Chronobiol. 2, 373-382 (1974)

TRIBUKAIT, B.: Die Aktivitätsperiodik der weißen Maus im Kunsttag von 16 bis 29 Stunden Länge. Z. Vergl. Physiol. 38, 479-490 (1956)

UEBELMESSER, E.R.: Über den endogenen Tagesrhythmus der Sporangienträgerbildung von Pilobolus. Arch. Mikrobiol. 20, 1-33 (1954)

WEVER, R.: Zum Mechanismus der biologischen 24-Stunden-Periodik. Kybernetik 1, 139-151 (1962)

WEVER, R.: Virtual synchronization towards the limits of the range of entrainment. J. Theoret. Biol. 36, 119-132 (1972)

WEVER, R.: Zur Zeitgeber-Stärke eines Licht-Dunkel-Wechsels für die circadiane Periodik des Menschen. Pflügers Arch. 321, 133-142 (1970)

WEVER, R.: The circadian multi-oscillator system of man. Int. J. Chronobiol. 3, 19-55 (1975a)

WEVER, R.: Die Bedeutung der circadianen Periodik für den alternden Menschen. Verh. Deut. Ges. Path. 59, 160-180 (1975b)

WEVER, R.: The circadian system of man. Berlin-Heidelberg-New York: Springer, 1978

8. Effects of Ahemeral Environmental Periodicities on the Rhythms of Adrenocortical and Locomotor Functions in Rats and Japanese Quail

A. SZAFARCZYK, J. BOISSIN, J. NOUGUIER-SOULÉ, and I. ASSENMACHER

In the view of modern concepts in chronobiology, the diurnal biologic rhythms result from the entrainment of endogenous rhythms by periodic environmental factors. The endogenous periodicities of "biologic clocks" which can be measured by exposing animals to nonrhythmic environments, usually extend within a circadian range, i.e., close to 24 h, so that most biologic rhythms are completely entrained by the natural environment.

Among other experimental approaches to the general mechanism of the endogenous oscillators that constitute the biologic clocks, one consists of the exploration of the plasticity or flexibility of endogenous periodicities, towards environmental Zeitgebers, with periods different from the endogenous periodicity, and different from the 24-h natural environmental period. Since the daily light-dark cycle provides the major Zeitgeber for a great variety of animal species, artificial, non-24-h light-dark cycles are commonly used in experimental studies involving the manipulation of biologic rhythms.

The following data relate to studies on two photoperiodically controlled animal models, the "nocturnal" Albino Rat, and the "diurnal" Japanese Quail. Two biologic rhythms considered were (1) the locomotor activity, as measured from actographic cages provided with piezoelectric transducers for the numerical recording of their oscillations, and (2) the closely related adrenocortical rhythm, as measured by the plasma concentrations of corticosterone (protein-binding assay). The periods of the locomotor rhythms were estimated by a spectral analysis, whereas Halberg's least-square method was used for the corticosterone rhythm.

Figure 1 illustrates the span of endogenous rhythms recorded for both species in different nonfluctuating environments ranging from constant darkness (DD) to constant light (LL) at various lighting levels.

Both species conform to "Aschoff's Rule" in that the endogenous period decreases (from 24.10 h to 21.30 h) with increasing light intensities in the "diurnal" quail, whereas the inverse relationship occurs in the "nocturnal" rat, i.e., increasing periods (from 24.2 h to 26.0 h) with increasing levels of light intensity.

Now if animals are exposed to environmental periods different from their endogenous periodicity, the spectral analysis indicates three possible responses (a) if entrainment is complete, the only period that appears in the power spectrum is the exogenous, environmental period; (b) if entrainment is incomplete, an endogenous periodicity "escapes" partially from the Zeitgeber, and two prominent periods, the exogenous and an endogenous, are present on the spectrum; (c) if entrainment is definitely impossible, the endogenous rhythm escapes completely from the exogenous Zeitgeber, and only the endogenous period is apparent on the spectrum.

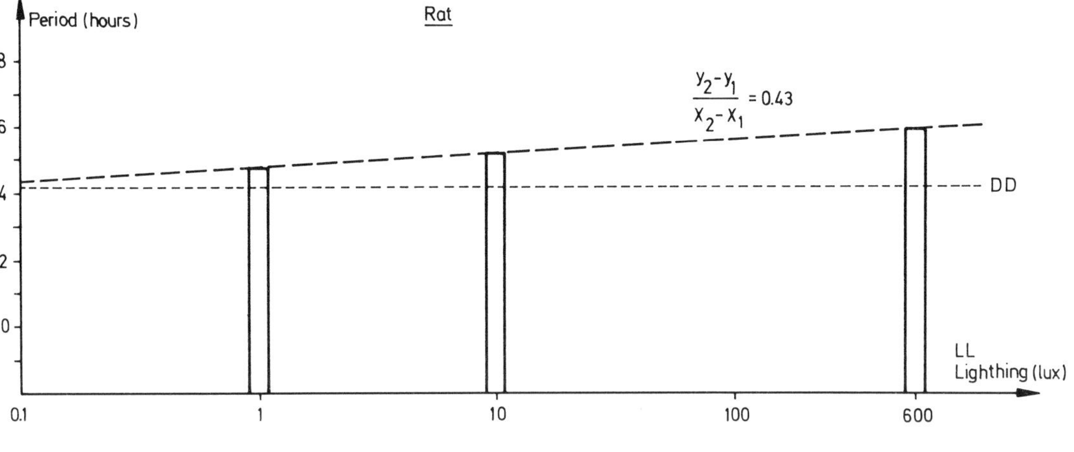

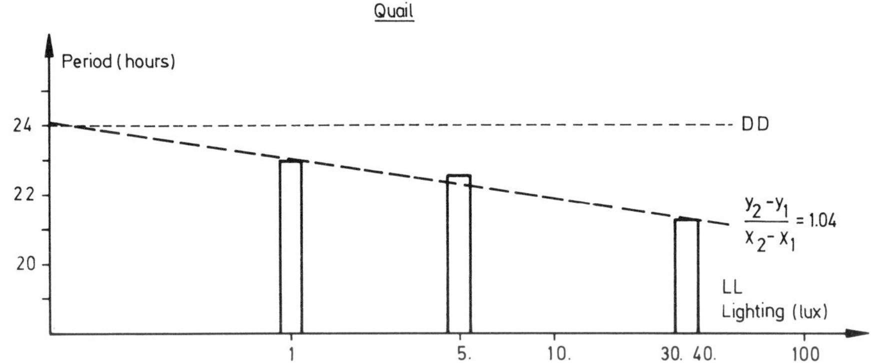

Fig. 1. Endogenous periods of locomotor activity rhythms in rats and Japanese Quail

Table 1, which summarizes the experimental data, shows that the plasticity of the endogenous rhythm of rats is rather low. Taking 25 h as the mean endogenous periodicity of rats (Fig. 1), it appears that lengthening or shortening the environmental period by 2 h (i.e., 27 h or 23 h respectively) was compatible with a full entrainment of the biologic rhythms. However, lengthening or shortening the exogenous period by 4 h (i.e., 29 h or 21 h respectively) led already to a partial escape of an endogenous rhythmicity. Finally, the only situation in which a biologic rhythm escaped completely was with an exogenous period of 13 h, in which no periodicity other than circadian could be detected in the corticosterone rhythm.

On the other hand, Japanese Quail display an amazing plasticity in endogenous rhythms, since entrainment was still complete for both biologic rhythms with environmental periods of either 35 h or 13 h. The corticosterone rhythm became free-running for an environmental period of 6 h, whereas the locomotor rhythm showed a partial escape for the extremely short environmental period of 3 h.

In conclusion, it can be stated that (1) The flexibility of endogenous rhythms towards environmental periodicities differs with respect to

Table 1. Plasticity of endogenous rhythms in rat and Japanese Quail

Period of environment	Photoperiodic regime	Prominent periodicities (h)			
		Locomotor activity		Plasma corticosterone	
		Exogenous	Endogenous	Exogenous	Endogenous
Rat					
48 h	28L-20D	48	25.5	48	Circadian
36 h	21L-15D	36	26	36	Circadian
29 h	14L-15D	29	25.8		
27 h	13L-14D	27	-	27	-
23 h	11L-12D	23	-	23	-
21 h	10L-11D	21	25.2		
13 h	6L- 7D	13	25.2	-	Circadian
Quail					
35 h	26L- 9D	35	-	35	-
13 h	6L- 7D	13	-	13	-
6 h	4L- 2D	6	-	-	Circadian
3 h	2L- 1D	3	24.3		

Nota: Dash means that no periodicity was detectable in this range.

species. Rats exhibit a particularly low palsticity that allows no more than ± 2 h range of environmental periodicity for a full entrainment of the endogenous periodicity; (2) The plasticity of different biologic rhythms in the same organism may be different. In the two biologic rhythms studied, the locomotor rhythm could be entrained farther from the endogenous period than the corticosterone rhythm, which could lead to an internal desynchronization between the two rhythms.

9. Problems of Re-entrainment of Circadian Rhythms: Asymmetry Effect, Dissociation and Partition

J. ASCHOFF

Entrained circadian rhythms maintain a more or less distinct phase-angle difference with respect to the Zeitgeber (ASCHOFF, 1965). After a sudden shift of the Zeitgeber, several periods are required to re-establish this phase relationship. Usually, the circadian system follows advance shifts of the Zeitgeber by advances, and delay shifts by delays. However, with 12-hour shifts of the Zeitgeber (= 180° shift), the circadian system may go through advance shifts despite the 50% lengthening of one Zeitgeber period. Further, within an organism, some rhythms may follow the Zeitgeber, while others move into the opposite direction: re-entrainment by "partition". There is, finally, the phenomenon of "asymmetry", in which the time necessary for re-entrainment differs between advance and delay shifts.

The Ambiguity of 12-Hour Shifts

A light-dark cycle (LD) of 12L 12D can be shifted by 180° by doubling either L or D once. The activity rhythm of Chaffinches (*Fringilla coelebs*) entrained to such a Zeitgeber follows a doubling of D by delay (ASCHOFF and WEVER, 1963). The pattern after a doubling of L is illustrated in Figure 1. In the lower record, the 24 h of L on the third day result

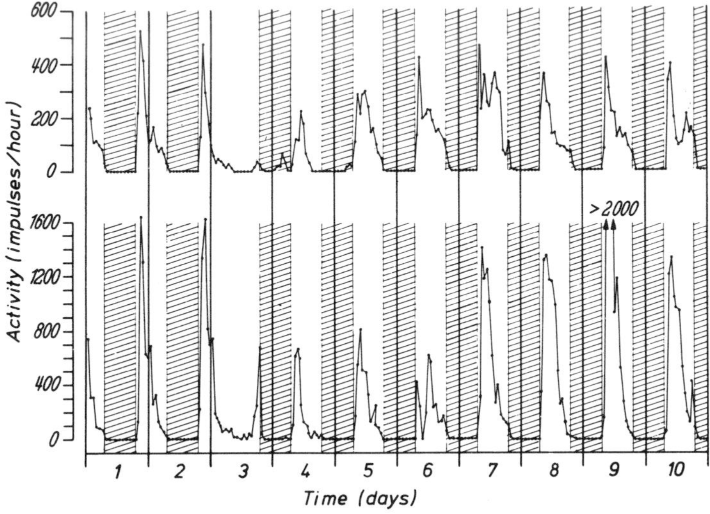

Fig. 1. Activity rhythms of two Chaffinches (*Fringilla coelebs*) kept in light-dark cycles and exposed to a 12-h phase shift at day 3. White area, 250 lux; shaded area, 0.5 lux. (From ASCHOFF and WEVER, 1963)

in two activity peaks of similar size which follow each other within about 13 h. The upper record shows three peaks of different sizes, the first two of which can hardly be interpreted as reflecting a true circadian period. The interpretation could then be that the lower diagram represents advance transients, the upper one a delay. A survey of the behavior of 22 finches is given in Figure 2. Onsets of activity are drawn for consecutive days after the shift of the Zeitgeber on

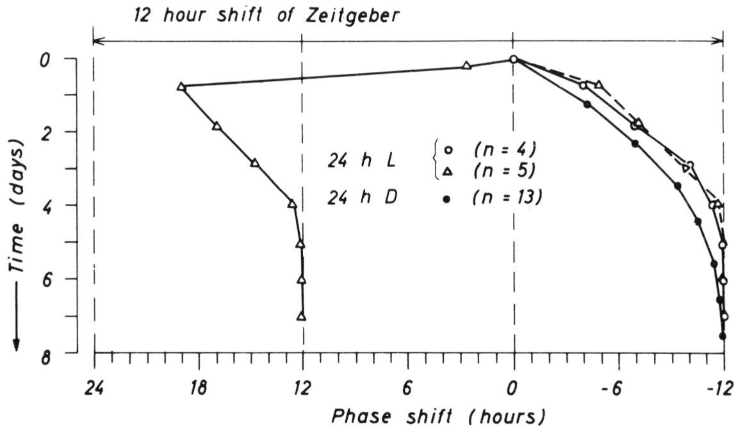

Fig. 2. Phase shift of the activity rhythms of Chaffinches (*Fringilla coelebs*) due to a 12-h shift of the entraining light-dark cycle at day zero, accomplished by either doubling one light-time (open symbols) or doubling one dark-time (closed circles). Zero on the abscissa: onset of activity before shift. Triangles connected by dashed line, replot of data from the left side after omission of first post-shift onset of activity. (Data from ASCHOFF and WEVER, 1963)

day zero. All 13 birds exposed to 24 D follow the Zeitgeber by a delay. Of the 9 exposed to 24 L, four had a pattern similar to that of the upper record in Figure 1, i.e., they showed clear delay shifts. The other five birds had a pattern similar to that of the lower record in Figure 1, and hence their data are plotted as advance shifts. However, considering the unusual shortness of the first post-shift period, as well as the overshoot of phase resulting from this interpretation, it may be justified to consider the first peak as an "artifact", and to omit it from the calculation of periods. If the data are replotted in this way the resulting delay shifts are indistinguishable from the "true" delay shifts. This example shows that there can be some arbitrariness in the interpretation of such experiments as to the part of the data that represents the real motion of the circadian system.

A somewhat more complex example has been provided by BOISSIN et al. (1975), who measured locomotor activity and plasma corticosteroids in the Japanese Quail (*Coturnix coturnix*). According to the analysis of the authors, the activity rhythm, unlike that of the finches, shows advance shifts after doubling of either L or D. The corticosteroid data, which are reproduced in Figure 3, are less easy to interpret. In the upper diagram (doubling of D) two short periods are followed by a very long one; lower diagram (doubling of L) either suggests an extreme long first period (i.e., a delay shift with an immediate resetting of the phase by more than 12 h) or, if the small intermediate elevation is taken into account, an advance shift. In Figure 4, the results obtained with quail are compared with those obtained with finches. The quail

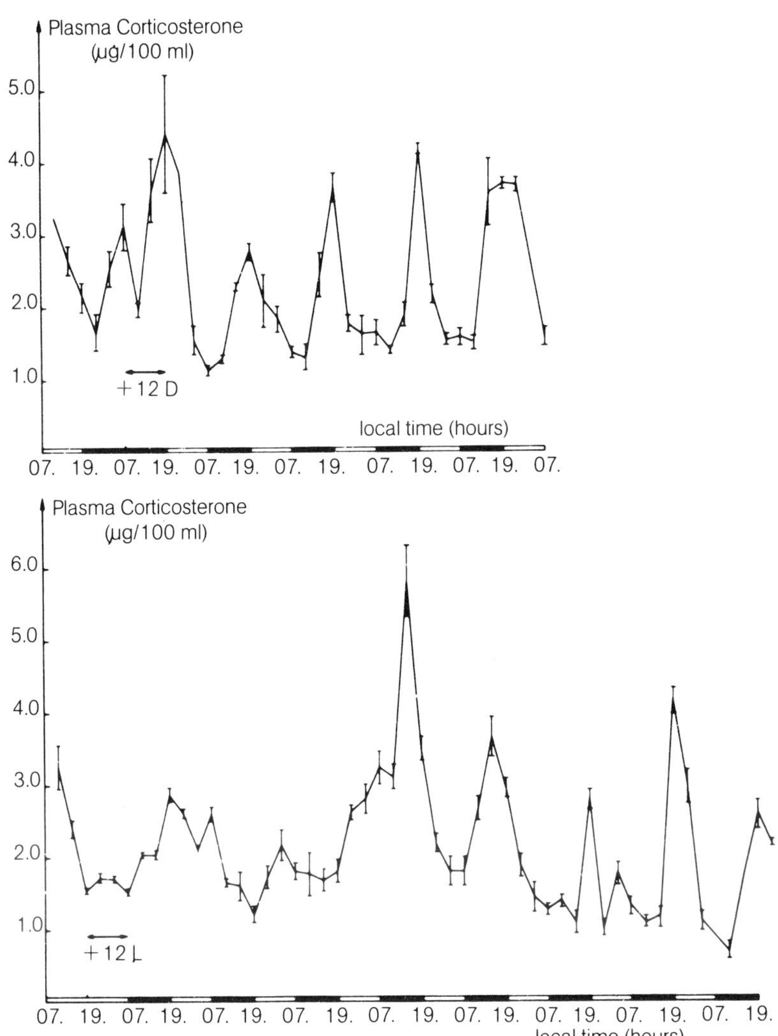

Fig. 3. Circadian rhythms of plasma corticosteroids in two Japanese Quail (*Coturnix coturnix*) kept in light-dark cycles (white and black bars, 4 and 0 lux) and exposed to 12-h phase shift by either doubling one dark-time (above) or one light time (below). (From BOISSIN et al., 1975)

data, although subject to alternative interpretations, at least permit assumption that after a Zeitgeber shift of 12 h, two components of the circadian system move into opposite directions. Further evidence for such a "partition" of the circadian system during re-entrainment is given below.

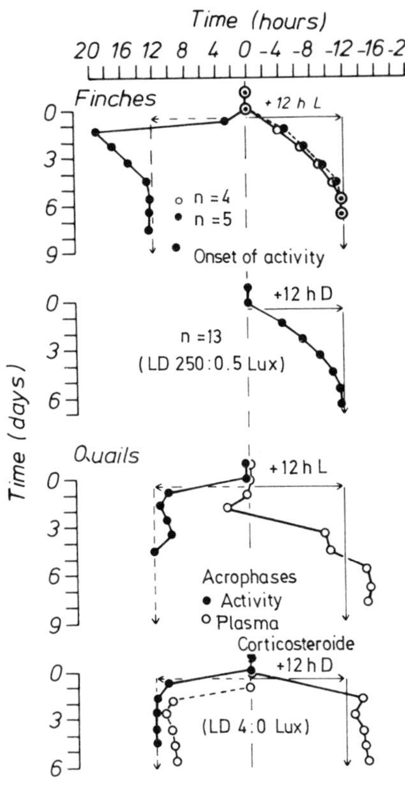

Fig. 4. Shift of circadian rhythms after 12-hour phase shifts of the entraining light-dark cycles at day zero, in Chaffinches (*Fringilla coelebs*) (above) and in Japanese Quail (*Coturnix coturnix*) (below). Zero on the abscissa is the phase of the rhythm before shift. Symbols connected by dashed lines are alternative interpretation of the data connected by solid lines. (Data for finches from ASCHOFF and WEVER, 1963; for quails from BOISSIN et al., 1975)

The Asymmetry Effect

After 6-h shifts of the Zeitgeber, rates of re-entrainment differ for advances and for delays. In experiments with chaffinches, 90% of re-entrainment was achieved within 2.5 days after the advance shift, and in 4.5 days after the delay shift (ASCHOFF and WEVER, 1963). Opposite results were obtained with rats: re-entrainment lasted 8.5 days after the advance, and 4.5 days after the delay shift (HALBERG et al., 1971). According to more recent publications, Japanese Quail agree with the finch pattern (BOISSIN et al., 1975), and Fruit Bats (*Rousettus aegyptiacus*) with the rat pattern (ERKERT, 1976; Fig. 5). The systematic difference in the asymmetry effect, either between birds and mammals, or between day-active and night-active species, must be related to differences in response curves, and most likely is related to differences in "prevailing" values of the circadian period τ, as indicated by the known relationship between shape of response curve and τ-values measured in DD (DAAN and PITTENDRIGH, 1976a), and by their dependence on light intensity in constant conditions (DAAN and PITTENDRIGH, 1976b).

For model oscillations, a strong dependence of the asymmetry effect on τ has been demonstrated by WEVER (1966). For τ-values shorter than 24.5 h, re-entrainment is more rapid after an advance than after a delay shift; the opposite holds for long τ-values. The hypothesis that it is not a difference between birds and mammals but between day and night activity that determines the asymmetry effect (ASCHOFF et al., 1975) is supported by the activity rhythm of a day-active lizard (*La-*

certa viridis) which follows the finch pattern (FISCHER, 1961), and by that of a night-active beetle (*Tribolim confusum*) which conforms to the rat pattern (CHIBA et al., 1973). [It should be noted, however, that an exception to the rule is in re-entrainment of the Golden Hamster (*Mesocricetus auratus*) which is slower after a 6-h delay than after an advance shift (POHL, 1978)]. The problem, of course, is closely related to the entrainment strategy of diurnal and nocturnal species in general (PITTENDRIGH and DAAN, 1976).

The average rate of re-entrainment differs generally between the two groups of animals by a factor of two, 102 min/day for day-active species, and 57 min/day for night-active species. This agrees with data summarized by HOFFMANN (1969), as well as with the observation that ranges of entrainment seem to be somewhat larger in (day-active) birds than with (night-active) mammals (ASCHOFF and POHL, 1978). The difference in mean re-entrainment time between the two groups cannot readily be explained on the basis of differences in light intensity used in the various experiments (Fig. 5; paranthesis); they therefore reflect differences either in oscillator characteristics, such as degree of persistance (KLOTTER, 1960), or in sensitivity to entraining signals (cf. the discussion in ASCHOFF and POHL, 1978).

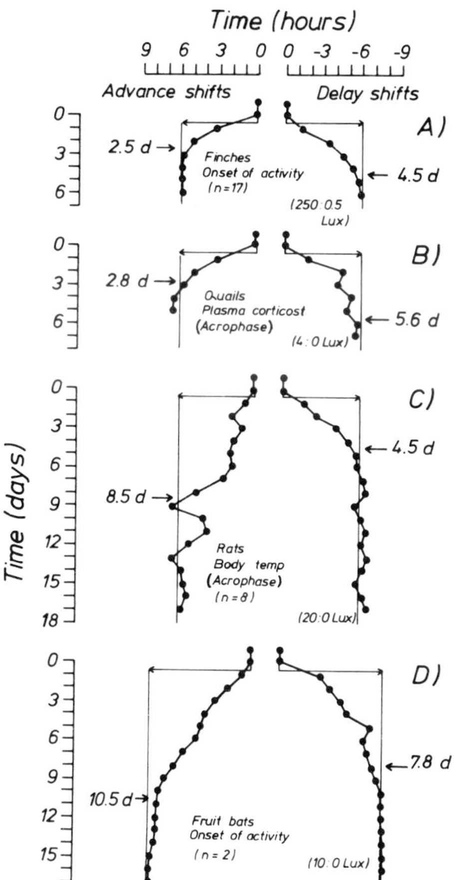

Fig. 5A-D. Shift of circadian rhythms after phase shifts of the Zeitgeber at day 0. Zero on the abscissa is phase of rhythm before shift. On the left and right margin, time (in days) for 90% re-entrainment. Species and source: A, *Fringilla coelebs* (ASCHOFF and WEVER, 1963), B, *Coturnix coturnix* (BOISSIN et al., 1975), C Sprague-Dawley rat (HALBERG et al., 1971), D, *Rousettus aegyptiacus*. (ERKERT, 1976)

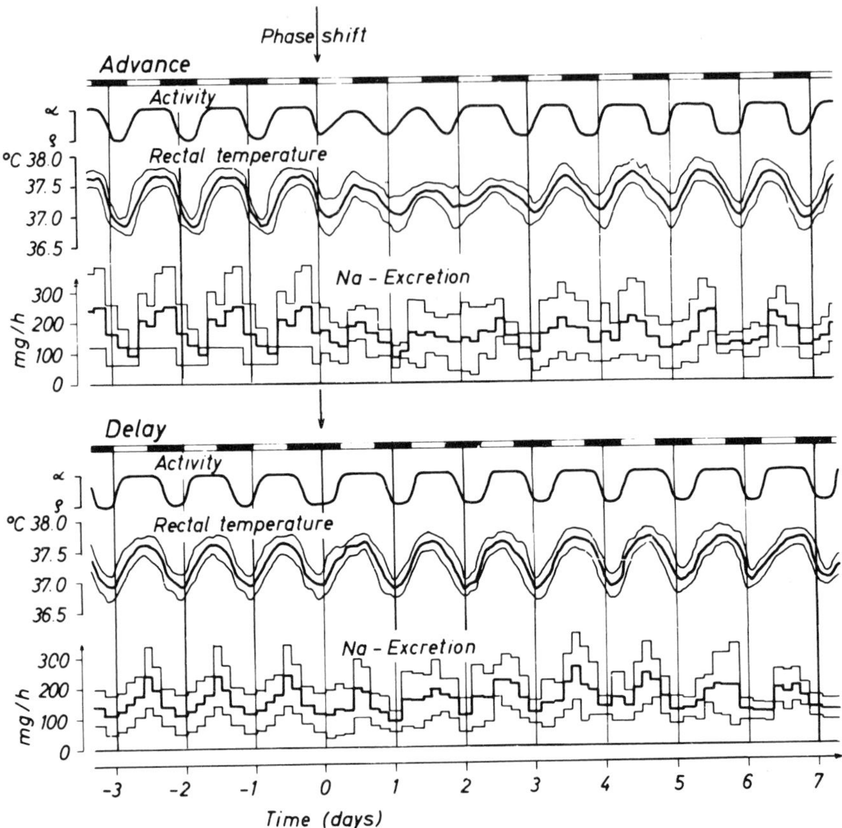

Fig. 6. Circadian rhythms of wakefulness (α) and sleep (ρ), of rectal temperature, and of urinary sodium excretion before and after a 6-h phase shift of the Zeitgeber (light and regular gong signals). Light and dark indicated by white and black bars (additional reading lamps available). Means and standard deviations (envelopes) from six subjects (4 kept singly, 2 as a group). (From WEVER, 1977)

Phase shifts of human circadian rhythms have been studied after trans-meridianal flights, after a shift of sleep-time in the laboratory or in field conditions, and after exposure to shifts of artificial Zeitgebers in isolation units (Fig. 6; for references, cf. ASCHOFF et al., 1975). The results (Fig. 6) can be summarized as follows (1) in all variables measured, an advance shift of 6 h is followed by advances, a delay shift of 6 h by delays, (2) the various rhythmic functions are re-entrained at different rates, resulting in transitory temporal disorder within the organism. This phenomenon, known from animal experiments as well (for references, cf. ASCHOFF et al., 1975), has been called "internal dissociation", and should not be confused with true "internal desynchronization" (ASCHOFF and WEVER, 1976); (3) the mean shift rate is greater after the advance shift (80 min/day, averaged from all variables) than for the delay shift (57 min/day); (4) the amplitudes of the rhythms are drastically reduced during advances, but not during delays.

With regard to the asymmetry effect, the results obtained in the isolation unit contrast with those obtained in flight experiments. If the measurements from seven studies are averaged (Fig. 7) the mean shift rate is 57 min/day after an east-bound flight, but 92 min/day after a

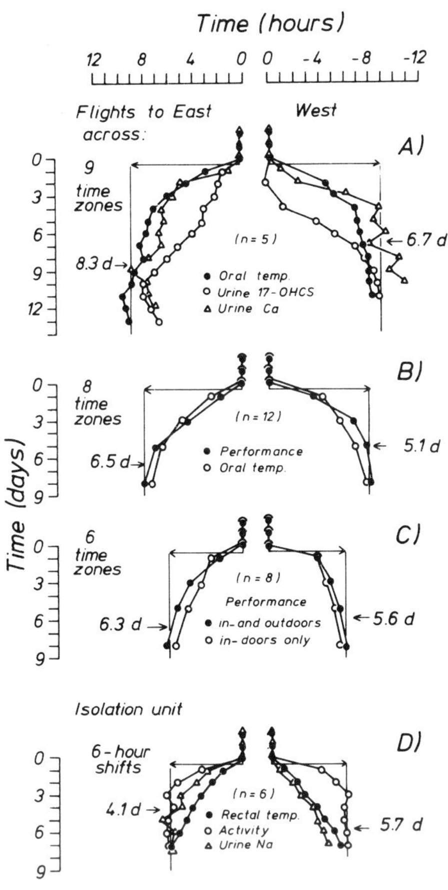

Fig. 7A-D. Shift of human circadian rhythms after transmeridianal flights or after shifts of the Zeitgeber in an isolation unit at day 0. Zero on the abscissa is phase of the rhythm before flight or shift. On the left and right margin, time (in days) for 90% re-entrainment (averaged from all variables). Sources: A, HALBERG et al. (1970, 1971); B, KLEIN et al. (1970); C, KLEIN and WEGEMANN (1974); D, WEVER (1977)

west-bound flight (ASCHOFF et al., 1975). Two of the graphs in Figure 7 illustrate the differences in rate of re-entrainment between variables. This figure also shows that in none of the experiments, including flight across nine time zones, was partition observed. (That this may occur is demonstrated by other experiments; cf. Fig. 9.) Furthermore, rate of re-entrainment depends on the schedule on which the subjects live after the flight. As has been shown by KLEIN and WEGMANN (1974), re-entrainment is slower when subjects are confined to their hotel rooms, as compared to conditions in which they are allowed to leave their rooms every second day (Fig. 7, third diagram from top). These observations emphasize the importance of social Zeitgebers for the entrainment of human circadian rhythms. Possible reasons for the difference in asymmetry effects found in the isolation unit and after flights are discussed in an earlier publication (ASCHOFF et al., 1975).

Re-entrainment by Partition

Usually, after a 6-h phase shift of the Zeitgeber or after a flight across six time zones, all rhythmic functions are shifted into the same direction. However, there is at least one exception to this rule. In addition to the six subjects who were studied in the isolation unit

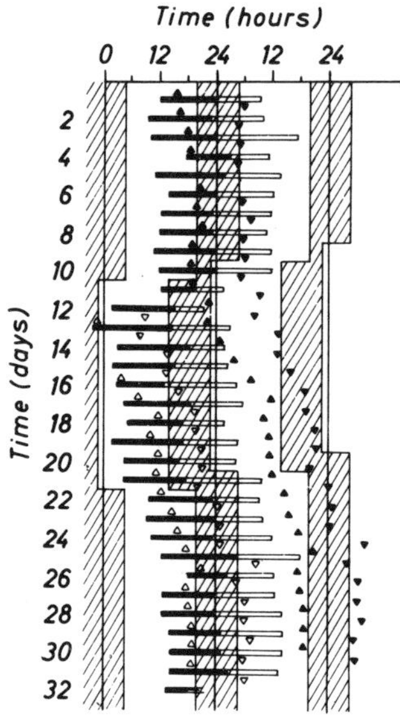

Fig. 8. Shift of circadian rhythms in a subject exposed in the isolation unit to a light-dark cycle and to regular gong signals (reading lamps available). Shaded area, darkness. Black and white bars, wakefulness and sleep. Closed triangles above and below bars, maxima and minima of rectal temperature. (Open triangles, double plot). (From WEVER, 1970)

(lowermost diagram of Fig. 7), there was one subject whose behavior deserves special attention (WEVER, 1970). As can be seen in Figure 8, his activity rhythm follows the Zeitgeber after both the advance and the delay shift. The rhythm of rectal temperature, however, indicated by the position of maxima and minima (closed triangles above and below bars) goes through a 18-h delay shift after the 6-h advance shift of the Zeitgeber. In flight experiments, such a partition between the activity rhythm and the rhythm of body temperature has been observed after an east-bound flight across nine time zones (KLEIN et al., 1977). There is finally a report of a 12-h shift of sleep-time in the hospital in which analysis of urine constituents from this subject indicates an advance shift for the rhythm of potassium excretion, and a delay shift for the 17-OHCS (LEVINE, 1976).

A summary of the studies cited (Fig. 9) conveys one clear message: partition phenomena have been observed after advance shifts of the Zeitgeber, after east-bound flights and after a 12-hour shift of the sleep-time; no partition has been found after delay shifts or after west-bound flights. It further is noteworthy that partition occurred in 1 out of 7 subjects after the 6-h advance of the Zeitgeber, but in four out of eight subjects after the east-bound flight across 9 time zones. It seems that the probability for partition increases with the extent of Zeitgeber shift, or with the number of time zones crossed, respectively, and that the lower limit is about 6 h. These findings are in agreement with data recently published by MINORS and WATERHOUSE (1976) from experiments, in which 24 subjects were exposed in an isolation unit to 8-h advance and delay shifts. From their measurements of urine constituents and of rectal temperature, the authors conclude that a Zeitgeber delay is always followed by a delay shift, while an 8-h Zeitgeber advance may result in an 8-h advance of the rhythms or in a 16-h delay.

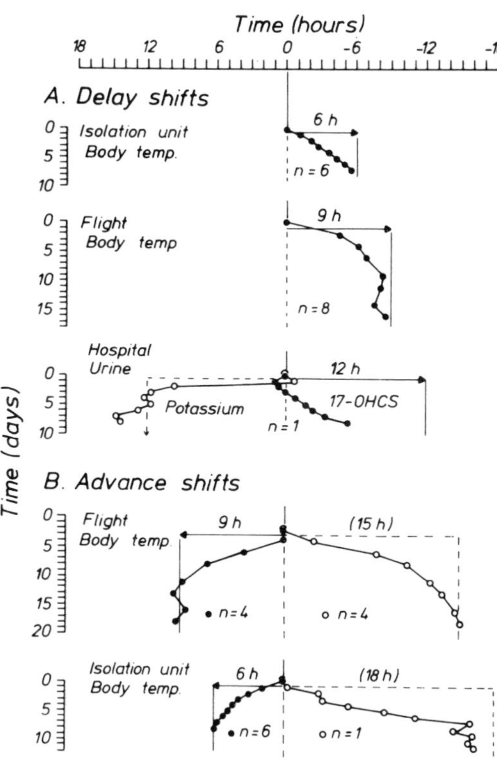

Fig. 9. Shift of human circadian rhythms after shift of Zeitgeber or after flights, respectively, at day 0. Zero on the abscissa is phase of rhythm before shift or flight. Sources: Isolation unit, WEVER (1978); flight, KLEIN et al. (1977); hospital, LEVINE (1976)

Conclusions

Although the preceding discussion was necessarily based largely on recordings of variables other than hormones, it can be taken for granted that the principles mentioned apply to the endocrine system as well. This certainly holds for the transitory temporal disorder that characterizes re-entrainment independent of whether it occurs with or without partition of rhythms. Such disorder probably contributes to the loss in performance during post-flight days in man (KLEIN and WEGMANN, 1974), and it may have immediate effects on health. Although in mice, after one 12-h shift, no increase in susceptibility to deleterious drugs has been found (NELSON and HALBERG, 1973), a shortening of life due to a life-long repetition of shifts has been described in both Blowflies (*Phormia terraenovae*; ASCHOFF et al., 1971) and Codling Moths (*Laspeyresia pomonella*; HAYES, 1976) and also in mice with weekly shifts beginning at 1 year of age (HALBERG et al., 1975). The extent to which less frequently experienced shifts could affect the well-being of man is still an open question. In this context, attention should be paid to the endocrine system which, on the one hand, seems to play an integrating role within the circadian system (GWINNER, 1974; MOORE-EDE et al., 1976), and for parts of which, on the other hand, extremely slow rates of re-entrainment have been observed (cf. Figs. 7 and 9). Shift experiments may well become a tool for analyzing interactions within the endocrine system.

References

ASCHOFF, J.: The phase angle difference in circadian periodicity. In: Circadian Clocks. Aschoff, J. (ed.). Amsterdam: North-Holland, 1965, pp. 263-276

ASCHOFF, J., HOFFMANN, K., POHL, H., WEVER, R.: Re-entrainment of circadian rhythms after phase shifts of the zeitgeber. Chronobiologia 2, 23-78 (1975)

ASCHOFF, J., POHL, H.: Phase-relations between a circadian rhythm and its zeitgeber within the range of entrainment. Naturwissenschaften 65, 80-84 (1978)

ASCHOFF, J., SAINT-PAUL, U.v., WEVER, R.: Die Lebensdauer von Fliegen unter dem Einfluß von Zeit-Verschiebungen. Naturwissenschaften 58, 574 (1971)

ASCHOFF, J., WEVER, R.: Resynchronisation der Tagesperiodik von Vögeln nach Phasensprung des Zeitgebers. Z. Vergl. Physiol. 46, 321-335 (1963)

ASCHOFF, J., WEVER, R.: Human circadian rhythms: a multi-oscillator system. Federation Proc. 35, 2326-2332 (1976)

BOISSIN, J., NOUGUIER-SOULE, J., ASSENMACHER, I.: Free-running, entrained and resynchronized circadian rhythms of plasma corticosterone and locomotor activity in the quail. Int. J. Chronobiol. 3, 89-125 (1975)

CHIBA, Y., CUTKOMP, L.K., HALBERG, F.: Circadian oxygen consumption rhythm of the flour beetle, *Tribolium confusum*. J. Insect. Physiol. 19, 2163-2172 (1973)

DAAN, S., PITTENDRIGH, C.S.: A functional analysis of circadian pacemakers in nocturnal rodents. II. The variability of phase response curves. J. comp. Physiol. 106, 253-266 (1976a)

DAAN, S., PITTENDRIGH, C.S.: A functional analysis of circadian pacemakers in nocturnal rodents. III. Heavy water and constant light: Homeostasis of frequency? J. Comp. Physiol. 106, 267-290 (1976b)

ERKERT, H.G.: Der Einfluß der Schwingungsbreite von Licht-Dunkel-Cyclen auf Phasenlage und Resynchronisation der circadianen Aktivitätsperiodik dunkelaktiver Tiere. J. Interdiscipl. Cycle Res. 7, 71-91 (1976)

FISCHER, K.: Untersuchungen zur Sonnenkompassorientierung und Laufaktivität von Smaragdeidechsen (*Lacerta viridis* Laur.). Z. Tierpsychol. 18, 450-470 (1961)

GWINNER, E.: Testosterone induces 'splitting' of circadian locomotor activity rhythms in birds. Science 185, 72-74 (1974)

HALBERG, F., HALBERG, E., MONTALBETTI, N.: Premesse e sviluppi della cronofarmacologia. Quaderni di medicina quantitativa 8, 7-5- (1970)

HALBERG, F., NELSON, W., CADOTTE, L.: Increased mortality in mice exposed to weekly 180° shifts of lighting regime LD 12:12 beginning at 1 year of age. Chronobiologia 2, Suppl. 1, 26 (1975)

HALBERG, F., NELSON, W., RUNGE, W.J., SCHMITT, O.H. et al.: Plans for orbital study of rat biorhythms. Results of interest beyond the biosatellite program. Space Life Sci. 2, 437-471 (1971)

HAYES, D.K.: Survival of the codling moth, the pink bollworm and the tobacco budworm after 90° phase-shifts at varied regular intervals throughout the life span. In: Shift Work and Health. Rentos, P.G., Shephard, R.D. (eds.). Washington: US Dept. Health, Ed. and Welfare, 1976, pp. 48-50

HOFFMANN, K.: Die relative Wirksamkeit von Zeitgebern. Oecologia 3, 184-206 (1969)

KLEIN, K.E., BRÜNER, H., HOLTMANN, H., REHME, H., STOLZE, J., STEINHOFF, W.D., WEGMANN, H.M.: Circadian rhythm of pilots' efficiency and effects of multiple time zone travel. Aerospace Med. 41, 125-132 (1970)

KLEIN, K.E., HERRMANN, R., KUKLINSKI, P., WEGMANN, H.M.: Circadian performance rhythms: Experimental studies in air operation. NATO-Conference Series (III-Human Factors) Vol. 3 (Vigilance). New York: Plenum Press, 1977, pp. 111-132

KLEIN, K.E., WEGMANN, H.M.: The resynchronization of human circadian rhythms after transmeridian flights as a result of flight direction and mode of activity. In: Chronobiology. Scheving, L.E., Halberg, F., Pauly, J.E. (eds.). Tokyo: Igaku Ltd., 1974, pp. 564-570

KLOTTER, K.: General properties of oscillating systems. Cold Spring Harbor Symp. Quant. Biol. 25, 185-187 (1960)

LEVINE, H.: Health and work shifts. In: Shift Work and Health. Rentos, P.G., Shephard, R.D. (eds.). Washington: US Dept. Health, Ed. and Welfare, 1976, pp. 57-69

MINORS, D.S., WATERHOUSE, J.M.: How do rhythms adjust to time shifts? J. Physiol. 265, 23 (1976)

MOORE-EDE, M.C., SCHMELZER, W.S., KASS, D.A., HERD, J.A.: Internal organization of the circadian timing system in multicellular animals. Federation Proc. 35, 2333-2338 (1976)

NELSON, W., HALBERG, F.: Effects of a synchronizer phase-shift on circadian rhythms in response of mice to ethanol or ouabain. Space Life Sci. 4, 249-257 (1973)

PITTENDRIGH, C.W., DAAN, S.: A functional analysis of circadian pacemakers in nocturnal rodents IV. Entrainment: pacemakers as clocks. J. Comp. Physiol. 106, 291-331 (1976)

POHL, H.: Comparative aspects of circadian rhythms in homeotherms. Re-entrainment after phase shifts of the zeitgeber. Int. J. Chronobiol. (1978, in press)

WEVER, R.: The duration of re-entrainment of circadian rhythms after phase shifts of the zeitgeber. J. Theoret. Biol. 13, 187-201 (1966)

WEVER, R.: Zur Zeitgeber-Stärke eines Licht-Dunkel-Wechsels für die circadiane Periodik des Menschen. Pflügers Arch. 321, 133-142 (1970)

WEVER, R.: The Circadian System of Man. Berlin-Heidelberg-New York: Springer, 1978 (in press)

10. Rapid Re-entrainment of the Estrous Cycle of Hamsters to Reversal of Scotophase and Photophase

C. S. CAMPBELL and J. S. FINKELSTEIN

Over the years an extensive literature has accumulated, showing that environmental phase-shifts result in a gradual re-entrainment of circardian rhythms involving several days of transient cycles (ASCHOFF et al., 1975). As Chapter II.7 shows, phase-shifts of the LD cycle can be successfully used as a tool for studying the functional relationships between circadian rhythms that normally maintain predictable phase relationships. This tool can also be utilized to examine such relationships between noncircadian rhythms, such as that complex of behavioral and endocrine rhythms that constitutes the estrous cycle.

An excellent external marker for hormonal rhythms in the female hamster is the onset of behavioral receptivity. This behavior, which requires a surge of progesterone following priming by estradiol, begins approximately 1 h (0.89 ± 0.17) before the offset of light on the evening of proestrus. In a first experiment, female hamsters were kept in 12L 12D (illumination level of 400 lux; dim red light during the dark) and their receptive and wheel-running behavior were monitored through several estrous cycles. On a day of estrus, the light-dark Zeitgeber phase was reversed (shifted) 12 h by 12 additional h of light. The onset of the daily activity period gradually advanced and required 7 days to re-entrain to the new offset of lights. In contrast, the onset of receptivity re-entrained within the first estrous cycle after reversal of photo- and scotophase by delaying 12 h, occurring 1.43 ± 0.12 h before light offset. Thus the activity and receptivity rhythms were dissociated in that first estrous cycle, with the onset of activity occurring before the onset of receptivity. The rapid re-entrainment of receptivity was confirmed by observations during the second and third estrous cycles after reversal, when the onset of receptivity showed no further shifts (0.94 ± 0.22 and 1.25 ± 0.41 h before light offset, respectively).

These observations were extended to an examination of the underlying hormonal rhythms. Serum levels of estradiol and progesterone were measured at three critical times in proestrus and estrus (see legend to Fig. 1) in animals before reversal of Zeitgeber phase and at the same clock times for animals in the first, second, and third estrous cycles after reversal. Data obtained were all consistent with a 12-h delay in these hormones. Serum levels of estradiol in pre-reversal control animals were low at all time points, as would be expected on the evening of proestrus, morning of estrus and evening of estrus. In animals subjected to reversal of Zeitgeber phase, the estradiol rhythm was delayed, since levels of the hormone were still high at the first time sampled (similar to levels normally seen on the morning of proestrus), and only later began to decline (Fig. 1). Progesterone levels in pre-reversal control animals were high on the evening of proestrus and on the morning of estrus, and then declined on the evening of estrus, while reversed animals initially had low serum titers and did not show high levels until the second time point sampled (Fig. 2). In both hormones, as in receptivity, there were no further changes during the second and third cycles after reversal. Thus these rhythms had re-entrained within the first estrous cycle after phase reversal of the

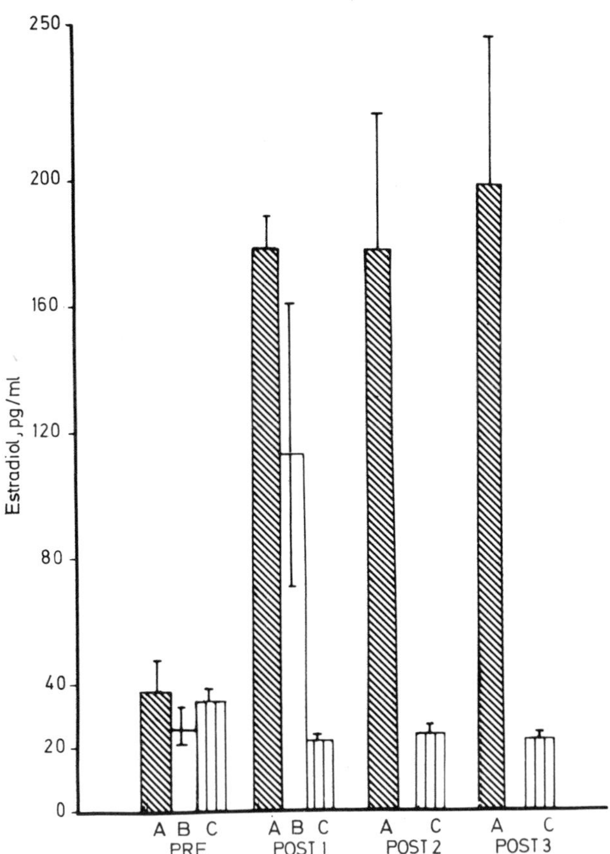

Fig. 1. Serum estradiol (pg/ml) in female hamsters autopsied either before reversal of Zeitgeber phase (PRE) or in the first, second, or third estrous cycles following reversal (POST 1, 2, 3). Diagonally hatched bars represent groups autopsied at time A, which was 3 h after the offset of lights (evening of proestrus) before reversal, and 9 h before the offset of lights after reversal. Open bars represent groups autopsied at time B, which was at the onset of lights (morning of estrus) before reversal, and at the offset of lights after reversal. Vertically hatched bars represent groups autopsied at time C, which was 1 h after the onset of lights (evening of estrus) before reversal, and 11 h before the offset of lights after reversal. Means and SEM are shown; each point represents five animals

Zeitgeber. Data on serum FSH, organ weights and timing of ovulation were all consistent with this rapid 12-h delay (FINKELSTEIN and CAMPBELL, 1977).

Of particular importance was that all of these variables maintained their normal temporal relationships and appeared to have shifted rapidly as a unit. For example, estradiol and progesterone maintained their normally inverse relationship described in Chapter II.5, and receptivity occurred only when serum progesterone and FSH levels were high and estradiol was low. These rhythms, then, all appear to be tightly coupled; there was no evidence of the dissociation of hormonal and behavioral relationships reported for the estrous cycle of rats under constant conditions (CAMPBELL and SCHWARTZ, 1974).

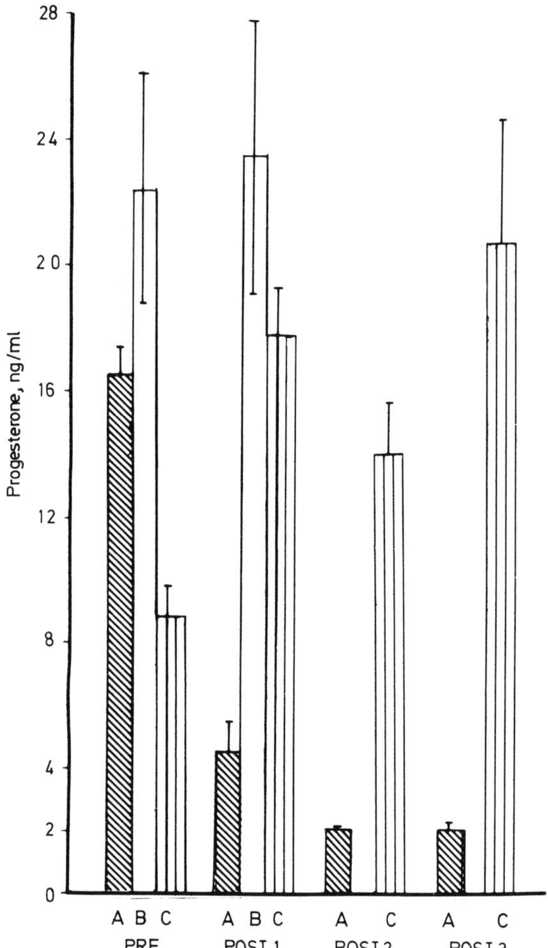

Fig. 2. Serum progesterone (ng/ml) in the hamsters described in the legend to Figure 1

In conclusion, estrous rhythms of hamsters are more labile than might have been predicted, since previous work has suggested that ovulation in the hamster requires 15-60 days to re-entrain to a 6-h phase-shift (ALLEVA et al., 1968). Perhaps, as BÜNNING (1973) has suggested, an inversion of the rhythm (180° phase-shift) may result in a "total reset" in some cases, whereas a change of a few hours may involve a genuine phase-shift with transients.

References

ASCHOFF, J., HOFFMANN, K., POHL, H., WEVER, R.: Re-entrainment of circadian rhythms after phase-shifts of the Zeitgeber. Chronobiologica 2, 23-78 (1975)

ALLEVA, J.J., WALESKI, M.V., ALLEVA, F.R., UMBERGER, E.J.: Synchronizing effect of photoperiodicity on ovulation in hamsters. Endocrinology 82, 1227-1235 (1968)

BÜNNING, E.: The Physiological Clock. 3rd ed. Berlin-Heidelberg-New York: Springer, 1973, p. 93

CAMPBELL, C.S., SCHWARTZ, N.B.: Timing of the events of the second estrous cycle of the rat in constant light (LL). Soc. Study of Reprod. Program (1974)

FINKELSTEIN, J.S., CAMPBELL, C.S.: Rapid re-entrainment of the hamster estrous cycle to photoperiod reversal. Soc. Study of Reprod. Program (1977)

11. Responses of the Diurnal Locomotor and Adrenocortical Rhythms in Rats exposed to a Weekly 8-Hour Phase-Shift of the Zeitgeber

A. SZAFARCZYK, J. NOUGUIER-SOULÉ, and I. ASSENMACHER

Two groups of female rats were kept in a regimen of 8 h light (08.00-16.00) and 16 h darkness. The first group was killed after 1 month to serve as controls for the diurnal corticosterone rhythm (Fig. 1a). Corticosterone was measured by a thin-layer chromatography-fluorimetric method for six rats at each sampling time. The second group remained thereafter at 8L 16D, but was then exposed for 9 weeks to repetitive 8-h phase-shifts of the photophase, by lengthening once a week a single photophase by 8 h (+ 120°). The locomotor rhythm was continuously recorded from four actographic cages housing three rats each. The daily position of the estimated acrophase (Halberg's least square method) compared with the Zeitgeber is plotted in Figure 1b. The graph shows that after each phase-shift of the synchronizer, the progressive resynchronization of the locomotor rhythm required almost one full week. In order to check the response of the adrenocortical rhythm that is usually closely coupled with the locomotor rhythm, the levels of plasma corticosterone were measured over a 48-h span (Fig. 1c, 6 rats per point) beginning on the second day of the fourth week of the experiment (indicated at T_1 on Fig. 1b). The comparison of Fig. 1c with the controls (Fig. 1a) shows that (1) the corticosterone rhythm displayed a marked phase advance with respect to the Zeitgeber through the two days of measurements, and that (2) the phase advance was reduced from one to the other day, thus indicating a trend towards a progressive resynchronization of the rhythm to the Zeitgeber. In conclusion, the data indicate that a weekly 8-h phase-shift in the photophase induced a state of permanent external desynchronization for both the locomotor and the adrenocortical rhythms. In addition it must be stated that after 9 weeks of repetitive phase-shifts the body weight of the rats was 20% less than in the controls.

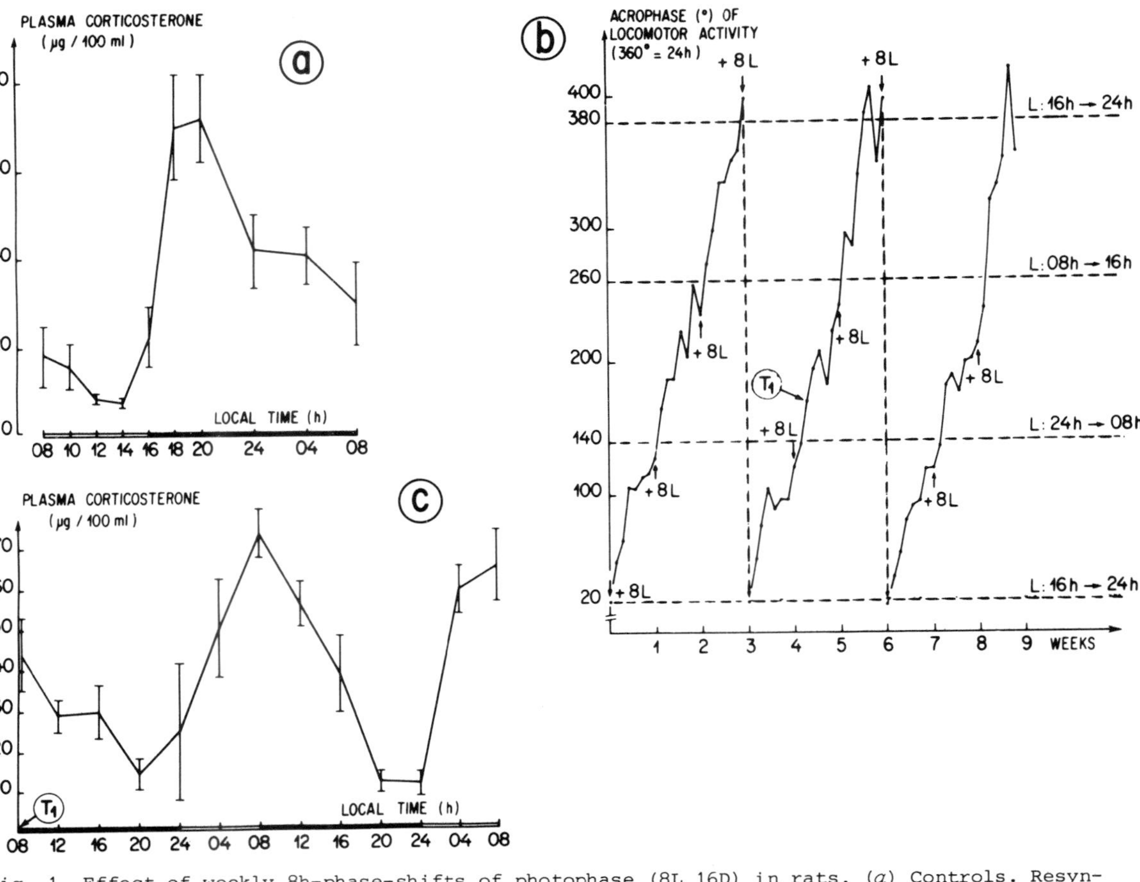

Fig. 1. Effect of weekly 8h-phase-shifts of photophase (8L 16D) in rats. (*a*) Controls. Resynchronization of (*b*) locomotor activity, and (*c*) corticosterone rhythms

Chapter III. Endocrine Functions in Osmoregulation

1. Hormonal Control of Sodium Transport by the Gills of Teleost Fish

D. H. Evans

Introduction

Teleost fish maintain ionic concentrations (predominantly NaCl) of body fluid that are distinctly different from their freshwater or marine environment. The mechanisms for osmotic and ionic regulation by teleost fish have recently been reviewed by MAETZ (1974, 1976) and EVANS (1978), and it is clear that various pathways exist to balance the net osmotic and diffusional movements of water and NaCl. These pathways include the renal complex (kidney and urinary bladder), as well as extrarenal tissues such as the branchial and intestinal epithelia. It is well established that several hormones play roles in the control of the rates of movements of water and NaCl through these pathways (for a recent discussion see JOHNSON, 1973). This review deals solely with our present knowledge of the hormonal control of Na transport by branchial epithelium.

A precautionary note is necessary. Studies of the hormonal control of branchial transport of Na in teleosts are complicated by the potential hemodynamic effects of various hormones. The teleost gill is an extremely complex tissue with vessels and sinuses that may permit the differential shunting of blood to or away from sites of high salt permeability or active transport. Such changes in patterns of blood flow could result in alterations in the measured fluxes of Na simply by changing the surface area of permeable membranes, or the blood flow to an actively transporting cell without direct effects on metabolically driven active transport. Two recent studies (PAYAN et al., 1975; GIRARD, 1976) have shown that hemodynamic effects of adrenaline on isolated, perfused heads of trout (*Salmo gairdneri*) could be separated from the effects on active transport of Na, but these types of controlled study have not as yet been utilized in other experiments. Therefore, one must approach with caution the conclusions drawn in most of the studies to be discussed in this paper. It is hoped that this review will promot the investigation of some of the phenomena described, using more rigorous techniques, in order to separate hemodynamic effects from effects on permeability or transport of teleost hormones.

Active Extraction of Na from Fresh Water

Many hormones have been suggested as potentiators of active Na transport in the freshwater teleost gill. DHARMAMBA and MAETZ (1972) showed in *Tilapia mossambica* that hypophysectomy was followed by a slight decrease (significant at the 5% level) in the rate of Na influx. MAETZ et al. (1967b) had found that hypophysectomy of *Fundulus heteroclitus* was followed by a significant decline in the rate of Na uptake (expressed as influx/external Na concentration). On the other hand, hypophysectomy of *Anguilla anguilla* was followed by a very significant stimulation of Na uptake (MAETZ et al., 1967a). Thus it appears that, at least in two species, hypophysial hormones may be involved in maintaining active Na uptake. The hormones involved may be those from the neurohypophysis since MAETZ et al. (1964b) have shown that injection of either isotocin or arginine vasotocin into intact *Carassius auratus* produced a significant stimulation of influx of radioactive Na. The latter, however, also produced an increase in Na efflux, presumably secondary to renal diuresis, and increased branchial permeability to Na (MAETZ and LAHLOU, 1974). In another series of experiments (MAETZ et al., 1964a), it was found that extracts from the urophysis also stimulated Na uptake by intact goldfish without affecting Na efflux. The urophysis, a neurohemal gland unique to teleosts, is situated below the caudal region of the spinal cord (see CHAN and BERN, 1976, for a recent review). These experiments should be repeated on hypophysectomized fish, and care should be taken to separate hemodynamic and transport effects, but the data can be treated as preliminary evidence that both the neurohypophysis and the urophysis may produce hormones that are able to stimulate Na uptake by freshwater teleosts.

There is some preliminary evidence that suggests that the interrenal gland (equivalent to the tetrapod adrenal cortex) of freshwater teleosts may also play a role in maintaining active Na uptake. Interrenalectomy of *Anguilla anguilla* was followed by a decline in Na uptake (CHESTER JONES et al., 1967; HENDERSON and CHESTER JONES, 1967; MAETZ, 1969) which could be reversed by injections of small doses of either aldosterone (HENDERSON and CHESTER JONES, 1967) or cortisol (CHESTER JONES et al., 1967).

By using an isolated, perfused head of the trout (*Salmo gairdneri*) PAYAN et al. (1975) have been able to demonstrate clearly that adrenaline can stimulate Na uptake from fresh water, a function distinct from its known hemodynamic effects. A ten-fold increase in the adrenaline concentration of the perfusion fluid (from 10^{-6} M to 10^{-5} M) was followed by an increase in the perfusion rate (presumably secondary to a fall in branchial vascular resistance), as well as an increase in the Na influx, net NH_4 efflux, and a reversal of the net Na flux, so there was a slight net uptake. The effects were reversible when the adrenaline concentration of the perfusion fluid was again reduced to 10^{-6} M. In an effort to separate hemodynamic effects from effects on active transport, PAYAN et al. (1975) added known alpha (phentolamine) and beta

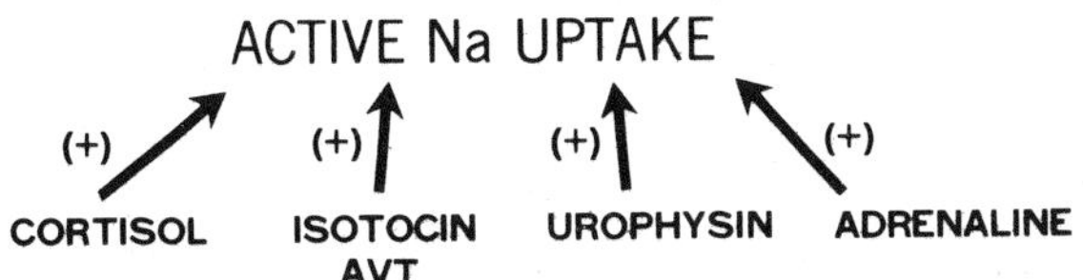

Fig. 1. Tentative summary of the interactions of hormones and Na transport in the gill of freshwater teleosts. +, stimulation

(propranolol) adrenergic blockers to the perfusion fluid. Propranolol increased the vascular resistance (decreased perfusion flow rate) significantly, and decreased the uptake of Na slightly (significant at the 5% level). However, addition of the two drugs together restored normal perfusion flow rate, but resulted in a significant reduction in Na influx. It is interesting that propranolol alone and the combination of propranolol and phentolamine also inhibited net efflux of NH_4. Since Na uptake is generally thought to be at least partially driven by a Na/NH_4 exchange mechanism (see MAETZ et al., 1976 and EVANS,

1978 for recent reviews), it is apparent that adrenaline is stimulatory to active Na uptake and is dependent upon a beta receptor for this effect.

Figure 1 summarizes the best assessment of the hormonal control of branchial Na transport in freshwater teleosts. However, it is obvious that further studies of this system must utilize techniques that permit separation of these effects from hemodynamic variations.

Active Extrusion of Na in Sea Water

Studies of the hormonal control of Na transport in the branchial epithelium of marine teleosts are, in addition to potential hemodynamic effects, complicated by the difficulty of separating the components of the Na fluxes across this tissue in vivo. With rare recent exceptions, studies of the hormonal control of Na fluxes in marine teleosts have assumed that changes in the total efflux (produced by removal of endocrine gland or hormonal injection) can be correlated with changes in the rate of active efflux of Na (see MAETZ, 1969; FORREST et al., 1973). We now know that the total efflux is actually composed of a rather substantial Na/Na exchange-diffusion and passive leak of Na superimposed on a rather small active efflux component (probably Na/K exchange) and a renal component (see EVANS, 1978, for a recent review). The renal component is so small that it can usually be ignored, but it is obvious that the total efflux could be significantly altered (by changes in Na/Na and leak components) without any appreciable change in the actual rate of active extrusion. One should therefore approach data based on total Na effluxes with caution.

Hypophysectomy of euryhaline teleosts acclimated to sea water resulted in a very significant decline in the total Na efflux (MAETZ, 1969; FLEMING and BALL, 1972; MACFARLANE and MAETZ, 1974). Prolactin injection of hypophysectomized fish usually resulted in a further decline (MAETZ, 1969; FLEMING and BALL, 1972); however, injection of ACTH restimulated Na efflux from two species of *Fundulus* (MAETZ, 1969; FLEMING and BALL, 1972). Bearing in mind the problems discussed above, one can tentatively conclude from these experiments that prolactin is inhibitory to active Na extrusion, while some hormone from the fish interrenal gland is stimulatory. The role of the interrenal gland (and cortisol in particular) is further emphasized by the finding (MAYER et al., 1967) that in *A. anguilla* hypophysectomy or interrenalectomy was followed by a significant decline in Na efflux, that was reversed by injections of cortisol but not by prolactin.

There is some evidence that supports the conclusion that at least a portion of this cortisol-stimulated Na efflux is indeed the due to the active component rather than to the Na/Na or leak components. MILNE et al. (1971) found that hypophysectomy of *A. anguilla* was followed by a 58% reduction in the Na/K-activated ATPase activity of homogenates of gill filaments, but that injection of ACTH into the fish restored the enzyme activity to control levels. PICKFORD et al. (1970b) had described similar results in hypophysectomized *F. heteroclitus* after injection with cortisol. Other studies (FORREST et al., 1973) indicate that when freshwater-acclimated *Anguilla rostrata* were injected with cortisol before being transferred to sea water, both the total Na efflux and the Na/K-activated ATPase activity of gill homogenate increased more rapidly than in uninjected controls after the transfer. In addition, SCHEER and LANGFORD (1976) showed that gills of hypophysectomized *A. anguilla* transferred from fresh water to sea water did not develop the normal, high Na/K-activated ATPase activity that characterizes this species in sea water, unless the animals were previously injected with cortisol. Since Na/K-activated ATPase is probably involved in the active extrusion of Na from marine teleosts (MAETZ and BORNANCIN, 1975), it appears that cortisol was acting directly on the active transport component. Unfortunately, no data exist on the effect of hypophysectomy or cortisol injection on the K-dependent Na efflux that is thought to be the physiologic indicator of active Na extrusion (EVANS et al., 1974; MAETZ and PIC, 1975; EVANS and COOPER, 1976).

It appears that the inhibition of Na efflux from hypophysectomized marine teleosts treated with prolactin may be via inhibition of the active extrusion of Na. PICKFORD et al. (1970a) found that injection of prolactin into hypophysectomized *F. heteroclitus* acclimated to freshwater reduced the Na/K activity of gill homogenates by 66%. This experiment should be repeated on seawater-acclimated fish, but it does indicate that prolactin may be inhibitory to active Na extrusion.

The isolated, perfused trout head has also been utilized to investigate the role of adrenaline in controlling Na efflux from seawater-acclimated animals (GIRARD, 1976). Addition of adrenaline to the perfusion fluids was followed by a significant reduction in the total Na efflux, as well as in the K-stimulated Na efflux. This indicates that adrenaline was probably inhibiting Na/K exchange and thereby active extrusion of Na, but the lack of measurements of the transepithelial electrical potential under these conditions precludes a definite statement. The fact that addition of adrenaline also reduced the Na efflux in freshwater baths after rapid changing of the medium indicates that there may also be a permeability effect, but, again, data on changes in electrical potential are lacking. However, GIRARD (1976) was able to demonstrate that these effects of adrenaline on Na effluxes were probably independent of hemodynamic effects by showing that the efflux of radioactive Na was not altered by a drastic reduction in the rate of experimental perfusion. Thus, it appears unlikely that changes in blood flow can account for the observed alteration of Na efflux produced by the addition of adrenaline to the perfusion fluid.

Figure 2 summarizes what is presently thought to be the hormonal control of active Na extrusion by marine teleosts.

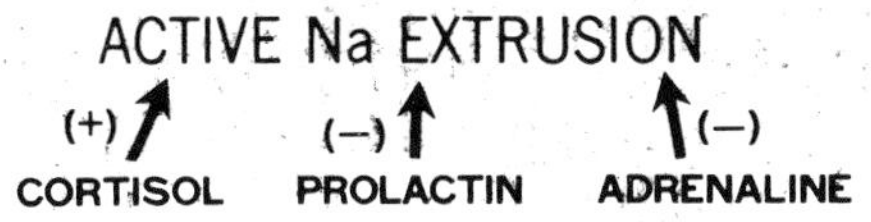

ACTIVE Na EXTRUSION

(+) ↗ CORTISOL (−) ↑ PROLACTIN ↑ (−) ADRENALINE

Fig. 2. Tentative summary of the interactions of hormones and Na transport in the gill of marine teleosts. +, stimulation; -, inhibition

Conclusions

This rather brief review of the hormonal control of Na transport by the branchial epithelium of teleosts indicates the relative paucity of critical data. It is clear that such studies must utilize techniques that can evaluate these parameters independently of hemodynamic effects. In addition, investigation of the hormonal control of active-transport mechanisms must be certain to separate experimentally the active component from passive and Na/Na-exchange diffusion. Thus definitive statements on the hormones that control this effector system of teleost osmoregulation await experimentation utilizing techniques described in the past three years. It is hoped that this review will prompt the use of such techniques in future investigations.

Acknowledgment and Dedication. This review was written while the author was supported by NSF grants, BMS 75-0091 and PCM 77-03914. It is dedicated to the memory of Dr. JEAN MAETZ, Villefranche-sur-Mer, France. His tragic death is an immeasurable loss to science and to those of us lucky enough to have been his friends.

References

CHAN, D.K.O., BERN, H.A.: The caudal neurosecretory system. A critical evaluation of the two-hormone hypothesis. Cell Tiss. Res. 174, 339-354 (1976)

CHESTER JONES, I., HENDERSON, I.W., CHAN, D.K.O., RANKIN, J.C.: Steroids and pressor substances in bony fish with special reference to the adrenal cortex and corpuscles of Stannius of the eel (*Anguilla anguilla* L.). Proc. 2nd Int. Congr. Steroid Hormones, Milan, Excerpta Med. 132, 136-145 (1967)

DHARMAMBA, M., MAETZ, J.: Effects of hypophysectomy and prolactin on sodium balance of *Tilapia mossambica* in fresh water. Gen. Comp. Endocrinol. 19, 175-183 (1972)

EVANS, D.H.: Ionic and osmotic regulation in fish. In: Comparative Physiology of Ionic and Osmotic Regulation in Animals. Maloiy, G.M.O (ed.). London: Academic Press, 1978, in press

EVANS, D.H., CARRIER, J.C., BOGAN, M.B.: The effect of external potassium ions on the electical potential measured across the gills of the teleost *Dormitator maculatus*. J. Exp. Biol. 61, 277-283 (1974)

EVANS, D.H., COOPER, K.: The presence of Na-Na and Na-K exchange in sodium extrusion by three species of fish. Nature (London) 259, 241-242 (1976)

FLEMING, W.R., BALL, J.N.: The effect of prolactin and ACTH on the sodium metabolism of *Fundulus kansae* held in deionized water, sodium-enriched freshwater, and concentrated sea water. Z. Vergl. Physiol. 76, 125-134 (1972)

FORREST, J.N. Dr., COHEN, A.D., SCHON, D.A., EPSTEIN, F.H.: Na transport and Na-K-ATPase in gills during adaptation to seawater: effects of cortisol. Am. J. Physiol. 224, 709-713 (1973)

GIRARD, J.P.: Salt excretion by the perfused head of trout adapted to sea water and its inhibition by adrenaline. J. Comp. Physiol. 111, 77-91 (1976)

HENDERSON, I.W., CHESTER JONES, I.: Endocrine influences on the net extrarenal fluxes of sodium and potassium in the European eel (*Anguilla anguilla* L.). J. Endocrinol. 37, 319-325 (1967)

JOHNSON, D.W.: Endocrine Control of hydromineral balance in teleosts. Am. Zool. 13, 799-818 (1973)

MACFARLANE, N.A.A., MAETZ, J.: Effects of hypophysectomy on sodium and water exchanges in the euryhaline flounder, *Platichthys flesus* (L.). Gen. Comp. Endocrinol. 22, 77-89 (1974)

MAYER, N., MAETZ, J., CHAN, D.K.O., FORSTER, M., CHESTER JONES, I.: Cortisol, a sodium excreting factor in the eel (*Anguilla anguilla* L.) adapted to seawater. Nature (London) 214, 1118-1120 (1967)

MAETZ, J.: Observations on the role of the pituitary-interrenal axis in the ion regulation of the eel and other teleosts. Gen. Comp. Endocrinol. Suppl. 2, 299-316 (1969)

MAETZ, J.: Aspects of adaptation to hypo-osmotic and hyper-osmotic environments. In: Biochemical and Biophysical Perspectives in Marine Biology, Vol. I. Malins, D.C., Sargent, J.R. (eds.). London: Academic Press, 1974, pp. 1-167

MAETZ, J.: Transport of ions and water across the epithelium of fish gills. In: Lung Liquids, Ciba Foundation Symposium 38 (new series). Amsterdam: Elsevier, Excerpta Medica, 1976, pp. 133-159

MAETZ, J., BORNANCIN, M.: Biochemical and biophysical aspects of salt excretion by chloride cells in teleosts. Forts. der. Zool. Band 23, Heft 2/3, 322-362 (1975)

MAETZ, J., BOURQUET, J., LAHLOU, B.: Urophyse et osmorégulation chez *Carassius auratus*. Gen. Comp. Endocrinol. 4, 401-414 (1964a)

MAETZ, J., BOURQUET, J., LAHLOU, B., HOURDRY, J.: Peptides neurohypophysaires et osmorégulation chez *Carassius auratus*. Gen. Comp. Endocrinol. 4, 508-522 (1964b)

MAETZ, J., LAHLOU, B.: Actions of neurohypophysial hormones in fishes. Handbook of Physiology-Endocrinology IV. Part 1, 521-544 (1974)

MAETZ, J., MAYER, N., CHARTIER-BARADUC, M.M.: La balance minérale du sodium chez *Anguilla anguilla* en eau de mer, en eau douce et au cours du transfert d'un milieu à l'autre: Effets de l'hypophysectomie et de la prolactine. Gen. Comp. Endocrinol. 8, 177-188 (1967a)

MAETZ, J., PAYAN, P., DE RENZIS, G.: Controversial aspects of ionic uptake in freshwater animals. In: Perspectives in Experimental Biology, Vol. I, Zoology. Spencer Davies, P. (ed.). Oxford and New York: Pergamon Press, 1976, pp. 77-92

MAETZ, J., PIC, P.: New evidence for a Na/K and Na/Na exchange carrier linked with Cl^- pump in the gill of *Mugil capito* in sea water. J. Comp. Physiol. 102, 85-100 (1975)

MAETZ, J., SAWYER, W.H., PICKFORD, G.E., MAYER, N.: Evolution de la balance minérale du sodium chez *Fundulus heteroclitus* au cours du transfert d'eau de mer en eau douce: Effets de l'hypophysectomie et de la prolactine. Gen. Comp. Endocrinol. 8, 163-176 (1967b)

MILNE, K.P., BALL, J.N., CHESTER JONES, I.: Effects of salinity, hypophysectomy and corticotrophin on branchial Na- and K-activated ATPase in the eel., *Anguilla anguilla* L. J. Endocrinol. 49, 177-178 (1971)

PAYAN, P., MATTY, A.J., MAETZ, J.: A study of the sodium pump in the perfused head preparation of the trout *Salmo gairdneri* in freshwater. J. Comp. Physiol. 104, 33-48 (1975)

PICKFORD, G.E., GRIFFITH, R.W., TORRETTI, J., HENDLER, E., EPSTEIN, F.H.: Branchial reduction and renal stimulation of (Na^+, K^+) -ATPase by prolactin in hypophysectomized killifish in fresh water. Nature (London) 228, 378-379 (1970a)

PICKFORD, G.E., PANG, P.K.T., WEINSTEIN, E., TORRETTI, J., HENDLER, E., EPSTEIN, F.H.: The response of the hypophysectomized cyprinodont, *Fundulus heteroclitus*, to replacement therapy with cortisol: Effects on blood serum and sodium-potassium activated adenosine triphosphatase in the gills, kidney, and intestinal mucosa. Gen. Comp. Endocrinol. 14, 524-534 (1970b)

SCHEER, B.T., LANGFORD, R.W.: Endocrine effects on the cation-dependent ATPases of the gills of European eels (*Anguilla anguilla* L.) and efflux of Na. Gen. Comp. Endocrinol. 30, 313-326 (1976)

2. Environment and Osmoregulation among Lungfishes and Amphibians

W. H. SAWYER, P. K. T. PANG, and S. M. GALLI-GALLARDO

Transition from an aquatic to a semiterrestrial environment early in amphibian evolution required drastic readjustments of osmoregulatory mechanisms. Studies on the endocrinology of osmoregulation among living lungfishes and amphibians allow us to explore some of the evolutionary adaptations that occurred among early amphibians. The lungfishes are of particular interest, since they are the closest surviving freshwater relatives of the sarcopterygian ancesters of the amphibians. Living amphibians are of interest, since they occupy environments ranging from the totally aquatic to almost wholly terrestrial. Studies on amphibian species from differing environments may enable us to distinguish osmoregulatory adaptations simply reflecting environmental conditions from those resulting from more fundamental and possibly irreversible evolutionary changes. Unfortunately relatively few studies on lungfish endocrinology have been reported, and only a few amphibian species have received detailed endocrine scrutiny.

Many endocrine systems are undoubtedly involved in osmoregulation among lungfishes and amphibians. Prolactin, adrenocortical steroids and the renin-angiotensin system all probably influence osmoregulation among amphibians, but we know almost nothing about their possible functions among lungfishes. Since time and space are limited, we will confine ourselves at a discussion of the actions of the neurohypophysial hormones on water balance, since this is a subject on which we have sufficient information to allow some speculation concerning how these changed during evolution of the early amphibians.

Neurohypophysial Hormones

The active peptides found in the neurohypophyses of both amphibians and lungfishes are arginine-vasotocin (AVT) and mesotocin (MT) (ACHER, 1974). There is much information on responses by amphibians to neurohypophysial hormones (BENTLEY, 1974), but less is known about responses by fishes (MAETZ and LAHLOU, 1974). Exogenous neurohypophysial hormones may influence water uptake or water excretion in a variety of ways (Table 1). We will first examine the distribution of these varied responses among amphibians, and attempt to relate this to their environments. Then we will describe some studies on responses by lungfishes to AVT and attempt to compare these to responses by amphibians, and make some conjectures concerning how AVT responses may have arisen during amphibian evolution.

Anuran Amphibians. Responses by common anurans of the genera *Bufo* and *Rana* to neurohypophysial hormones have been studied extensively (BENTLEY, 1974). We will not attempt a detailed review of this subject. In most frogs and toads, AVT exerts hydroosmotic effects on skin, urinary bladder and renal tubule, and a glomerular antidiuretic effect. In addition, MT increases glomerular filtration rate (GFR) and urine flow in frogs (JARD, 1966; PANG and SAWYER, 1976; PANG, 1977). This occurs

Table 1. Actions of exogenous neurohypophysial hormones that may influence water balance

A. Primarily vascular

1. Systemic vasoconstriction, hypertension and glomerular diuresis
2. Systemic vasodilation, hypotension and glomerular antidiuresis?
3. Glomerular vasoconstriction and antidiuresis
4. Glomerular vasodilation and diuresis

B. Increased water permeability

1. Hydroosmotic effect on skin
2. Hydroosmotic effect on urinary bladder
3. Hydroosmotic effect on renal tubules

despite a transient decrease in arterial blood pressure (PANG, 1977), indicating that it cannot be a pressure diuresis. This is further confirmed in experiments on frog kidneys arterially perfused at constant pressure. In these MT is also diuretic and reduces total renal vascular resistance. This strongly implies that MT dilates the afferent glomerular vessels. In similarly perfused kidneys, AVT decreases GFR and increases renal vascular resistance (PANG, 1977). This is consistent with the conclusion that AVT constricts the afferent glomerular arterioles originally based on direct visualization and clearance measurements (SAWYER, 1951).

Hydroosmotic responses by anuran urinary bladders have been observed repeatedly in vivo (SAWYER and SCHISGALL, 1956) and in vitro (BENTLEY, 1958; SAWYER, 1960). Both AVT and MT have a hydroosmotic effect on frog bladders, but AVT is about 40 times more active (SAWYER, 1966a).

Hydroosmotic responses by the renal tubule have been more difficult to demonstrate unequivocally. Previous evidence has been indirect and not wholly convincing. AVT usually reduces GFR which can reduce excretion of osmotically free water in two ways, directly, by reducing the volume of filtrate and indirectly, by decreasing flow rate through the renal tubules. The first effect of lowered GFR can be compensated for by calculating the "relative free water clearance", the free water clearance factored by the GFR (SAWYER, 1957). This cannot compensate for the possible effects of reduced flow rates. Reduced flow rates alone can, in dogs, sharply reduce excretion of free water even in the absence of ADH (BERLINER and DAVIDSON, 1957). Thus the assumption that a reduced relative free water clearance indicates a tubular hydroosmotic response (SAWYER, 1957; JARD, 1966) is not altogether safe despite the observation that antidiuresis occasionally occurs without an evident fall in GFR (SAWYER, 1957).

We have recently reexamined the tubular antidiuretic response in frogs by a different approach. It is possible to perfuse the kidneys by both arterial and renal portal circulations. Appropriate adjustment of the relative pressures of the perfusions allows one to exclude the portal perfusate from access to the glomerular circulation, while allowing it access to the peritubular capillaries. AVT added to the arterial perfusate in such a preparation causes both glomerular and tubular antidiuresis. When added to the renal portal perfusion, AVT causes tubular antidiuresis but does not reduce GFR. This evidence, although not absolutely conclusive, provides strong support for the conclusion that AVT can exert a tubular hydroosmotic effect in anuran amphibians, as it can in mammals.

A totally aquatic anuran, *Xenopus*, does not show a detectable change in body weight when injected with neurohypophysial hormones (EWER, 1952). This is consistent with the weak (MAETZ, 1963) or absent (BENTLEY, 1969a) hydroosmotic response by *Xenopus* skin in vitro. Adaptation by *Xenopus* to its aquatic environment is believed to be secondary. This was apparently accompanied by suppression of the hydroosmotic response of the skin.

Although EWER (1952) and MCBEAN and GOLDSTEIN (1970) reported that injections of neurohypophysial hormones into the dorsal lymph sac of *Xenopus* failed to cause consistent antidiuresis HENDERSON et al. (1972) found that intravenous AVT produces a dose-related antidiuresis. They could not detect any tubular effect. We have also found *Xenopus* to be highly sensitive to the antidiuretic effect of intravascular AVT (PANG and GALLI-GALLARDO, unpublished). The largely aquatic Chilean toad, *Calyptocephallela*, also shows antidiuresis in response to AVT (PANG, 1977; GALLI-GALLARDO, E. MARUSIC and PANG, unpublished). BENTLEY (1969b) has shown that plasma hydroosmotic activity, presumed due to AVT, increases in *Xenopus* immersed in hypertonic NaCl. Thus a mechanism exists for release of AVT in response to an osmotic stress in this aquatic species. This may be physiologically useful in case these aquatic animals encounter dehydrating conditions. It is also possible that the ability to release AVT and to show an antidiuretic response may merely be a reflection of the more terrestrial habitats of their ancestors.

MT causes a clear diuretic response in *Calyptocephallela* (PANG, 1977; GALLI-GALLARDO, MARUSIC and PANG, unpublished). This response to MT may be an adaptation allowing an aquatic animal to excrete excess water when necessary.

Urodeles. Some salamanders can respond to injected neurohypophysial hormones by increased water uptake across the skin (HILLMAN, 1974; BROWN and BROWN, 1977), but hydroosmotic responses by isolated skins have not been detected. Many urodeles, however, do not show increased water uptake when injected with AVT (BENTLEY, 1971). Urinary bladders from some urodeles also show typical hydroosmotic responses in vitro (BENTLEY and HELLER, 1965; BROWN and BROWN, 1977). Hydroosmotic responses of skin and bladder are not observed in more aquatic species, such as *Necturus*, *Siren* or *Amphiuma*. Hydroosmotic responses among urodeles, therefore, appear to be adaptations to more terrestrial environments.

Most of the urodeles that have been studied respond to AVT with an antidiuresis. This is primarily due to a reduction in GFR (ALVARADO and JOHNSON, 1965; BENTLEY, 1971, 1973). GARLAND et al. (1975), however, recently concluded that AVT had a tubular antidiuretic action in *Necturus*, although the basis for this was not evident from their published data. We have recently attempted to demonstrate the presence of a tubular antidiuretic response by doubly perfusing *Necturus* kidneys (PANG and GALLI-GALLARDO, unpublished). AVT added to the arterial perfusion decreases GFR, and increases renal vascular resistance (GALLI-GALLARDO et al., 1977). Creatinine U/P concentration ratios remained unchanged, providing no evidence for increased tubular water reabsorption. When AVT was added to the portal perfusate creatinine U/P ratios remained unchanged (unpublished). These experiments provide no evidence that AVT can modify renal tubular permeability in *Necturus*. Thus tubular antidiuretic responses remain to be clearly identified among urodeles, although the species studied are few.

ALVARADO and JOHNSON (1965) found that large doses of oxytocin caused a slow loss of weight in larval *Ambystoma*. Although they failed to find an initial diuresis, they considered that weight loss meight reflect a delayed diuretic effect of oxytocin. MT has an acute diuretic effect in *Necturus* (PANG and C. OGURO, unpublished). Such a response could be physiologically useful to an aquatic organism such as *Necturus* as a mechanism for hastening excretion of excess water.

Although AVT can cause antidiuresis in aquatic urodeles, BENTLEY (1973) questions its physiologic significance. These species descended from semi-terrestrial ancestors and antidiuretic responses may merely represent relics of their ancestry. Studies on more primitive aquatic urodeles such as *Cryptobranchus* are badly needed.

Lungfishes. It is not clear whether lungfishes can respond to neurohypophysial hormones by increasing the rate at which they absorb water or electrolytes from their environments. HELLER and BENTLEY (1965) reported that intraperitoneal injections of large doses of AVT did not cause a weight gain in *Protopterus*. Since subsequent experiments (SAWYER, 1966b) showed that even smaller intraperitoneal doses of AVT cause a marked diuresis and natriuresis in this species, the lack of a weight loss in HELLER and BENTLEY'S (1965) lungfish suggests that the rate of water uptake may have increased after AVT. Whether this does indeed occur and whether it reflects drinking or increased permeability of gill or skin is a question that deserves exploration. It is possible that the water-balance response was not, as is usually thought, an original invention of the early amphibians.

Renal responses by lungfishes to AVT have been explored in some detail. *Protopterus* (SAWYER, 1970), *Lepidosiren* (SAWYER and PANG, 1972 and unpublished data) and *Neoceratodus* (SAWYER et al., 1976) all respond to AVT with a brisk diuresis and natriuresis. The question remains as to whether this reflects a direct effect of AVT on the glomerular circulation (SAWYER, 1972) or an indirect response to elevated systemic blood pressure (SAWYER et al., 1976).

We have recently reexamined the question of whether AVT exerts a direct glomerular diuretic effect by arterially perfusing *Lepidosiren* kidneys (GALLI-GALLARDO et al., 1977). When perfusion pressure is constant, AVT markedly reduces perfusion rate, indicating vasoconstriction in the perfused tissues, that include tail muscles as well as kindeys. Under these circumstances AVT may actually cause a glomerular antidiuresis, quite opposite from the response seen in the intact fish. When the kidneys are perfused at a constant rate, AVT markedly increases perfusion pressure and evokes a glomerular diuresis. These experiments, and those on *Neoceratodus*, do not require that we assume that AVT has a specific and direct diuretic action on the glomerular circulation. It will be important to reexamine responses by *Protopterus* to see whether earlier indications of a direct diuretic effect of AVT can be substantiated.

It is possible that AVT first evolved as a vasopressor hormone concerned with cardiovascular regulation. Highly sensitive vascular receptors exist among cyclostomes (SOMLYO and SOMLYO, 1968) and teleosts (HOLDER and GUERNÉ, 1976) as well as among lungfishes. If AVT participates in blood pressure regulation among fishes one might expect it to be released by volume depletion or hypotension, as renin appears to be released in fishes (NISHIMURA et al., 1977). Sensitive assay methods must be developed and applied in an attempt to define those changes in circulating AVT levels that occur when circulating volumes and pressures are experimentally manipulated.

Evolution of the Osmoregulatory Functions of Neurohypophysial Hormones

If we accept the hypothesis that the primitive functions of AVT among fishes may relate to cardiovascular regulation rather than osmoregulation, we should then consider how this hormone became adapted to serve as a water-retaining hormone among amphibians. Considering the vasoconstrictor effects of AVT, we can easily see how a systemic vasopressor and a secondary diuretic response, as seen in lungfishes, could be changed into a glomerular antidiuretic response in amphibians. Merely shifting the density or sensitivity of vasoconstrictor receptors in the peripheral and renal vasculature could accomplish this. We have seen that the systemic circulation of lungfishes appears much more sensitive to AVT than the glomerular circulation. In frogs, however, we have been able to show that the afferent glomerular circulation responds to doses of AVT much lower than those that cause detectable vasoconstriction in the isolated perfused leg (PANG and GALLI-GALLARDO, unpublished). It would actually be a disadvantage to an amphibian if antidiuretic levels of AVT raised systemic blood pressure, since the increased renal perfusion pressure would oppose the effects of afferent glomerular vasoconstriction. Thus the relative insensitivity of the systemic vasculature to AVT may be as much an adaptation to terrestrial environments as is the enhanced sensitivity of the afferent glomerular arteriole.

Whether AVT functions to maintain blood pressure, fluid volumes, or both, the same type of physiologic stimuli should cause its release. These would be hypotension or volume depletion. In fishes, such release may serve to preserve blood pressure. In amphibians, release would primarily serve to increase water uptake and inhibit urine flow. In extreme instances, such as hemorrhage, when large amounts of AVT are released (BENTLEY, 1969b; SAWYER and PANG, 1975; PANG, 1977), it may also serve to sustain systemic blood pressure by causing general vasoconstriction.

It is a long-standing belief among biologists that old hormones acquire new functions when these can confer some adaptational advantage. If AVT were first adapted by early amphibians as a glomerular antidiuretic hormone released in response to volume depletion, it would seem to make sound teleologic sense that other appropriate responses to this hormone should also evolve. Receptors capable of mediating increased permeability of the urinary bladder, skin, and renal tubules are present among amphibians. Increased permeability of these membranes contributes to rehydration and restoration of fluid volumes by encouraging reabsorption of water from the bladder and renal tubules and enhancing water uptake from the surrounding environment. Whenever the hydroosmotic responses may have first evolved, they persist in the renal tubules of higher tetrapods as the single most important endocrine factor in maintaining water balance.

Conclusions

During the early evolution of the amphibians, preexistent hormones became adapted to serve new needs related to the maintenance of body fluid and its composition, despite the repeated stresses of water loss imposed by the newly invaded terrestrial environment. Apparently new adaptations included the use of neurohypophysial hormones to control GFR. Hydroosmotic responses of skin, urinary bladder and renal tubule also appeared early in amphibian evolution and assumed an important role in controlling water balance. The relatively few studies of osmoregulation among lungfishes fail to suggest that any of the endocrine osmoregulatory mechanisms typical of amphibians preexisted in their sarcopterygian ancestors.

Acknowledgments. Previously unpublished work by the authors has been supported by Research Grants from the National Science Foundation (PCM76-18689 and TCM76-82239) and the National Institutes of Health (AM 01940).

References

ACHER, R.: Chemistry of the neurohypophysial hormones: an example of molecular evolution. In: Handbook of Physiology, Section 7: Endocrinology, Vol. IV, Part 1. Knobil, E., Sawyer, W.H. (eds.). Washington, D.C.: Am. Physiol. Soc., 1974, pp. 119-130

ALVARADO, R.H., JOHNSON, S.R.: The effects of arginine vasotocin and oxytocin on sodium and water balance in *Ambystoma*. Comp. Biochem. Physiol. 16, 531-546 (1965)

BENTLEY, P.J.: The effects of neurohypophysial extracts on water transfer across the wall of the isolated urinary bladder of the toad *Bufo marinus*. J. Endocrinol. 17, 201-209 (1958)

BENTLEY, P.J.: Neurohypophyseal hormones in Amphibia: A comparison of their actions and storage. Gen. Comp. Endocrinol. 13, 39-44 (1969a)

BENTLEY, P.J.: Neurohypophysial function in Amphibia: hormone activity in the plasma. J. Endocrinol. 43, 359-369 (1969b)

BENTLEY, P.J.: Endocrines and Osmoregulation. A Comparative Account of the Regulation of Water and Salt in Vertebrates. New York-Heidelberg-Berlin: Springer, 1971, p. 300

BENTLEY, P.J.: Osmoregulation in the aquatic urodeles *Amphiuma means* (the Congo eel) and *Siren lacertina* (the mud eel). Effects of vasotocin. Gen. Comp. Endocrinol. 20, 386-392 (1973)

BENTLEY, P.J.: Actions of neurohypophysial peptides in amphibians, reptiles, and birds. In: Handbook of Physiology, Section 7: Endocrinology, Vol. IV, Part 1. Knobil, E., Sawyer, W.H. (eds.). Washington, D.C.: Am. Physiol. Soc., 1974, pp. 545-563

BENTLEY, P.J., HELLER, H.: The water-retaining action of vasotocin on the fire salamander (*Salamandra maculosa*): The role of the urinary bladder. J. Physiol. 181, 124-129 (1965)

BERLINER, R.W., DAVIDSON, D.G.: Production of hypertonic urine in the absence of pituitary antidiuretic hormone. J. Clin. Invest. 36, 1416-1427 (1957)

BROWN, P.S., BROWN, S.C.: Water balance responses to dehydration and neurohypophysial peptides in the salamander *Notophthalmus viridescens*. Gen. Comp. Endocrinol. 31, 189-201 (1977)

EWER, R.F.: The effects of posterior pituitary extracts on water balance in *Bufo carens* and *Xenopus laevis*, together with some general considerations of anuran water economy. J. Exp. Biol. 29, 429-439 (1952)

GALLI-GALLARDO, S.M., PANG, P.K.T., SAWYER, W.H.: Arginine-vasotocin actions on arterially perfused kidneys of bullfrogs, mudpuppies and South American lungfish. Federation Proc. 36, 593 (Abstract) (1977)

GARLAND, H.O., HENDERSON, I.W., BROWN, J.A.: Micropuncture study of the renal responses of the urodele amphibian *Necturus maculosus* to injections of arginine vasotocin and an anti-aldosterone compound. J. Exp. Biol. 63, 249-264 (1975)

HELLER, H., BENTLEY, P.J.: Phylogenetic distribution of the effects of neurohypophysial hormones on water and sodium metabolism. Gen. Comp. Endocrinol. 5, 96-108 (1965)

HENDERSON, I.W., EDWARDS, B.R., GARLAND, H.O., CHESTER JONES, I.: Renal function in two toads, *Xenopus laevis* and *Bufo marinus*. Gen. Comp. Endocrinol. Suppl. 3, 350-359 (1972)

HILLMAN, S.S.: The effect of arginine vasopressin on water and sodium balance in the urodele amphibian *Aneides lugubris*. Gen. Comp. Endocrinol. 24, 74-82 (1974)

HOLDER, F.C., GUERNÉ, J.M.: Une preparation particulierement sensible à l'action de la vasotocine: le bulbe aortique de l'Anguille d'eau douce. C.R. Acad. Sci. (Paris) 283D, 1767-1769 (1976)

JARD, S.: Étude des effets de la vasotocin sur l'excrétion de l'eau et des électrolytes par la rein de la grenouille *Rana esculenta* L.: analyse à l'aide d'analogues artificiels de l'hormone naturelle des caratères structuraux requis pour son activité biologique. J. Physiol., Paris, Suppl. 15, 1-124 (1966)

MAETZ, J.: Physiological aspects of neurohypophysial function in fishes with some reference to the Amphibia. Symp. Zool Soc. London 9, 107-140 (1963)

MAETZ, J., LAHLOU, B.: Actions of neurohypophysial hormones in fishes. In: Handbook of Physiology, Section 7: Endocrinology, Vol. IV, Part 1. Knobil, E., Sawyer, W.H. (eds.). Washington, D.C.: Am. Physiol. Soc., 1974, pp. 521-544

MCBEAN, R.L., GOLDSTEIN, L.: Renal function during osmotic stress in the aquatic toad *Xenopus laevis*. Am. J. Physiol. 219, 1115-1123 (1970)

NISHIMURA, H., LUNDE, L.G., ZUCKER, A.: Renin response to hemorrhage in the aglomerular toadfish, *Opsanus tau*. Federation Proc. 36, 459 (Abstract) (1977)

PANG, P.K.T.: Osmoregulatory functions of neurohypophysial hormones in fishes and amphibians. Am. Zool. 17, 739-749 (1977)

PANG, P.K.T., SAWYER, W.H.: Diuretic and vascular responses to mesotocin by *in situ* and arterially perfused bullfrog (*Rana catesbiana*) kidneys. Federation Proc. 35, 690 (Abstract) (1976)

SAWYER, W.H.: Effect of posterior pituitary extracts on urine formation and glomerular circulation in the frog. Am. J. Physiol. 164, 457-466 (1951)

SAWYER, W.H.: Increased renal reabsorption of osmotically free water by the toad (*Bufo marinus*) in response to neurohypophysial hormones. Am. J. Physiol. 189, 564-568 (1957)

SAWYER, W.H.: Increased water permeability of the bullfrog (*Rana catesbiana*) bladder in vitro in response to synthetic oxytocin and arginine vasotocin and to neurohypophysial extracts from nonmammalian vertebrates. Endocrinology 66, 112-120 (1960)

SAWYER, W.H.: Relations of chemical structures to functions of posterior pituitary hormones. Proc. Assn. Res. Nervous and Mental Disorders, 43rd Ann. Mtg. pp. 45-58 (1966a)

SAWYER, W.H.: Diuretic and natriuretic responses of the lungfish (*Protopterus aethiopicus*) to arginine vasotocin. Am. J. Physiol. 210, 191-197 (1966b)

SAWYER, W.H.: Vasopressor, diuretic and natriuretic responses by the lungfish to arginine vasotocin. Am. J. Physiol. 218, 1789-1794 (1970)

SAWYER, W.H.: Neurohypophysial hormones and water and sodium excretion in the African lungfish. Gen. Comp. Endocrinol. Suppl. 3, 345-349 (1972)

SAWYER, W.H., BLAIR-WEST, J.R., SIMPSON, P.A., SAWYER, M.K.: Renal responses of Australian lungfish to vasotocin, angiotensin II and NaCl infusion. Am. J. Physiol. 231, 593-602 (1976)

SAWYER, W.H., PANG, P.K.T.: Neurohypophysial hormones and water and sodium balances in the South American lungfish (*Lepidosiren paradoxa*). Proc. 4th Int. Congr. Endocrinol. Abstracts, p. 137 (1972)

SAWYER, W.H., PANG, P.K.T.: Endocrine factors in osmoregulation by lungfishes and amphibians. Gen. Comp. Endocrinol. 25, 224-229 (1975)

SAWYER, W.H., SCHISGALL, R.M.: Increased permeability of the frog bladder to water in response to dehydration and neurohypophysial extracts. Am. J. Physiol. 187, 312-314 (1956)

SOMLYO, A.V., SOMLYO, A.P.: Vasotocin-magnesium interaction in vascular smooth muscle of the hagfish (*Eptatretus stoutii*). Comp. Biochem. Physiol. 24, 267-270 (1968)

3. Osmoregulation and Hormones in Reptiles

E. SKADHAUGE

A number of excellent reviews of various aspects of osmoregulation in reptiles have been published recently (BRADSHAW, 1975; BENTLEY, 1976; DANTZLER, 1976; DUNSON, 1976). This short survey will, therefore, after a general introduction, concentrate on the one subject that has been dealt with only briefly by other authors, i.e., the interaction of kidney and cloaca, or the role in osmoregulation of sojourn of ureteral urine in the lower end of the gut.

General Introduction

One difficulty occurs in the treatment of the hormonal aspects of osmoregulation in reptiles. We know something about effects of osmotic stimuli, i.e., the reaction to salt-loading or depletion, to hydration or dehydration, but relatively little about the role of hormones in these effects. This survey must accordingly deal with osmotic stimuli and the reaction to these, whereas the effects of hormones must to some extent be inferred from their actions in other vertebrates.

The routes for water loss in reptiles are evaporation, and excretion through kidney, intestine, and salt gland. Except for evaporation, these are also the routes for salt excretion.

Reptilian skin has been considered traditionally as "impermeable" to water, but this is not so. In crocodiles studied by P.J. BENTLEY up to 80% of the water lost by evaporation in non-heat-stressed animals was from the skin (BENTLEY, 1976). Evaporation may constitute up to 50% of the total water loss in desert lizards (BENTLEY, 1976). In a dehydrated desert snake, the Royal Snake, DMI'EL and ZILBER (1971) found that 85% of the total water loss occurred as evaporation. In nature, reptiles avoid evaporation by behavioral regulation such as burrowing in wet soil. No hormonal regulation of the evaporation is known.

A salt gland has evolved in turtles and lizards. It functions to excrete salt in a total osmotic concentration three- to six-fold of plasma osmolality. It can be responsible for excretion of up to 50% of an external salt load (DUNSON, 1976). Little is known about the activation of the salt gland in reptiles. It is not known whether it needs expansion of volume to function, or only higher plasma osmolality. The possible hormonal involvement is not certain (DUNSON, 1976). However, our ignorance goes even further. Some reptiles excrete predominantly K and less Na with a variable ratio depending upon the Na:K ratio of the salt load. How is this Na:K change regulated? It is not known.

Reptiles encounter various problems of osmoregulation. Most are terrestrial and must excrete salt and save water. There are, however, other patterns. Marine snakes depend entirely on the salt gland to survive. Freshwater turtles must take up sodium actively. A bladder is absent from all crocodiles and snakes, but present in turtles and in some lizards. The turtle bladder has been studied in some detail and, like the amphibian bladder, largely as a biophysical tool. It does not respond to arginine vasotocin, but aldosterone augments sodium transport (BENTLEY, 1976).

The renal function of reptiles is characterized by a fairly constant osmotic ratio of urine to plasma, often in the range of 0.6-0.9. Reptiles pass a fairly large fraction of filtered sodium and water as ureteral urine (BRADSHAW, 1975; DANTZLER, 1976). Antidiuresis during dehydration is induced by the release of arginine vasotocin (AVT) which acts both by reducing the glomerular filtration rate, and increasing the permeability to water and to sodium reabsorption by the tubules.

The similarity between reptiles and birds has been stressed. Birds have even been claimed to be only "glorified reptiles." Both are uricotelic, which allows renal excretion of nitrogen waste with little loss of water. They differ, however, in other important aspects of osmoregulation. First, reptiles have apparently no volume receptors (BRADSHAW, 1978). Crocodiles and lizards may be loaded with an isosmotic saline solution, which they will retain, and not excrete until they are given pure water which lowers blood osmolality. Second, some lizards have a remarkable tolerance to high concentration of sodium in the plasma. They can withstand a doubling of plasma sodium from 150 to 300 mEq/l. The salt is simply retained, if necessary for months, and not excreted until they can obtain water.

Third, crocodiles and lizards may respond to salt or water loading only after 2-3 weeks. This may occur even if they are kept at their preferred body temperature of 34-36°C.

Cloacal Absorption of Ureteral Urine

In a number of reptiles that possess no urinary bladder, the ureteral urine is stored in the coprodeum. Ureteral urine is fluid. Before "voiding" by defecation, this urine is transformed into semi-solid pellets of urates and uric acid. These pellets are not mixed with feces, which is stored in the rectum (or colon or large intestine) orad to the so-called coprodeum (which in spite of the name contains no feces). At "voiding" the "urine" and feces pellets are deposited one after the other (ROBERTS and SCHMIDT-NIELSEN, 1966). From these observations it is logical to assume that a transmural absorption of water from ureteral urine occurs. Since the osmotic ratio of urine to plasma in reptiles nearly always is below unity, the osmotic difference between coprodeum and plasma would favor a passive absorption of water. Furthermore, water might be absorbed as solute-linked water flow following an absorption of NaCl or absorption of other ions. Ion exchange pumps, Na^+ for K^+ or NH_4^+, and Cl^- for HCO_3^-, might also conserve NaCl at low energetic cost. Both by modifying the ureteral urine, and by resorbing salt and water from feces, the lower intestine in reptiles thus has a role in osmoregulation.

In spite of the obvious importance of the cloaca, few studies have been performed. Those available fall in three groups: First, a cloacal resorption has been inferred from a comparison of ureteral urine as collected directly and after sojourn in the cloaca. Second, the transmural difference in electric potential (PD) or the short circuit current (SCC) has been measured. Third, direct transport studies in vivo or in vitro have been performed to elucidate the transport parameters and mechanisms. This information provides a necessary background for comprehension of the role of hormones and possible adaptations and regulatory mechanisms.

Comparison of Ureteral Urine Flow Rate and Cloacal Excretion Rate. When the flow rate and ionic composition of ureteral urine are compared with the cloacal excreta, in order to assess cloacal resorption or secretion, two general remarks are appropriate. First, only ions and other molecules in solution are available for absorption. Ureteral urine contains spheres of amorphous concrements of urates, 8-10 μ in diameter (MINNICH, 1976), which in the cloaca, where a slight acidification takes place, coalesce into larger concrements. This insoluble part of the excreta may contain Na and K equivalent to a concentration of 2000 mEq/l. This ability to excrete cations as urate dihydrates without osmotic consequence allows the uricotelic vertebrates to excrete their cations and nitogen waste with as little water as only few mammals, the best concentrating desert rodents, can do. Concerning ion conservation or excretion, the greatest problem in the cloaca of uricotelic vertebrates is therefore presumably that of chloride.

Calculation of cloacal resorption from difference of ureteral and cloacal output depends on correct determinations of both parameters. Since the former can only be obtained after some interference with the animal, the question is whether the experimental situation induces changes in renal functions. This seems to be so. It has been observed in a lizard clearance study that glomerular filtration rate determined by collection of ureteral urine was larger than in undisturbed animals in which the urine was collected by natural voiding (BRADSHAW et al., 1972).

In snakes JUNQUEIRA et al. (1966) subjected some undisturbed individuals to dehydration, resulting in an average weight loss of 1.1% body weight per day. In dehydrated animals in which the ureters were cannulated surgically, the urine thus bypassing the cloaca, the average weight loss was 3.7% per day.

In the freshwater crocodile, *Crocodylus acutus*, SCHMIDT-NIELSEN and SKADHAUGE (1967) measured cloacal absorption by alternate collections of ureteral urine via a catheter inserted into the cloaca and evacuation of the cloacal contents after suitable intervals.

The osmotic ratio of urine to plasma in the crocodile ranged from the hydrated to the dehydrated state from 0.7 to 0.9; the rates of absorption of cloacal salt and water were approximately 100 μl H_2O/kgh and 20 μmol NaCl/kg h, respectively, at 25°C. The conservation of Na and Cl in the cloaca would seem to be at the expense of excretion of ammonium bicarbonate.

BRADSHAW (1975, 1978) has, by comparison of cloacal and ureteral discharge, estimated 80-90% cloacal water absorption in the lizard *Amphibolurus ornatus*. He found indication of regulation of cloacal sodium resorption. During long-term water loading, which led to NaCl depletion, the fractional Na absorption in the cloaca was 99%. During saline-diuresis only 58% of Na presented to the colon was absorbed. Experiments of animals with hypophysial lesions suggested that AVT is not essential for the cloacal absorption of water. Aldosterone may, however, influence absorption of sodium, and therefore also of water.

DUNSON (1967) studied the Na absorption in the cloaca of the freshwater turtle *Pseudemys scripta*. Sodium isotope uptake measurements were carried out with and without closure of the cloacal slit. The closure reduced the rate of uptake by 68%.

Measurements of Transmural PD and SCC in Snakes. JUNQUEIRA et al. (1966) demonstrated average transmural PD values of 20-64 mV, lumen negative, in vivo. In *Xenedon* snakes, in vitro measurements in Ussing chambers showed an average SCC of 19 $\mu A/cm^2$. These data suggest a vigorous salt absorption, presumably by active transport of Na. BENTLEY and BRADSHAW (1972) found in in vitro preparations of *Amphibolurus ornatus* and *inermis* a PD of 20-50 mV, lumen negative, and a SCC of 400-500 μA/100 mg cloaca-colon tissue. This corresponds to approximately 35 μEq Na/100 g lizard per day. They found no effect of AVT on these parameters.

Experiments Involving Perfusion in vivo and in vitro. BRAYSHER and GREEN (1970) introduced an isotonic solution in vivo in the isolated cloaca of *Varanus gouldii*. They observed an average fluid absorption of 8.4 ml/kg h at 30°C. The Na absorption was 1.88 mEq/kg h. These authors claim a large increase in water and Na absorption after injection of AVT into the blood stream, but they base their results on differences during a brief interval after the installation. SKADHAUGE and DUVDEVANI (1977) perfused the coprodeum of *Agama stellio* with a NaCl solution of an osmolality equal to that of ureteral urine in lizards with free access to water. This osmolality is 210 mOsm corresponding to a urine plasma osmotic ratio of 0.7. The cloacal contents collected from previously undisturbed animals were in osmotic equilibrium with plasma. The perfusion experiments indicated water absorption of 2.39 ml/kg h; NaCl absorption of 203 and 131 μEq/kg h, respectively, and K secretion of 45 μEq/kg h. (In the paper the unit was erroneously given as mEq). The absorption of NaCl and water represented approximately 80% of ureterally excreted water and NaCl. Since the absorbate had an ion concentration of 121 mEq/l, thus being hypoosmotic to plasma, water absorption is presumably due to a combination of osmotic and solute-linked water flow.

HOUSE (1974) perfused the cloaca of *Dipsosaurus dorsalis* in vivo with a salt solution very close to plasma osmolality. He found in dehydrated individuals an average water absorption of 56 μl/kg h. The osmolality of the perfusion fluid increased and K secretion of 19 μEq/kg h was measured. DUNSON (1967) measured in an in vitro preparation of the cloaca in *Pseudemys* the Na influx and the SCC. The mean Na uptake was 0.62 $\mu Eq/cm^2$ h, almost equal to the observed SCC of 17 $\mu A/cm^2$.

Conclusion. Cloacal absorption of NaCl and water from ureteral urine is import in reptiles, particularly as studied in crocodiles and lizards. About 80% of both NaCl and water is resorbed. The resorption is most likely regulated through aldosterone.

Mechanism of Cloacal Water Absorption. A cloacal absorption of water may arise from the difference in osmolality between lumen and plasma or be a consequence of electrolyte absorption, the so-called solute-linked water flow. MURRISH and SCHMIDT-NIELSEN (1970) have, however, suggested that the colloid-osmotic pressure created by the plasma protein concentration may give a sufficient driving force for withdrawal of water from the cloacal contents of reptiles. Although the presence of this force is unquestionable, there are serious reservations concerning its quantitative importance. The plasma colloid-osmotic pressure in dehydrated *Dipsosaurus dorsalis* was 267 cm H_2O. Since 20 mm Hg (272 cm H_2O) is equal to 0.026 atm and 1 atm equal to 39 mOsmol, the driving force of the colloid-osmotic pressure is only about 1 mOsmol. (In comparison, the limiting driving force for solute-linked water flow is usually around 1-3 atm.) If the osmotic permeability coefficient of the cloaca is high, about 10 μl H_2O/kgh mOsmol a water transport of only 10 μl/kg h can occur. This is small compared to the transmural flow observed in reptilan cloacae. It seems, therefore, unlikely that the proposed mechanism is of quantitative importance. It is, however, possible that the colloids may absorb a final minute fraction of water in the cloaca after solute-linked transport. Since the cloacal wall seems to have a reflection coefficient of unity for the major solutes of plasma and cloacal contents, the colloid-osmotic force will only be of value if the osmotic concentration in the cloaca is lower or equal to that of plasma.

References

BENTLEY, P.J.: Osmoregulation. In: Biology of the Reptilia, Vol. V. Gans, C., Dawson, W.R. (eds.). London: Academic Press, 1976, pp. 365-412

BENTLEY, P.J., BRADSHAW, S.D.: Electrical potential difference across the cloaca and colon of the Australian lizards *Amphibolurus ornatus* and *A. inermis*. Comp. Biochem. Physiol. 42A, 465-471 (1972)

BRADSHAW, S.D.: Osmoregulation and pituitary-adrenal function in desert reptiles. Gen. Comp. Endocrinol. 25, 230-248 (1975)

BRADSHAW, S.D.: Volume regulation in desert reptiles and its control by pituitary and adrenal hormones. In: Osmotic and Volume Regulation. Jørgensen, C.B., Skadhauge, E. (eds.). Copenhagen: Munksgaard, 1978

BRADSHAW, S.D., SHOEMAKER, V.H., NAGY, K.A.: The role of adrenal corticoids in the regulation of kidney function in the desert lizard *Dipsosauros dorsalis*. Comp. Biochem. Physiol. 43A, 671-735 (1972)

BRAYSHER, M., GREEN, B.: Absorption of water and electrolytes from an Australian lizard *Varanus gouldii* (Gray). Comp. Biochem. Physiol. 35, 607-614 (1970)

DANTZLER, W.H.: Renal function (with special emphasis on nitrogen excretion). In: Biology of the Reptilia, Vol. V. Gans, C., Dawson, W.R. (eds.). London: Academic press, 1976, pp. 447-503

DMI'EL, R., ZILBER, B.: Water balance in a desert snake. Copeia 1971, 754-755

DUNSON, W.A.: Sodium fluxes in fresh-water turtles. J. Exp. Zool. 165, 171-182 (1967)

DUNSON, W.A.: Salt glands in reptiles. In: Biology of the Reptilia, Vol. V. Gans, C., Dawson, W.R. (eds.). London: Academic Press, 1976, pp. 413-445

HOUSE, D.G.: Modification of urine by the cloaca of the desert iguana, *Dipsosaurus dorsalis*. M.S. Thesis, Univ. Mulwaukee, Wisconsin, 1974

JUNQUIERA, L.C.U., MALNIC, G., MONGE, C.: Reabsorptive function of the ophidian cloaca and large intestine. Physiol. Zool. 39, 151-159 (1966)

MINNICH, J.E.: Adaptations in the reptilian excretory system for excreting insoluble urates. Israel. J. Med. Sci. 12, 854-861 (1976)

MURRISH, D.E., SCHMIDT-NIELSEN, K.: Water transport in the cloaca of lizards: Active or passive? Science 170, 324-326 (1970)

ROBERTS, J.S., SCHMIDT-NIELSEN, B.: Renal ultrastructure and the excretion of salt and water by three terrestrial lizards. Am. J. Physiol. 211, 476-486 (1966)

SCHMIDT-NIELSEN, B., SKADHAUGE, E.: Function of the excretory system of the crocodile (*Crocodylus acutus*). Am. J. Physiol. 212, 973-980 (1967)

SKADHAUGE, E., DUVDEVANI, I.: Cloacal absorption of NaCl and water in the lizard *Agama stellio*. Comp. Biochem. Physiol. 56A, 275-279 (1977)

4. Hormonal Regulation of Salt and Water Balance in Granivorous Birds

E. SKADHAUGE

Introduction

This survey treats the involvement of hormones in osmoregulation in birds without salt glands. This restricts the target organs for hormonal action to the kidney and cloaca. "Granivorous" has been chosen to cover terrestrial birds that may face deficiencies in salt or water. Adaptation to xeric conditions as such is of less importance in birds in a hormonal context, since desert life depends on adaptation of structural and functional parameters without hormonal determining factors. Birds of prey can be excluded since, by flying at high altitudes, they are able to avoid the desert climate. They also have an inborn independence of water, since they feed on prey that contains two thirds water which provides adequately for their metabolic requirements.

This survey will deal first with renal excretion, then with cloacal absorption, and finally with the interaction between these two organs.

Hormonal Regulation of Renal Functions

The structure of the avian kidney shows reptilian and mammalian characteristics. There are typically reptilian nephrons, which lack loops of Henle, and typically mammalian nephrons with these loops (BRAUN and DANTZLER, 1972). Both types join in the collecting ducts, which pass through medullary cones into which the loops of Henle dip. The blood supply is arterial and portal from the legs. The portal flow constitutes roughly half the total flow in the domestic fowl (SKADHAUGE, 1973, p. 12). The portal blood perfuses the tubuli, but not the glomeruli. The blood flow in the vasa recta in the medullary cones is of post-glomerular origin.

The morphologic background would thus seem to permit a "reptilian" anti-diuresis with shut-down of glomeruli, and the formation of a concentrated urine due to a "mammalian" counter-current multiplier system operating in the medullary cones. Physiologic experiments confirm both of these predictions.

In a study on the domestic fowl (SKADHAUGE and SCHMIDT-NIELSEN, 1967a), and in the budgerigar (EMERY et al., 1972), hypertonicity and accumulation of Na and Cl were observed in the medullary cones. Maximal osmotic ratios of urine to plasma of 4-5 have been observed in birds, although 1.5-3 is most common even in desert birds (SKADHAUGE, 1974a). However, only relatively few species have been examined, particularly among birds of prey.

When birds pass from hydration to dehydration the urine flow is greatly reduced and the osmolality is increased. Some reduction of the glomerular filtration rate (GFR) is observed together with a small reduction of the excretion of "strong" electrolytes (SKADHAUGE and SCHMIDT-NIELSEN, 1967b). These changes can be mimicked by injections of arginine vasotocin (AMES et al., 1971), a naturally occurring octapeptide in the avian neurohypophysis. The effect of smaller doses of the hormone can largely be attributed to action on tubular permeability, whereas the higher doses seem to reduce GFR. This reduction has recently been demonstrated to involve the reptilian, and not the mammalian nephrons (BRAUN and DANTZLER, 1974). The mechanism of the reduction of GFR seems to be a contraction of the afferent glomerular arterioles (BRAUN, 1976).

The renal-concentrating ability in birds is related to the relative amount of medullary tissue (JOHNSON and SKADHAUGE, 1975; SKADHAUGE, 1976), presumably as a result of a larger fraction of mammalian nephrons being present in the good concentrators. Adaptation to desert conditions is not necessarily related to a good concentrating ability. Both good and less good concentrating abilities are found in well-adapted desert species (SKADHAUGE, 1974a). This may be due to the fact that the overall water conservation through the excreta is a combination of renal excretion and post-renal modification of ureteral urine by cloacal resorption of water (see later).

Concerning cloacal resorption of ureteral urine, it should be emphasized that only ions and molecules in solution will be resorbed. In birds the majority of renally excreted nitrogen is present as urate dehydrates of sodium and potassium (MCNABB et al., 1972) resulting in a precipitate that would correspond to around 2.000 mEq/l if these ions were in solution. More than 50% of the urine osmolality in dehydrated domestic fowls is accounted for by potassium-ammonium-phosphate. The fluid that moves into the intestine is thus of differing osmolality, depending upon the water balance, and of a very different composition from that which usually occurs in vertebrate intestines.

Hormonal Regulation of Cloacal Resorption

The ureteral urine moves retrogradely into the coprodeum and large intestine, as far as the ceca. The urine is stored in these parts of the gut, together with feces. In granivorous birds the yellow or white precipitate of urates sits like a cap on the outside of a central fecal core (SKADHAUGE, 1968; SKADHAUGE and BRADSHAW, 1974), whereas in some birds of prey the lowest end of the coprodeum contains urine alone. The epithelium of coprodeum and colon constitutes the main functional segment for resorption from ureteral urine (Fig. 1).

There are two major methods for studying the transport parameters for this resorption, and thus the role of hormones. The first is by in vivo intraluminal perfusion of the coprodeum and colon, the second by in vitro mounting of the isolated epithelial tissue in the so-called Ussing chamber (USSING and ZERAHN, 1951).

In vivo Experiments. In vivo perfusion studies have revealed a slight dependence of the cloacal transport parameters on the level of hydration of the animal, but a major adjustment due to the NaCl balance. Several studies have been performed on the domestic fowl, and some observations on desert birds are available (see below).

Hydration-Dehydration. The most important transport parameters are the V_{max} and the K_m for net sodium transport (which thus is describable by saturation kinetics), the osmotic permeability coefficient, and the

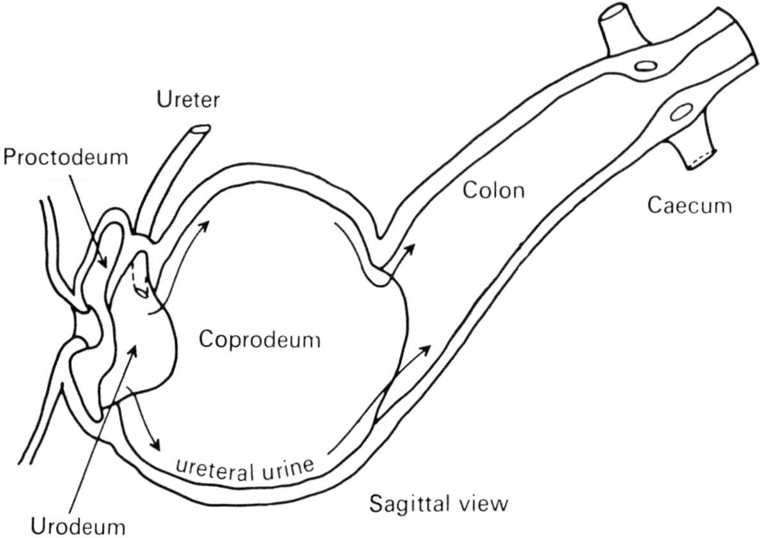

Fig. 1. A sagittal view of the coprodeum and colon of the domestic fowl. The retrograde movement of ureteral urine into the lower gut is shown. Coprodeum and colon are the main sites for postrenal modification of ureteral urine

so-called solute-linked water flow. The last is the number of water molecules that follow one sodium ion transported across the cloacal wall in the absence of an osmotic difference across the epithelium. From hydration to dehydration these parameters changed relatively little (BINDSLEV and SKADHAUGE, 1971a, b), but the changes are of significance. They can be shown by computer calculations to augment the fractional water absorption of ureteral urine from -6% to +14% of the ureteral urine water (SKADHAUGE and KRISTENSEN, 1972). No effect of arginine vasotocin (AVT) could be shown on the sodium transport by the cloaca in vivo (SKADHAUGE, 1967), nor in vitro (E. SKADHAUGE, unpublished).

Salt Loading/Depletion. The conditions cause major changes in the rate of sodium absorption and, correlated with the rate of sodium transport, changes in the transmural flow of chloride and potassium. Early in vivo experiments (SKADHAUGE, 1967) established (1) that a low luminal sodium concentration results in a decreased rate of sodium absorption, (2) that a high luminal potassium concentration reduces the rate of net sodium absorption, and (3) that external sodium loading prior to perfusion experiment almost halves the V_{max} for sodium absorption. Subsequent systematic perfusion experiments showed the net sodium absorption rate to be describable by saturation kinetics both in a desert species with a low sodium diet (SKADHAUGE, 1974b) and in the domestic fowl on a normal commercial sodium-containing diet, but which were starved for two days prior to experiment (BINDSLEV and SKADHAUGE, 1971b). In recent experiments on nonstarved birds (D.H. THOMAS and E. SKADHAUGE, in preparation) sodium loading reduced the net sodium absorption rate considerably and changed the kinetics from Michaelis-Menten type saturation kinetics to a linear relationship. The first type of kinetics is compatible with a carrier-mediated process, the second with diffusion limitation. Furthermore, in these experiments, which have been reported briefly (THOMAS et al., 1975), strong linear correlations were observed among the rates of net sodium absorption, the net absorption of chloride and secretion of potassium. The relationship among these rates (rounded values) is best illustrated by an example: a net sodium absorption rate of 40 μEq/kg h as observed in sodium-depleted birds at a luminal sodium concentration of 40 mEq/l is associated with a Cl absorption of 30 μEq/kg h, and a K secretion of 16 μEq/kg h. The unit base per kg body weight, has been chosen, since the same anatomical segment is perfused in each bird.

The major mineralo-corticoid hormones in birds are aldosterone and corticosterone (SANDOR and MEDHI, 1977). Although secretion rates and plasma concentrations of these hormones as functions of the NaCl balance are not well known in birds, NaCl depletion will be assumed to be associated with an increase in aldosterone production. D.H. THOMAS and E. SKADHAUGE (in preparation), therefore, investigated the influence of both acute and chronic injections of aldosterone on the cloacal transport parameters with an in vivo preparation in the domestic fowl. The acute effect on net sodium transport was a steep increase in the absorption rate after 1 h reaching a plateau of a five-fold higher transport rate after 5 h. In birds given an external sodium load, the absolute increase was only 60% of that in birds on a normal commercial chicken food. The potassium secretion was also augmented. Chronic injections resulted in qualitatively similar responses, but of lower magnitude. However, injections at frequent intervals were not tested. The conclusion to be drawn from these experiments is that aldosterone is involved in regulation of sodium absorption, but the role of other hormones remains to be investigated.

Absorption of Ions Other than NaCl. It has been noted recently that the strong electrolytes Na, K and Cl only account for a small fraction of osmolality of ureteral urine in granivorous birds (SKADHAUGE, 1974a). Furthermore, a few observations indicate that high concentrations of ammonium ion occur in ureteral urine, as observed in ducks (MCNABB et al., 1972). A systematic investigation of ureteral urine of dehydrated domestic fowls fed wheat and barley, thus being on a low sodium diet, showed Na and Cl to account for only 12% of the osmolality (SKADHAUGE, 1977), whereas ammonium, potassium and phosphate had mean concentrations of 120 mEq/l, 73 mEq/l and 130 mEq/l, respectively, accounting for 42% of the osmolality. The concentrations of divalent ions, calcium and magnesium were low, as were the concentrations of bicarbonate and urea.

Potassium is subjected to secretion in the cloaca, apparently linked to the Na absorption. Only very high luminal concentrations of potassium resulted in absorption (SKADHAUGE, 1967). Potassium also plays a major role in vitro in reducing the Na absorption rate in the domestic fowl. A physiologic potassium concentration of around 50 mEq/l reduced the net sodium absorption rate to roughly 1/4 of the Na transport rate observed in a Krebs phosphate buffer, 140 mEq/l Na (U. KATZ and E. SKADHAUGE, in preparation).

Ammonium ions undergo a limited absorption also linked with the net sodium absorption with only 12 mEq/kg h, absorbed for 40 mEq/kg h sodium. The absorptive capacity of the coprodeum-large intestine segment can be calculated to be 9% of the ureteral excretion of ammonium in a salt-depleted granivorous fowl. Phosphate undergoes little net transport across the cloacal wall.

In vitro Experiments. The study of the cloacal transport parameters was advanced when ways were found to mount the epithelium in vitro in the Ussing chamber (CHOSHNIAK et al., 1977). This permits the simultaneous measurement of the electrical parameters generated by the tissue, i.e., electric potential difference (PD), and the current necessary to short-circuit the tissue (SCC), and the unilateral transepithelial fluxes of ions as studied with isotopes. These tissues survive for 3-5 h in vitro at 38°C in an oxygenated Krebs-phosphate buffer with glucose as metabolic fuel. We first began measurement of the electrical parameters of the coprodeum of fowls reared on three diets: wheat and barley (low sodium), commercial chicken food (which includes some NaCl), and commercial food with additional oral NaCl loading (Table 1). Only

Table 1. Transport parameters of the isolated coprodeum of the domestic fowl

Diet:	Wheat + barley (low Na)	Commercial food (high Na)	
PD:	37.3 ± 2.2	4.7 ± 0.6	mV
SCC:	10.6 ± 0.4	0.6 ± 0.1	μEq/kg h
Sodium flux			
Mucosa-serosa	13.2 ± 0.5	1.5 ± 0.2	μEq/kg h
Serosa-mucosa	1.4 ± 0.2	1.4 ± 0.2	μEq/kg h

From CHOSHNIAK et al. (1977)
Means ± S.E. are reported.

the low sodium diet is associated with a high short-circuit current and PD, whereas even a medium sodium load leads to an almost complete suppression of both parameters. When the origin of the PD and SCC was sought by study of unilateral movements of Na and Cl, the flux ratio for chloride was unity, indicating passive transport, but the sodium fluxes demonstrated an active mucosa-to-serosa transport of sodium also giving rise to the PD. The net sodium flux was identical to the SCC. The concept of sodium transport as active (requiring metabolic energy closely associated with the cellular expenditure of ATP) is further strengthened by the finding that ouabain inhibited the transport only after application to the serosa side.

A very high sensitivity of the coprodeum epithelium to the NaCl balance of the animal is reasonable from an osmoregulatory point of view, since the coprodeum is the final meeting ground for ureteral urine and feces. The coprodeal resorption will thus be able to regulate the final Na balance very precisely.

The study of colonic transport has only recently been initiated, but some preliminary data are available (B.G. MUNCK and S. SKADHAUGE, in preparation). The chicken colon shows a pattern different from that of the coprodeum, but only in NaCl-loaded birds. In the NaCl-depleted birds the SCC of the colon is equal to or even higher than that of the coprodeum. The SCC is not dependent upon the presence of amino acids, and it is almost totally suppressed by Amiloride applied from the mucosal side. This agent is supposed to block the entry of sodium into the cells. In NaCl loading the PD and SCC are moderately reduced, but only when amino acids are present in the bathing solutions, otherwise the electrical parameters (and the unilateral sodium flux in the mucosa-to-serosa direction) are strongly reduced. Furthermore, this amino acid-stimulated sodium transport is not inhibited by Amiloride. Sodium loading is thus associated with the occurrence of a sodium pump similar to the carbohydrate-amino acid-stimulated sodium pump known from the mammalian small intestine. Sodium depletion causes this phenomenon to disappear, but activates a nonelectrolyte-independent, ATP-dependent sodium pump, presumably located at the baso-lateral membrane.

The ability of aldosterone to mimic the effects of sodium depletion has only recently been explored with in vitro preparation (D.H. THOMAS et al., in preparation). After addition of aldosterone in vitro, only small effects on SCC or PD were observed even after 5 h in the presence of several amino acids and glucose. In vivo injections of aldosterone produced a partial change to the pattern characteristic of sodium-depleted birds. This phenomenon was more marked in colon than in coprodeum. Suppression of adrenocorticoid production by Metopiron (Ciba) in Na-depleted birds, however, was without any effect on the electical parameters. Much more work is thus necessary before the role of hormones in the responses to sodium-loading or depletion is elucidated. The very large changes in SCC and unilateral sodium fluxes should make the bird cloaca ideal for the study of hormones.

Quantitative Interaction between Kidney and Cloaca. When flow rates and composition of ureteral urine are known for the most common osmotic situations, and the cloacal transport parameters are equally well determined, the interaction, that is the quantitative modification induced by the cloacal sojourn of ureteral urine can be elucidated. The interaction is best described by the fraction of salt and water saved during the storage of ureteral urine in the cloaca. Table 2 shows these relations for Na and H_2O in the domestic fowl. It appears that only in

Table 2. Cloacal absorption in birds

Species	Osmotic situation	Urine osmolality	Absorption
Fowl	Hydration	115 mosmol	H_2O: 2%
Fowl	Salt-loading	362 mosmol	Na : 1-2%
Fowl	Dehydration	538 mosmol	H_2O: 14% Na: 69%
Galah	Dehydration	982 mosmol	H_2O: 10-20% Na: 70%

Fractional absorption (in percent) of Na and water are calculated for the domestic fowl and the Galah. Based on findings reported in SKADHAUGE and SCHMIDT-NIELSEN (1967b), SKADHAUGE and KRISTENSEN (1972), SKADHAUGE (1974a, b)

the dehydrated state is water absorption critical, and except during salt loading, a large part of ureterally excreted sodium is reabsorbed in the cloaca. Since absorption of water from the originally hyperosmotic urine as produced in the dehydrated state requires NaCl absorption by solute-linked water flow, the storage of ureteral urine in the cloaca would seem to lead to a water loss, provided the urine osmolality is sufficiently high, and the sodium concentration of the urine sufficiently low (KRAG and SKADHAUGE, 1972). Such cloacal water loss would seem to threaten granivorous desert birds, since they are good concentrators and receive a low sodium diet (SKADHAUGE, 1974a). Such a bird the Australian Parrot *Cacatua roseicapilla*, has been investigated. Although this bird has a urine-concentrating ability that is 60% greater than that of the domestic fowl, it has a lower osmotic permeability coefficient of the cloacal wall, and a higher rate of solute-linked water flow. These factors, together with a lower rate of urine flow, permit a cloacal absorption of water almost identical to that of the domestic fowl (SKADHAUGE, 1974b; Table 2).

It was mentioned above that the renal-concentrating ability is not well correlated with desert adaptation, as both good and bad concentrators are well adapted to desert life (SKADHAUGE, 1974a). Computer calculations have shown that, ceteris paribus, a lower concentrating ability associated with a proportionally higher flow rate of urine should lead to a higher rate of cloacal resorption of water (SKADHAUGE and KRISTENSEN, 1972). This may explain the good desert adaptation of the emu, *Dromaius novae-hollandiae*, (SKADHAUGE, 1974a). Birds with a high urine-concentrating ability like the Galah, *Cacatua roseicapilla*, and the Budgerigar, *Melopsitticus undulatus*, may rely oppositely on a low cloacal osmotic permeability coefficient (SKADHAUGE, 1974b; KRAG and SKADHAUGE, 1972). Two adaptive strategies may accordingly be envisioned in birds: either a low renal-concentrating ability associated with a high rate of absorption in the cloaca, or a good renal-concentrating ability with an almost impermeable cloacal wall. The latter would also seem most appropriate for birds that suffer both dehydration and occasional salt loading, such as the Zebra Finch, *Taeniopygia castanotis* (SKADHAUGE and BRADSHAW, 1974).

Conclusion

The pattern or excretion and salt and water in birds is complex and fascinating. It involves both reptilian and mammalian components. The kidney has "reptilian" nephrons which reduce the rate of glomerular filtration in the presence of arginine vasotocin. There are also "mammalian" nephrons with loops of Henle, permitting hypertonicity in the medullary cone, that provides a counter-current system. Antidiuresis therefore occurs due to permeability-increasing effects of arginine vasotocin on the collecting ducts.

Ureteral urine passes retrogradely into the coprodeum and large intestine where sodium chloride is absorbed and potassium secreted. The quantitatively important ions of fluid ureteral urine are ammonium and phosphate. The former undergoes a slight absorption, partly coupled with sodium absorption; phosphate undergoes little net transport. In the dehydrated state, water is absorbed even from the originally hyperosmotic urine. Sodium transport by the cloacal wall is extremely sensitive to the sodium balance of the animal; a large fraction of ureterally excreted Na can be reabsorbed in the cloaca. The rate of sodium absorption is at least partly regulated by aldosterone.

References

AMES, E., STEVEN, K., SKADHAUGE, E.: Effects of arginine vasotocin on renal excretion of Na^+, K^+, Cl^-, and urea in the hydrated chicken. Am. J. Phys. 221, 1223-1228 (1971)

BINDSLEV, N., SKADHAUGE, E.: Salt and water permeability of the coprodeum and large intestine in the normal and dehydrated fowl (*Gallus domesticus*). In vivo perfusion studies. J. Physiol. 216, 735-751 (1971a)

BINDSLEV, N., SKADHAUGE, E.: Sodium chloride absorption and solute-linked water flow across the epithelium of the coprodeum and large intestine in the normal and dehydrated fowl (*Gallus domesticus*). In vivo perfusion studies. J. Physiol. 216, 753-768 (1971b)

BRAUN, E.J.: Intrarenal blood flow distribution in the desert quail following salt loading. Am. J. Phys. 231, 1111-1117 (1976)

BRAUN, E.J., DANTZLER, W.H.: Function of mammalian-type and reptilian-type nephrons in kidney of desert quail. Am. J. Phys. 222, 617-629 (1972)

BRAUN, E.J., DANTZLER, W.H.: Effects of ADH on single-nephron glomerular filtration rates in the avian kidney. Am. J. Phys. 226, 1-8 (1974)

CHOSHNIAK, I., MUNCK, B.G., SKADHAUGE, E.: Sodium chloride transport across the chicken coprodeum. Basic characteristics and dependence on sodium chloride intake. J. Phys. 271, 489-504 (1977)

EMERY, N., POULSON, T.L., KINTER, W.B.: Production of concentrated urine by avian kidneys. Am. J. Phys. 223, 180-187 (1972)

HOLMES, W.N., FLETCHER, G.L., STEWART, D.J.: The patterns of renal electrolyte excretion in the duck (*Anas platyrhynchos*) maintained on freshwater and on hypertonic saline. J. Exp. Biol. 48, 487-508 (1968)

JOHNSON, O.W., SKADHAUGE, E.: Structural-functional correlations in the kidneys and observations of colon and cloacal morphology in certain Australian birds. J. Anat. 120, 495-505 (1975)

KRAG, B., SKADHAUGE, E.: Renal salt and water excretion in the Budgerygah (*Melopsittacus undulatus*). Comp. Biochem. Phys. 41A, 667-683 (1972)

MCNABB, F.M.A., MCNABB, R.A., WARD, J.M.: The effects of dietery protein content on water requirements and ammonia excretion in pigeons, *Columbia livia*. Comp. Biochem. Phys. 43A, 181-185 (1972)

SANDOR, T., MEDHI, A.Z.: Adrenocortical function in birds. Proc. 1st Int. Symp. Avian Endocrinol. pp. 88-91 (1977)

SKADHAUGE, E.: In vivo perfusion studies of the water and electrolyte resorption in the cloaca of the fowl (*Gallus domesticus*). Comp. Biochem. Phys. 23, 483-501 (1967)

SKADHAUGE, E.: Cloacal storage of urine in the rooster. Comp. Biochem. Phys. 24, 7-18 (1968)

SKADHAUGE, E.: Renal and cloacal salt and water transport in the fowl, *Gallus domesticus*. Danish Med. Bull. 20, Suppl. 1, 1-82 (1973)

SKADHAUGE, E.: Renal concentrating ability in selected West Australian birds. J. Exp. Biol. 61, 269-276 (1974a)

SKADHAUGE, E.: Cloacal resorption of salt and water in the Galah (*Cacatua roseicapilla*). J. Phys. 240, 763-773 (1974b)

SKADHAUGE, E.: Water conservation in xerophilic birds. Israel J. Med. Sci. 12, 732-739 (1976)

SKADHAUGE, E.: Solute composition of the osmotic space of ureteral urine in dehydrated chickens (*Gallus domesticus*). Comp. Biochem. Phys. 56A, 271-274 (1977)

SKADHAUGE, E., BRADSHAW, S.: Saline drinking and cloacal excretion of salt and water in the Zebra Finch. Am. J. Phys. 227, 1263-1267 (1974)

SKADHAUGE, E., KRISTENSEN, K.: An analogue computer simulation of cloacal resorption of salt and water from ureteral urine in birds. J. Theor. Biol. 45, 473-487 (1972)

SKADHAUGE, E., SCHMIDT-NIELSEN, B.: The renal medullary electrolyte and urea gradient in roosters and turkeys. Am. J. Phys. 212, 1313-1318 (1967a)

SKADHAUGE, E., SCHMIDT-NIELSEN, B.: Renal function in domestic fowl. Am. J. Phys. 212, 793-798 (1967b)

THOMAS, D.H., SKADHAUGE, E., READ, M.W.: Steroid effects on gut function in birds. Biochem. Soc. Trans. 3, 1164-1168 (1975)

USSING, H.H., ZERAHN, K.: Active transport of sodium as the source of electric current in the short-circuited isolated frog skin. Acta Phys. Scand. 23, 119-127 (1951)

5. Endocrine Response in Osmoregulation: Hormonal Adaptation in Aquatic Birds

W. N. HOLMES

The maintenance of steady-state homeostatic conditions requires that the mean daily intakes of water and electrolytes are equivalent to the mean daily losses. Thus, the volume of water absorbed from the gastrointestinal tract (I) of a bird living in an environment where freshwater is always available must equal the sum of the volumes of water lost through excretion as urine (V) and feces (F), and through evaporation from the respiratory surfaces (R). This general relationship may be expressed as

$$I = V + F + R \qquad (1)$$

Similarly, the daily intake of any osmotically active substance (x) must balance the sum of the amounts lost via all pathways. Since the water lost via the respiratory tract does not contain dissolved electrolytes, all of the electrolytes ingested by an organism lacking sweat glands must be excreted in the urine and feces. The osmotic balance of such an organism may therefore be represented as follows:

$$i_x I = (u_x V + f_x F) \qquad (2)$$

where i_x represents the concentration of substance x in the volume of water reabsorbed from the gut (I) and u_x and f_x represent the concentrations of x in the volumes of water excreted as urine and feces respectively.

Although birds can produce hypertonic urine, most species probably discharge a hypotonic fluid into the cloaca as long as adequate amounts of fresh drinking water are available. Indeed, experiments on the freshwater-maintained Mallard have suggested that the birds rarely, if ever, excrete hypertonic cloacal fluid, even under conditions of extreme antidiuresis (HOLMES and ADAMS, 1963; HOLMES et al., 1968; BRADLEY et al., 1971). When fresh drinking water is replaced by either hypertonic saline or seawater, however, they do produce cloacal urine that is hyperosmotic with respect to plasma (HOLMES et al., 1968; STEWART et al., 1969). But, even under these circumstances, approximately half of the total cation concentration in the urine consists of ammonium ion, and the limiting isorrheic concentration of Na^+ is always less than that which could be necessary to permit all of the ingested Na^+ to be excreted by the kidneys (Table 1). In these birds, therefore, the limited excretory capability of the kidney must be augmented by an extrarenal excretory mechanism. Thus, the general equation representing osmotic balance in these birds must be modified:

$$i_x I = (u_x \cdot V + f_x \cdot F_x + e_x \cdot E) \qquad (3)$$

where e_x = the concentration of substance x in the extrarenal excretory fluid.

The nasal or "salt" gland located in each orbit has developed into an extrarenal excretory organ in those avian species living in environments in which an abundance of osmotically free water is not always

Table 1. A comparison of the relative proportions of the major cations in the cloacal discharge of freshwater- and seawater-maintained Mallards, *Anas platyrhynchos*. (Adapted from FLETCHER and HOLMES, 1968)

	Total cation concentration (mM)	Percentage of total cation concentration		
		Na^+	K^+	NH_4^+
Freshwater-maintained	172	6	30	64
Seawater-maintained	246[a]	16[a]	29	55

[a] Significantly different from corresponding value for freshwater-maintained Mallards.

available. When stimulated by an osmotic load, these glands discharge a concentrated solution of electrolytes, and in this way a marine bird, for example, may excrete more than 90% of the Na^+ and Cl^- and 70% of the K^+ in its diet (FLETCHER and HOLMES, 1968).

Although some species of birds live continuously in the marine environment, others only visit coastal habitats during a portion of their life histories. In these species, adaptation to a coastal environment may involve changes in the absorptive properties of the small intestine. For example, within a few hours of being given hypertonic saline drinking water, Mallard ducklings that have been raised on fresh drinking water show increases in the rates of uptake of water and Na^+ across the intestinal mucosa. Within 48 h, the rates become maximal along the entire length of the small intestine, and this high rate is sustained as long as the birds drink hypertonic water. On return to fresh drinking water, the mucosal transfer rates soon decline, and within three days return to normal (CROCKER and HOLMES, 1971). However, if these birds are treated with spironolactone before they are given hypertonic drinking water, the increases in mucosal transfer do not occur (Fig.

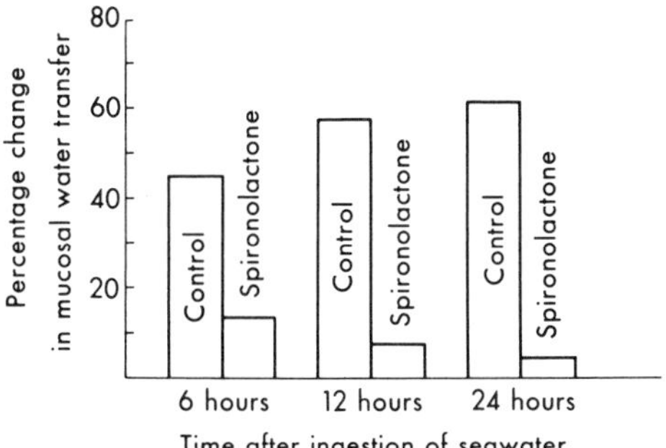

Fig. 1. The effect of spironolactone on mucosal water transfer in ducklings during adaptation to a diet containing seawater. The mucosal transfer rates were measured in vitro in everted sacs prepared from the small intestine. Spironolactone (5 mg) was administered orally to the experimental birds 24 h before they were given seawater to drink. The mean values were derived from determination on at least 6 individuals of both control and experimental groups at each interval after initial exposure to seawater. The suppression of the increase in mucosal water transfer by spironolactone was significant ($P < 0.01$) at the end of each time interval. (From CROCKER and HOLMES, 1976)

1). Inhibition of endogenous corticosteroidogenesis by treatment with metyrapone also prevents development of this adaptive response in the intestinal mucosa (CROCKER and HOLMES, 1976). Furthermore, increases similar to those occurring in the birds given hypertonic saline can be induced in freshwater ducklings by treating them with corticosterone; as in the case of birds given hypertonic saline, this response can be effectively blocked by an oral dose of spironolactone prior to injection of the corticosterone (CROCKER and HOLMES, 1971, 1976).

Development of increased rates of mucosal transfer of water seems to be essential for sustained function of the nasal gland in birds that are continuously exposed to hypertonic drinking water; if the development is blocked by treatment with either spironolactone or metyrapone, then the nasal glands do not appear to secrete fluid in response to the ingestion of seawater (CROCKER and HOLMES, 1971). Thus, the initiation and continuation of nasal gland function in coastal marine birds may depend on the establishment of increased absorptive properties in the intestinal mucosa, and the development of these properties seems to depend on an adrenocortical hormone, probably corticosterone (CROCKER and HOLMES, 1976).

In response to uptake of the osmotically active material in the drinking water, a sequence of events leading to the onset of secretion by the nasal gland is initiated. The first step in this secretory reflex involves the stimulation of an osmoreceptor. This receptor is located in the extracellular compartment outside of the central nervous system, and is probably associated with either the heart or the cardiac circulation (HANWELL et al., 1972). Sustained nasal gland function seems to depend upon the stimulation of two motor pathways; one involving visceral motor impulses that stimulate the glands directly, and the other consisting of efferent impulses that stimulate the secretion of corticotropin-releasing hormone from the median eminence. This latter reflex is of particular interest to the endocrinologist, since it leads to an activation of the adenohypophysio-adrenocortical axis (for review, see HOLMES and PHILLIPS, 1976).

When Mallards are given loads of hypertonic saline, immediate four- to fivefold increases in plasma corticosterone concentration occur and are sustained for 2 to 3 h (Fig. 2). Similar increases in adrenocortical activity have been observed in Pekin Ducks that have been given hypertonic saline loads (DONALDSON and HOLMES, 1965; MACCHI et al., 1967). Removal of the adenohypophysis prevents this increase in plasma corticosterone concentration, and the secretion of nasal gland fluid in response to the saline load is reduced to only 5% of normal (Fig. 3). Conversely, treatment of the adenohypophysectomized birds with ACTH increases corticosterone concentrations in peripheral blood and restores a normal extrarenal excretory response (Fig. 3; WRIGHT et al., 1966; BRADLEY and HOLMES, 1972; HOLMES et al., 1972). The imposition of partial adrenocortical insufficiency through either acute discontinuance of ACTH replacement therapy in adenohypophysectomized birds, or by unilateral adrenalactomy on the previous day, causes the extrarenal response to decrease significantly (Figs. 3, 4). Removal of both adrenal glands almost totally abolishes the secretion of nasal gland fluid, and a normal response can be restored by corticosteroid replacement therapy (Fig. 4; THOMAS and PHILLIPS, 1975). The attenuation of adrenocortical function by treatment with metyrapone also diminishes nasal gland secretion in ducks given hypertonic saline, and normal extrarenal excretion may be restored following the administration of corticosterone (Fig. 5). Finally, augmentation of the endogenously produced corticosteroids by injection of cortisol, deoxycorticosterone, 18-OH-corticosterone and ACTH significantly enhances excretion in ducks given hypertonic saline loads (HOLMES et al., 1961;

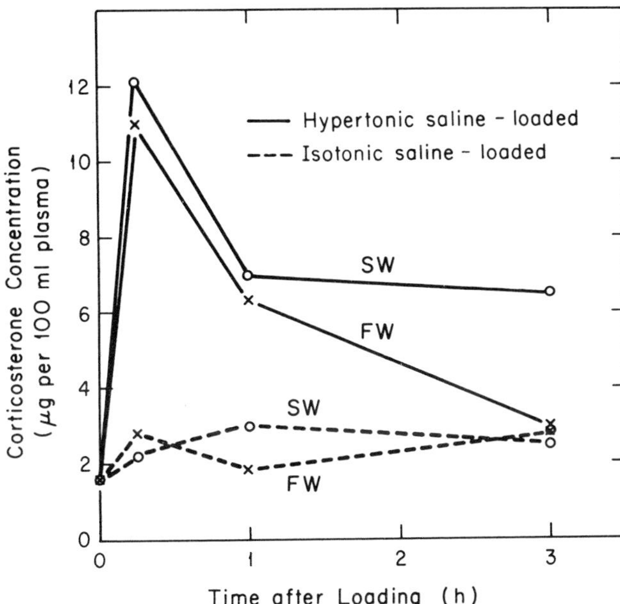

Fig. 2. Changes occurring in the plasmic concentrations of corticosterone in fresh- water- and seawater-maintained Mallards (*Anas platyrhynchos*) following the oral administration of either isotonic or hypertonic saline loads. (Drawn from data published by ALLEN et al., 1975a)

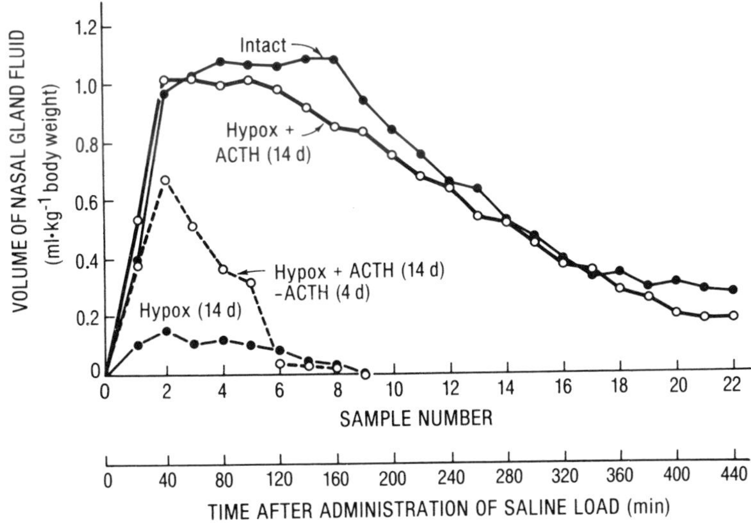

Fig. 3. Effect of adenohypophysectomy and replacement therapy with ACTH on the discharge of nasal gland fluid by the Mallard (*Anas platyrhynchos*). A group of adenohypophysectomized birds were given saline loads after ACTH replacement therapy for 14 days and another group were similarly treated with ACTH for 14 days but were saline-loaded four days after the last dose of ACTH. Each bird received a single intravenous load (20 ml/kg body wt) of hypertonic saline (470 mM NaCl, 10 mM KCl) at zero time. (From HOLMES et al., 1972)

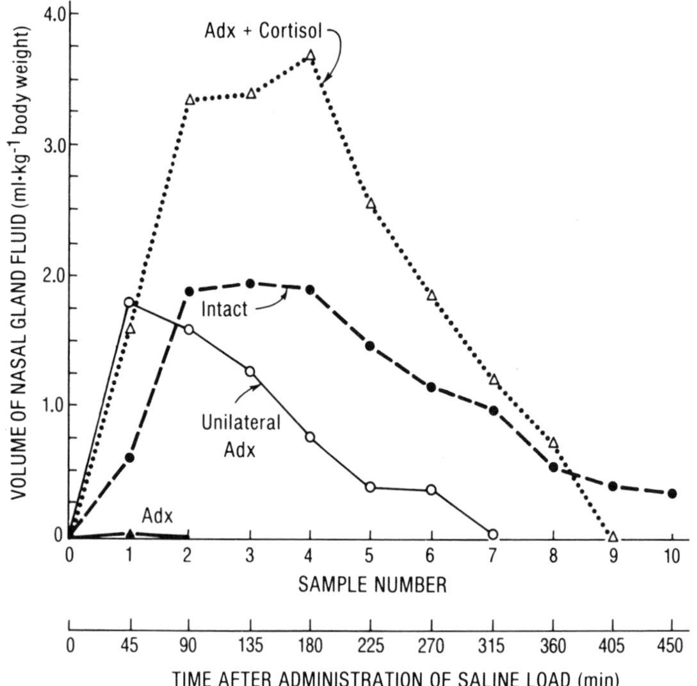

Fig. 4. Effect of total and subtotal adrenalectomy on the discharge of nasal gland fluid by the duck (*Anas platyrhynchos*). Each bird received a single oral load of 20 ml of 20% NaCl solution. The unilaterally adrenalectomized birds were examined 12 hours after surgery, total adrenalectomy was done in two stages on successive days and the birds were tested 6-12 hours after removal of the second gland. The totally adrenalectomized birds maintained on cortisol were tested after receiving four daily 5 mg doses intramuscularly. (From PHILLIPS et al., 1961)

PHILLIPS and BELLAMY, 1962; LANTHIER and SANDOR, 1973). Aldosterone has no effect on nasal gland secretion; this is not surprising, however, since the hypernatremia that precedes nasal gland secretion is not consistent with the stimulation of aldosterone release from the adrenal cortical tissue (PHILLIPS and BELLAMY, 1962).

The stimulatory effects of corticosterone on the nasal gland appear to be mediated by a direct intracellular action. The intravenous administration of labeled corticosteroids at the time that the birds are loaded with hypertonic saline has shown that an intracellular accumulation of radioactivity occurs in the cells of the nasal gland, but not in the cells of the adjacent Harderian gland (PHILLIPS and BELLAMY, 1966, 1967; SANDOR and FAZEKAS, 1973; ALLEN et al., 1975b). The secretory cells of the nasal glands, therefore, appear to be specific targets for the direct action of circulating corticosteroids. This has been further substantiated through the identification of specific corticosteroid receptors in both the cytoplasm and the nuclei of nasal gland cells (SANDOR and FAZEKAS, 1973; ALLEN et al., 1975b; SANDOR et al., 1977). Studies in vitro have shown that both high affinity-low capacity and low-affinity high-capacity receptors are present in the cytosolic fraction of nasal gland cells. Each type of receptor has a greater affinity for corticosterone than either aldosterone or deoxycorticosterone, and incubation of the cytosolic fraction of nasal gland

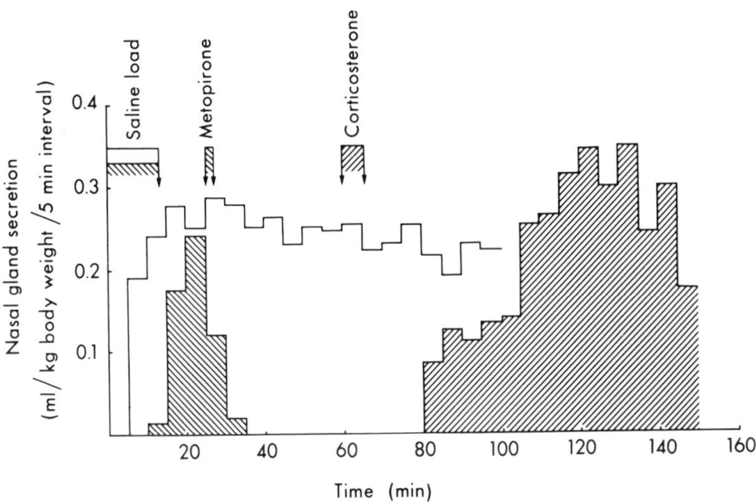

Fig. 5. The effect of metyrapone and corticosterone on the pattern of nasal gland secretion by Mallards, *Anas platyrhynchos*, (n = 7) loaded with hypertonic saline. During the indicated intervals intravenous infusions (1 ml/min) or 10% NaCl solution (5.5 ml/kg body weight), 80 mg/kg body weight of metyrapone dissolved in propylene glycol (100 mg/ml) and 0.5 mg corticosterone in isotonic saline (0.05 mg/ml) were administered. (From CHEESEMAN, PHILLIPS and CHEESEMAN, in HOLMES and PHILLIPS, 1976)

tissue with trypsin causes an almost total loss of the binding properties (SANDOR and FAZEKAS, 1973; ALLEN et al., 1975b). The high-affinity receptors in the cytosolic fraction have an apparent dissociation constant (k_D) of 10^{-9} M and the number of binding sites in both active and quiescent tissue is equivalent to approximately 10^{-12} mol/mg protein (SANDOR et al., 1977). In common with receptors isolated from other target tissues, isolated cytosolic receptors from nasal gland cells bind efficiently with labeled aldosterone only at 0°C; at 25°C, only 10% of the initial binding at 0°C is observed. The physiologic significance of receptors that have much greater affinity for the hormonal ligand at such low temperatures is not clear, particularly when the receptors have been isolated from responsive tissues in homeothermic vertebrates. Studies in vitro have shown that when labeled corticosterone is added to the cytosolic fraction from nasal gland cells, it becomes associated with a heavy (9-11 S) and a light (3-4 S) protein fraction. The peak of heavy protein is sensitive to high ionic concentrations, and in 0.4 M KCl shifts to the 4 S region when isolated by centrifugation in a linear sucrose gradient. Recombination studies show that when a cytosolic fraction containing labeled corticosterone complexes is incubated in the presence of nuclei that have not been exposed to labeled corticosterone, the receptors in the cytosolic fraction become depleted of labeled material, and the ligand becomes associated with the nuclei (SANDOR et al., 1977).

In the nuclei, the labeled material becomes associated with a Tris-soluble macromolecule and with a Tris-insoluble macromolecule that is soluble in 0.4 M KCl; this latter macromolecule is believed to be associated with chromatin in the nuclei (TAKEMOTO et al., 1975; SANDOR et al., 1977). It is important to note, however, that most of the tritiated material associated with these nuclear receptors is in the form of tritiated 11-dehydrocorticosterone. This conversion of labeled hormone probably occurs in the cytoplasm prior to transfer of the labeled ligand to the nuclear receptors. Thus, after incubating a cytosolic fraction from actively secreting nasal gland cells for 120 min in the presence of ^{3}H-corticosterone, 95% of the original radioligand is converted to ^{3}H-11-dehydrocorticosterone. Cytosolic and nuclear fractions isolated from the adjacent Harderian gland, and from more remote tissues such as lung and liver, do not possess the same abilities either to bind or to metabolize significant amounts of labeled corticosterone.

A similar metabolic conversion of labeled corticosterone appears to occur in vivo, for 20 min following the intravenous injection of ^{3}H-corticosterone, the ratio of labeled 11-dehydrocorticosterone:labeled corticosterone in the cytosolic fraction of nasal tissue is about 11:1 (SANDOR et al., 1977). Although the relative amount of labeled metabolite is consistently greater in both in vivo and in vitro experiments, there remains nevertheless a small quantity of unaltered tritiated corticosterone bound to the cytosolic receptors. One cannot overlook the possibility, therefore, that either one or both of these corticosteroids may play a crucial role in the physiologic response of the nasal gland. In view of these observations, any indirect stimulation of nasal gland function through the gluconeogenic action of corticosterone would appear to be minor (cf. PEAKER et al., 1971; HOLMES et al., 1972).

The inhibitory effects of spironolactone on the uptake of Na^{+} and water out of the intestinal lumen in seawater-maintained ducklings suggests that this drug may occupy hormonal binding sites in the mucosa. Thus, the transfer of Na^{+} and water may also be stimulated by a cellular interaction between corticosterone and macromolecular receptors in the cells of the intestinal mucosa.

The proposed sequence of physiologic events leading to the initiation and continuation of nasal gland function in marine birds are outlined in Figure 6. In summary, this sequence proposes that the uptake of ingested seawater will initiate a sensory input to an osmoreceptor located in either the heart or the cardiac circulation (HANWELL et al., 1972). Afferent impulses from this receptor are then relayed along two motor pathways. The first of these involves a cholinergic visceral motor pathway that is believed to stimulate directly the initial secretion of electrolytes from nasal gland cells (FÄNGE et al., 1958; HOKIN and HOKIN, 1960; SCHMIDT-NIELSEN, 1960; BORUT and SCHMIDT-NIELSEN, 1963; HOKIN, 1963; VAN ROSSUM, 1966; ASH et al., 1969).

The second set of motor impulses is believed to pass along a neurosecretory pathway with neurons terminating in the median eminence. These impulses probably cause the release of corticotropin-releasing hormone from the median eminence, and as a result the hypophysio-adrenal axis is activated (STAINER and HOLMES, 1969). The increased synthesis, and the release of corticosterone from the adrenal gland cause the plasma concentration of corticosterone to increase and the hormone may then act simultaneously at at least three sites (DONALDSON and HOLMES, 1965; MACCHI et al., 1967; ALLEN et al., 1975a). Under conditions of chronic exposure to seawater, corticosterone may stimulate increases in the rates of transfer of Na^{+} and water across the mucosa of the small intestinal; this will not only facilitate the uptake of a sufficient volume of ingested water, but will also accelerate stimulation of the osmoreceptor in birds that are fully adapted to a marine environment (CROCKER and HOLMES, 1971, 1976). Corticosterone may also act on the kidney to cause an increase in the urinary excretion of K^{+}; this may complement the excretion of K^{+} by the nasal glands, but the simultaneous enhancement of Na^{+} retention in the distal nephron will tend to offset slightly the excretion of Na^{+} by the nasal gland (HOLMES and ADAMS, 1963). Finally, corticosterone may enter the nasal gland

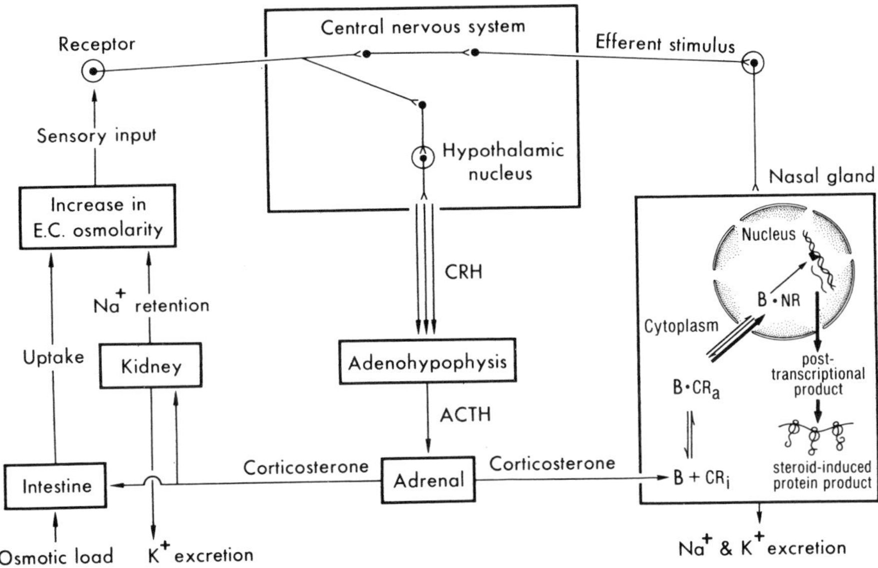

Fig. 6. A schematic representation of the pathways believed to be involved in the regulation of secretion by nasal glands in marine birds. The representation of the interactions between corticosterone (B) and the intracellular receptors (CR_i and CR_a = inactive and active cytoplasmic receptors respectively) in the nasal gland cells are similar to those described for other steroid-sensitive tissues; the indicated model, therefore, may be equally applicable to responsive cells in the intestinal mucosa and the kidney tubule

cells and, after reacting with specific receptors in the cytoplasm and the nucleus, induce the synthesis of a protein that may be related to the enhancement of excretion of Na^+ and K^+ (SANDOR and FAZEKAS, 1973; ALLEN et al., 1975b; TAKEMOTO et al., 1975; SANDOR et al., 1977).

Acknowledgments. Financial support for this research was provided by the National Science Foundation, Washington, D.C., and the Committee for Research, University of California, Santa Barbara. I am also grateful to Mrs. ILENE HAMES who assembled the bibliography and typed the manuscript.

References

ALLEN, J.C., ABEL, J.H., TAKEMOTO, D.J.: Effect of osmotic stress on serum corticoid and plasma glucose levels in the duck (*Anas platyrhynchos*). Gen. Comp. Endocrinol. 26, 209-216 (1975a)

ALLEN, J.C., ABEL, J.H., TAKEMOTO, D.J.: Uptake and binding of labeled corticosterone by the salt gland of the duck (*Anas platyrhynchos*). Gen. Comp. Endocrinol. 26, 217-225 (1975b)

ASH, R.W., PEARCE, J.W., SILVER, A.: An investigation of the nerve supply to the salt gland of the duck. Quart. J. Exp. Physiol. 54, 281-295 (1969)

BORUT, A., SCHMIDT-NIELSEN, K.: Respiration of avian salt-secreting glands in tissue slice experiments. Am. J. Physiol. 204, 573-581 (1963)

BRADLEY, E.L., HOLMES, W.N.: The role of the nasal glands in the survival of ducks (*Anas platyrhynchos*) exposed to hypertonic saline drinking water. Can. J. Zool. 50, 611-617 (1972)

BRADLEY, E.L., HOLMES, W.N., WRIGHT, A.: The effects of neurohypophysectomy on the pattern of renal excretion in the duck *Anas platyrhynchos*. J. Endocrinol. 51, 57-65 (1971)

CROCKER, A.D., HOLMES, W.N.: Intestinal absorption in ducklings (*Anas platyrhynchos*) maintained on freshwater and hypertonic saline. Comp. Biochem. Physiol. 40A, 203-211 (1971)

CROCKER, A.D., HOLMES, W.N.: Fators affecting intestinal absorption in ducklungs (*Anas platyrhynchos*). Proc. Soc. Endocinol., May (1976)

DONALDSON, E.M., HOLMES, W.N.: Corticosteroidogenesis in the freshwater and saline-maintained duck (*Anas platyrhynchos*). J. Endocrinol. 32, 329-336 (1965)

FÄNGE, R., SCHMIDT-NIELSEN, K., ROBINSON, M.: Control of secretion from the avian salt gland. Am. J. Physiol. 195, 321-326 (1958)

FLETCHER, G.L., HOLMES, W.N.: Observations on the intake of water and electrolytes by the duck (*Anas platyrhynchos*) maintained on freshwater and on hypertonic saline. J. Exp. Biol. 49, 325-339 (1968)

HANWELL, A., LINZELL, J., PEAKER, M.: Nature and location of the receptors for salt-gland secretion in the goose. J. Physiol. 226, 453-472 (1972)

HOKIN, L.E., HOKIN, M.R.: Studies on the carrier function of phosphatidic acid in sodium transport. I. The turnover of phosphatidic acid and phophoinositide in the avian salt gland on stimulation of secretion. J. Gen. Physiol. 44, 61-85 (1960)

HOKIN, M.R.: Studies on a Na^{+}+K^{+}-dependent, ouabain-sensitive adenosine triphosphatase in the avian salt gland. Biochim. Biophys. Acta 77, 108-120 (1963)

HOLMES, W.N., ADAMS, B.M.: Effects of adrenocortical and neurohypophysial hormones on the renal excretory pattern of the water-loaded duck (*Anas platyrhynchos*). Endocrinology 73, 5-10 (1963)

HOLMES, W.N., FLETCHER, G.L., STEWART, D.J.: The patterns of renal electrolyte excretion in the duck (*Anas platyrhynchos*) maintained on freshwater and on hypertonic saline. J. Exp. Biol. 48, 487-508 (1968)

HOLMES, W.N., LOCKWOOD, L.N., BRADLEY, E.L.: Adenohypophysial control of extrarenal excretion in the duck (*Anas platyrhynchos*). Gen. Comp. Endocrinol. 18, 59-68 (1972)

HOLMES, W.N., PHILLIPS, J.G.: The adrenal cortex of birds. In: Genral, Comparative and Clinical Endocrinology of the Adrenal Cortex. Chester Jones, I., Henderson, I.W. (eds.). London: Academic Press, 1976, pp. 293-420

HOLMES, W.N., PHILLIPS, J.G., BUTLER, D.G.: The effect of adrenocortical steroids on the renal and extra-renal responses of the domestic duck (*Anas platyrhynchos*) after hypertonic saline loading. Endocrinology 69, 483-495 (1961)

LANTHIER, A., SANDOR, T.: The effect of 18-hydrocorticosterone on the salt-secreting gland of the duck (*Anas platyrhynchos*). Can. J. Physiol. Pharmac. 51, 776-778 (1973)

MACCHI, I.A., PHILLIPS, J.G., BROWN, P.: Relationship between the concentration of corticosteroids in avian plasma and nasal gland function. J. Endocrinol. 38, 319-329 (1967)

PEAKER, M., PEAKER, S.J., PHILLIPS, J.G., WRIGHT, A.: The effects of corticotrophin, glucose and potassium chloride on secretion by the nasal salt gland of the duck (*Anas platyrhynchos*). J. Endocrinol. 50, 293-299 (1971)

PHILLIPS, J.G., BELLAMY, D.: Aspects of the hormonal control of nasal gland secretion in birds. J. Endocrinol. 24, vi-vii (1962)

PHILLIPS, J.G., BELLAMY, D.: The control of nasal gland function with special reference to the role of adrenocorticosteroids. Proc. 2nd Int. Congr. Hormone Steroids. Excerpta Med. Int. Congr. (Series No. 1321), p. 1065 (1966)

PHILLIPS, J.G., BELLAMY, D.: The control of nasal gland function, with special reference to the role of adrenocorticoids. Proc. 2nd Int. Symp. Hormonal Steroids. Excerpty Med. Int. Congr. (Series No. 132), pp. 877-881 (1967)

PHILLIPS, J.G., HOLMES, W.N., BUTLER, D.G.: The effect of total and subtotal adrenalectomy on the renal and extra-renal response of the domestic duck (*Anas platyrhynchos*). Endocrinology 69, 958-969 (1961)

ROSSUM, G.D.V. VAN: Movements of Na^{+} and K^{+} in slices of herring-gull salt gland. Biochim. Biophys. Acta 126, 338-349 (1966)

SANDOR, T., FAZEKAS, A.G.: Corticosteroid binding macromolecules in the nasal gland of the domesticated duck. 7th Conf. Eur. Comp. Endocrinol. (Budapest), Abstr. 71 (1973)

SANDOR, T., MEHDI, A.Z., FAZEKAS, A.G.: Corticosteroid-binding macromolecules in the salt-activated nasal gland of the domestic duck (*Anas platyrhynchos*). Gen. Comp. Endocrinol. 32, 348-359 (1977)
SCHMIDT-NIELSEN, K.: The salt secreting gland of marine birds. Circulation 21, 955-967 (1960)
STAINER, I.M., HOLMES, W.N.: Some evidence for the presence of a corticotrophin releasing factor (CRF) in the duck (*Anas platyrhynchos*). Gen. Comp. Endocrinol. 12, 350-359 (1969)
STEWART, D.J., HOLMES, W.N., FLETCHER, G.L.: The renal excretion of nitrogenous compounds in the duck (*Anas platyrhynchos*) maintained on freshwater and hypertonic saline. J. Exp. Biol. 50, 527-539 (1969)
TAKEMOTO, D.J., ABEL, J.H., ALLEN, J.C.: The metabolism of corticosterone in the salt gland of the duck, *Anas platyrhynchos*. Gen. Comp. Endocrinol. 26, 226-232 (1975)
THOMAS, D.H., PHILLIPS, J.G.: Studies in avian adrenal steroid function. IV. Adrenalectomy and the response of the domestic ducks (*Anas platyrhynchos* L.) to hypertonic NaCl loading. Gen. Comp. Endocrinol. 26, 427-439 (1975)
WRIGHT, A., PHILLIPS, J.G., HUANG, D.P.: The effect of adenohypophysectomy on the extra-renal and renal excretion of the saline-loaded duck (*Anas platyrhynchos*). J. Endocrinol. 36, 249-256 (1966)

6. Hormones and Mammalian Osmoregulation

W. V. MACFARLANE

As dry land was invaded by vertebrate tetrapods, their integuments became less permeable to water, so that renal osmoregulation became more important. On mammals, skin glands for sweat, sebum and milk secretion evolved, and vasopressin was exchanged for vasotocin. Renal-concentrating capacity for recycling of water increased, without dependence on the cloaca. In the arid cold of the Cretaceous, mammals kept warm and secreted isotonic milk under a barrage of hormones (estrogen, prolactin, progesterone, thyroxine, insulin, oxytocin and cortisol) to feed young in a dry climate. Behavioral skills also developed with larger cerebral cortices, enhancing tactics for survival.

Osmotic forces are exerted across membranes lying between the outside world and the interstitial fluid (IF) - skin, lungs, gut, nephron, bladder, and reproductive tracts; between IF and plasma across capillary and lymphatic walls; between IF and intracellular fluid (ICF) across cell membranes, and across choriodal-type gland cells in the formation of the transcellular fluids of CSF, eye, and gut (Fig. 1). There are two main components to osmolality in all of these spaces: crystalloid and electrolyte osmotic pressures (OP), and onchotic pressure deriving from macromolecules, mainly protein.

Mammals have been conservative in maintaining an intracellular osmolality around 300 mosmol/l (5100 torr), with an onchotic component of about 70 torr (ROBINSON, 1965). Extracellular fluid concentrations are regulated to 280-450 mosmol/l, but are usually about 300 mosmol/l with an onchotic protein pressure of 25 torr.

The synthesis of proteins is regulated in part by hormones, through steroid and thyroid action on DNA and RNA. Liver RNA is activated by cortisol to produce more protein and fat, but in muscle cortisol increases catabolism of protein. Testosterone and growth hormone are anabolic, increasing protein, and decreasing fat, in muscle and most tissues (MUNRO, 1970). Estradiol brings about a fairly specific increase of protein synthesis in uterine muscle, with some effect also on mammary glands. All hormones that induce enzymes in cells (insulin, thyroxine, steroids) increase the onchotic potential of cells. While hormones acting on the liver may increase plasma proteins, there seems also to be direct stimulation of the liver by low osmotic pressure to synthesize albumin.

Osmoregulation takes place in a flow system (MACFARLANE and HOWARD, 1972). Body water turns over at rates of 10% to 35% daily (MACFARLANE, 1976) according to ecotype. Sodium and K pools turn over more slowly, at 1% to 10% each day; turnover of proteins varies, but those in plasma are replaced at 1% to 5% daily. Among mammals there are different ecotypes that move osmotic components through living systems at rates proportional to the metabolic rate. Jungle mammals (cattle, pigs) turn over water, energy, protein, and the other constituents two or three-times more rapidly than desert or fossorial animals (camel, *Notomys*). These rates determine the degree of regulatory precision, as well as the tolerance to osmotic maladjustment that may occur. Hormones inter-

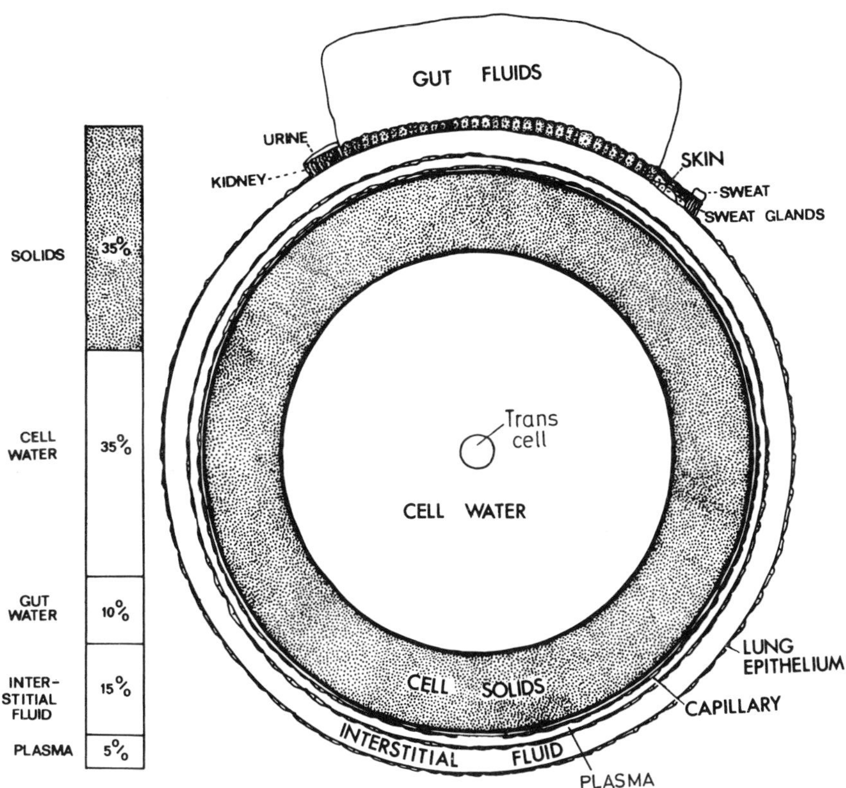

Fig. 1. The body composition of mammals by weight (left column) shows 65% water content with osmotic processes acting between cells, gut, interstitial, and plasma divisions. Urine, gut fluids and sweat are shown (right) as extracorporeal fluids osmotically related to the interstitial fluid (IF). The IF has large surface contacts with gut, capillaries and lung alveoli, as well as with cell membranes of tissues, across which osmotic exchanges occur.
Diagrammatic surface areas (proportional to actual areas) are larger for capillaries and alveoli, smaller for gut and least for skin and renal tubules

vene to alter the amount, timing, or duration of genetically determined cell action, usually with adaptive effects. There are both upper and lower limits, however, to the effectiveness of adjustment by hormones.

Surfaces. In mammals the tradition of high intracellular K concentrations in an extracellular Na medium is maintained by specific ion-pumping systems at cell surfaces. A mammal is, however, a complex set of surfaces, both of cells and tissues. In a 50-kg sheep or man there are about 1.3 m^2 of largely impermeable skin surface. This area is however, more than doubled by sweat, sebaceous, milk, and lachrymal glands, which produce somewhat hypotonic secretions from the interstitial fluid (OP 5100 torr and VP 757). The vapor pressure (VP) of water in the air is only 10-20 torr, so there is a large gradient between the IF and air across 1 mm of squamous epithelium, or 10 μm of gland cell wall. There are also 50 m^2 of alveoli and bronchi in a 50-kg animal. This epithelium, 1-2 μm thick, has 37 torr of water VP on the outside. Loss of water by diffusion from these surfaces raises the osmotic pressure of the IF that remains behind, and the kidney adjusts the electrolytes. The OP of the extracorporeal medium in the alimentary tract fluctuates widely as food, fluid, saliva, and secretions mix. Saliva, with an OP of 295-350 mosmol/l, is regulated in composition by aldosterone acting on acini and ducts (BLAIR-WEST et al., 1967; SCHNEYER et al., 1972). After drinking water, this may be diluted ten times. In ruminants the copious saliva (10 l per day in sheep) and fermentation products of pasture plants mix in the rumen to reach an OP of 200-450 mosmol/l. The fluid passing on to the omasum and abomasum is near 300 mosmol/l, but a sheep drinking 3 l of water may hemolyze its fragile red blood cells by absorbing hypotonic fluid too rapidly. It then excretes rosé urine. In the rumen of cattle (and presumably other ruminants) water moves across to the IF along an osmotic gradient generated by CO_2 movement to the blood (DOBSON et al., 1972).

Gland cells and brush borders in the gut greatly increase the surface area across which pump action and osmotic forces act. In the colon, Na is reabsorbed, and with it water passes back to the ECF, while K and Ca are secreted into the lumen. Adrenal hormones and vasopressin influence the feces-drying function of the colon, which is best developed in desert animals (camel, goat) and least powerful in swamp species (cattle, buffalo).

A further major surface is the kidney. The 2 million tubules of man or sheep, or 8 million in cattle, filter and secrete to produce urinary fluids with osmolalities from 100 to 3800 mosmol/l. The nephric gland cells respond to adrenal, pituitary, thyroid and gonadal hormones, though the basic secretory-absorptive capacities are genetic and intrinsic to a species. Man and swine, as tropical animals, achieve low urinary concentrations (1000-1300 mosmol/l) while sheep, oryx or *Dipodomys* and *Notomys* from arid areas range from 3800 to 9200 mosmol/l (64690 to 156620 torr) maxima. No addition of vasopressin, however, will concentrate human urine much above 1200 mosmol/l, nor does excess aldosterone dilute urine much below 100 mosmol/l. In the pig nephron, the OP changes from 5100 torr in the glomeruli to 17,000 torr at the loop of Henle and collecting duct; or in those regions of a desert mouse, to 150,000 torr. Yet at the end of the distal tubule, the fluid remains iso-osmotic with plasma. Secretion of Cl and Na by the ascending loop concentrate the local IF, which through the countercurrent mechanism concentrates the urine (WIRZ et al., 1951). Urine, although outside the body, is modified in the bladder as water is attracted to hypertonic bladder urine, and as some electrolytes and urea diffuse back into the blood.

Mechanisms and Adaptations. Osmotic concentrations are modified by diffusion, by facilitated or active transport, by hormone-assisted movement of solutes, and by protein synthesis. Hormones contribute to each of these.

Diffusion along gradients is basic to all water movements. Urea diffuses throughout the body, though it is not moved only by solvent drag. Yet there is no clinching evidence of urea being actively transported by mammalian nephrons. The resistance of the epidermis to diffusion has evolved genetically. Diffusion is high in animals with high water and energy turnover (cattle, *Sminthopsis*), and low in desert forms with low turnover rates (*Dasyurus*, *Notomys*), probably as a result of the rate at which water must move through epithelial cells (HAINES et al., 1974; MACFARLANE, 1976). Vasopressin increases back-diffusion of water in the nephron.

Faciliated and active transport systems use carrier molecules or energy from ATP to move solutes. From the intestine, transport of Na, K, Ca, amino acids, glucose, fatty acids, or vitamins is increased by adrenal steroids and thyroxine (T_4) or T_3. Movement across cell membranes into liver, muscle, gland and nerve is largely by active transport. In excitable tissues, however, Na and Ca move into, and K out from cells along diffusion gradients, while restoration of those ions is active, consuming ATP. Secretion of milk, sweat, tears, and gut fluids requires energy, and is on uphill gradients, as is absorption and secretion in the kidney, for most molecules other than water and urea (SCHNEYER et al., 1972). Hormones regulating use of energy (growth hormone, insulin, thyroxine, glucocorticoids, adrenalin) influence the amount of active transport that generates osmotic gradients.

Osmotic forces act across capillary endothelia which in gut villi have many 50 nm fenestrae (17 × 10" holes in 13 km of capillary/100 g) associated with slow protein diffusion. This yields a relative onchotic pressure; but in smooth muscle there are fewer fenestrae, so that protein movement by pinocytosis or passage through intercellular spaces is involved. There is much more capillary bed in skeletal muscle (260 km/100 g) with tight junctions and little passage of protein to IF. The osmotic forces across capillaries are largely due to protein distribution, which is highest in plasma, lower in lymphatics, and least in IF. However, plasma Ca^{2+} is needed to maintain the resistance to leak from arterioles and capillaries that prevents edema (so calcitonin and parathormone are background regulators of ECV).

Hormone Activities. Endocrine substances contribute to osmoregulation by changing the amount of water, solute, or protein in body fluids.

1. Water input to mammals comes from drinking, food or metabolic water. Thirst is a complex function in which neurohumors take part. Adrenalin in the hypothalamus increases thirst, and in pharmacologic doses at least, thirst is increased by angiotensin II (FITZSIMONS, 1971). Uptake of water from the gut follows osmotic flow gradients created by electrolytes (aldosterone, calcitonin) or by absorption of metabolites, aided by thyroxine, cortisol and insulin.

2. Water output control is partly endocrine. Arginine vasopressin in marsupials and eutheria is the background to normal water output. Lysine and arginine vasopressins both occur in warthogs, hippopotami, and peccaries (FERGUSON and HELLER, 1965) while pigs have only the lysine form. Vasopressins are unique to mammals. In most mammals their plasma concentration is less than 2 μU/ml, which is sufficient to prevent diabetes insipidus. Responses to additional vasopressin are poor in the fetus and neonate. Lambs respond less to lysine than to arginine vasopressin, but by 8 weeks of age there is no clear difference. The Desert Spiny Mouse *Acomys* has high concentrations of vasopressins at rest, but in most other mammals the plasma levels are low.

Vasopressin is released by increased plasma osmolality arising from evaporation of water, increments of electrolytes, or by low plasma volume (blood loss) when baroreceptors in heart and carotid sinuses respond. Syncope or poor venous return to the left atrium, pain or limbic cortical activation of the supraoptic cells, may also release the hormone, so that circulating vasopressin rises to 30-200 μU/ml.

Vasopressin usually reduces urine volume and increases its concentration, but does not alter electrolyte excretion. There are, however, exceptions:

a) Sodium excretion is increased in dogs by vasopressin (BROOKS and PICKFORD, 1958).

b) In hydropenic animals vasopressin increases Na, K, PO_4 and Cl excretion with water, in an osmotic diuresis (KURTZMAN and ROGERS, 1972). A direct hormone action reducing tubular reabsorption seems likely.

c) Ruminants respond to vasopressins by increased excretion of K, which in hydropenia is associated with higher urine flow rates - a diuresis. In hydrated sheep or camels, vasopressin decreases urine output but still increases K, Cl, and sometimes Na excretion (KINNE et al., 1961; CROSS et al., 1963; GANS, 1964; KUHN and PEETERS, 1967; KURTZMAN and BOONJARERN, 1975). The effects are not explicable by changes of filtration. The secretion of K during dehydration is probably valuable to ruminants in which food K is high, since increased plasma K would lead to dysrhythmias.

Probably vasopressins change water permeability of the apical membrane of cells partly by the action of cyclic AMP on kinases, partly by direct peptide action on membrane lipids. Microtubules may also alter the number of pores for water passage. The calculated changes in pore size (up to 20-30 Å) do not show in electron micrographs, so either opening of more small pores, or vesicle transport would be needed to allow water (not urea) back to the IF.

Vasopressins in osmoregulation are adaptive, in the context of water, salts, food, heat, and seasonal changes. Depletion of ECV is proportional to plasma vasopressin concentration above 8% loss of volume in rats. However, sheep in the desert showed no increments of plasma vasopressin until 3 days of dehydration at 38-42°C reduced plasma volume by 20% (unpublished), although urine flow fell within a few hours. Carotid sinus, left atrial and pulmonary receptors for blood pressure activate vasopressin release to help restore circulating plasma. Noradrenalin suppresses this by altering the sensitivity of the baroreceptor system (SCHRIER et al., 1975). Angiotensin II may act in the hypothalamus to release vasopressin by action on the supraoptic nuclei. Thus, several hormones converge through central and peripheral mechanisms to modulate the amount of vasopressin in circulation, and thus the body water content.

Extracellular Electrolytes. Electrolytes are regulated by both gut and kidney cells. Active uptake of Na from the gut is reduced by lack of thyroxine or cortical steroids. Salt-loading induces synthesis of NaK ATPase in gut and kidney to increase Na and K exchange within cells. Glucocorticoids release K, PO_4 and SO_4 from cells to the ECF. The main control of ECV is, however, through renal responses to aldosterone. Initiation of aldosterone release from adrenal glomerular cells comes about (DENTON, 1965) by four main mechanisms:

1. Raised plasma Na or lowered K concentration act directly on the adrenal cortex glomerular cells, to release aldosterone.

2. Low pressure in renal vessels or low Na concentration, act through juxtaglomerular and macula densa cells on renal arterioles, to release granules of renin which react with α_2-globulin to produce angiotensin I, which then loses two amino acid residues in the lungs to become the octapeptide angiotensin II, which releases aldosterone. This induces enzymes in proximal tubule cells which bring about Na reabsorption. Sweat, salivary, gut, and mammary glands respond particularly to aldosterone by reducing Na output. Retained Na osmotically retains water to restore or increase ECV.

3. Decrease in blood pressure, postural change, and blood loss all act through central mechanisms to raise plasma aldosterone. Vagal afferents from the heart take part in this. The efferent route is probably along

renal nerves to the juxtaglomerular cells, bringing about the release of renin, and thus of aldosterone.

4. ACTH releases aldosterone, though this is not a major control. There is also an elusive central nervous component in these controls.

In animals other than ruminants, aldosterone increases K excretion, but not in sheep and cattle (MACFARLANE et al., 1967). Instead, vasopressin increases renal K excretion. Herbivores (ingesting large amounts of K with plants) produce high concentrations of K from sweat and muzzle glands. When water supplies are low, they remove K by renal action.

Mountain or tropical grasses grow on soil leached of Na by heavy rainfall. Herbivores on those pastures produce aldosterone to retain Na (DENTON, 1965), so that the ingested Na is recycled. There is no evidence that sustained high levels of aldosterone have deleterious effects on man or beast. The vegan Melanesians of the New Guinea mountains ingest only 10-30 mEq of Na daily from sweet potato or taro, with 500-700 mEq of K. They have low Na concentrations in urine, sweat, saliva, and milk, with correspondingly raised K levels (Table 1). Blood

Table 1. Concentrations of electrolyte and aldosterone in vegan Melanesians and European omnivores

	Na mEq/l		K mEq/l		K/Na	
	M	E	M	E	M	E
Urine	27	182	224	70	8.3	0.38
Sweat	12	93	9	6	0.7	0.06
Saliva	9	33	30	19	3.3	0.58
Milk	3	11	10	14	3.3	1.3
Aldosterone (blood) ng/dl	23	4.5				

M, Melanesian adults in a minimally acculturated Tsenda vegan village.
E, Europeans on mixed diet, in New Guinea.

Typical average values illustrate the general pattern of electrolyte response to low Na, High K intake.

aldosterone is five to ten times higher in concentration than among Europeans. Plasma renin activity and ECV are also raised in Melanesians. However, arterial blood pressures are low (90/60 torr down to 73/45 in healthy, aged adults). Pressures rise as acculturation leads to salt intake, and blood aldosterone falls (MACFARLANE et al., 1968).

Plasma electrolytes ranged from Na 122-145 mEq/l and K 4-6 mEq/l. The ratio K:Na is an index of aldosterone activity, and this was 3 to 22 times greater among the Melanesians than in Europeans, while the average aldosterone concentration in blood was five times greater in Melanesians. Adaptation of cells and fluids to low Na, high K intake is achieved, with no apparent ill effect, since the Melanesians are overall physically fit. They suffer hypokalemia and muscle weakness, however, when suddenly exposed to high Na, low K European foods.

There are no very clear hormonal regulators of K other than steroids. Muzzle glands of cattle (BREWER and MACFARLANE, 1967) and sweat glands of camels or sheep secrete excess K. Plasma Ca concentration however, is the result of uptake from the gut (calciferol) balanced by deposition in bone (calcitonin) and Ca mobilization with excretion (parathormone). Chloride is in some degree regulated independently of Na, since there are Cl pumps in the stomach and other gland cells. However, mainly Cl^- appears to follow the charge of Na^+. Bicarbonate forms from CO_2 and H_2O as needed to meet cationic concentrations.

Natriuresis. The long search over 30 years for hormonal mechanisms that promote removal of excess Na (MILLS, 1963; KLAHR and RODRIGUEZ, 1975) has yielded pituitary and renal peptides that are active physiologically, and prostaglandins PGA_2 and PGE_2 that increase Na excretion (LEE and ATTALLAH, 1975). The PGA_2 seems a strong candidate, acting by renal cortical vasodilatation. A substance extracted from Na-loaded rat kidneys inhibits NaK ATPase, and comes near to meeting the specifications of a natriuretic hormone to reduce edema. Elimination of excess Na is needed after salt ingestion or expansion of ECV, and when this fails the basis for high blood pressure and edema is laid.

Environmental Impacts on Osmoregulation.

Heat. Heat, exercise, dehydration, and electrolyte loading all disturb osmotic balance. Extracellular fluid increases in mammals during summer (to provide water for evaporative cooling) and there is a lower ECV in winter. Hormones take part in these seasonal adjustments. Men and sheep heated for 4 h at 41°C in summer and winter evaporated the same amount of water in each season. In summer, the already raised PV and ECV were reduced, while Na concentration, osmolality and vasopressin concentrations increased (MACFARLANE and ROBINSON, 1957). In winter there was little change in any of these values, though PV and ECV were about 25% less than in summer. A possible explanation was that bouts of Na retention (by aldosterone) occurring in spring, could change the sensitivity of neurons for vasopressin release. Injection of deoxycorticosterone into sheep in winter was therefore undertaken. At 41°C, concentration of sheep plasma took place in winter, while plasma vasopressin rose to high levels (MACFARLANE et al., 1958), for a month after the steroid treatment. It appears that mineralocorticoids influence cellular responses, as well as the distribution of body fluid loss. Without the steroids, fluid in winter was mobilized, presumably from cells and gut, to keep the PV, ECV, and OP unchanged while fluid was lost for evaporative cooling. Expansion of the ECV, from the raised renin-angiotensin content of plasma after evaporative cooling, takes place in Aboriginal desert people during summer and in Melanesians. Both groups have larger ECV (250-280 ml/kg) than Europeans (180-200 mg/kg), and higher renin activity in plasma.

In sheep there is a reduction of excretion of 17-ketosteroid and 17-OHCS in summer, relative to winter (ROBINSON et al., 1955). Aldosterone is released in spring and summer heat, both by reduction of ECV during sweating, and by hypostatic fluid accumulation. There is a seasonally reciprocal relation between excretion of 17-ketosteroids and aldosterone, which may influence the cell-extracellular balance of electrolytes. Acute heating also reduces 17-KS and 17-OHCS excretion.

Exercise. The effects of exercise on fluid and electrolytes, particularly in the heat, are considerable. Four h of work at 38°C result in 4 days reduced 17-ketosteroid output, aldosterone increment, Na retention, and reduction of output of urine water (MACFARLANE, 1963). Standard tread-mill exercise leads to plasma vasopressin increments 70% greater in summer than in winter, among the same human subjects (MACFARLANE and ROBINSON, 1957).

In the desert during summer, Aboriginal and European men walked together (MACFARLANE, 1973) for 1 h. The Aboriginals sweated at nearly twice the rate of Europeans, but there was a reduction of 60 to 82% in Na excretion among the Europeans, while the Aboriginal men increased Na output by up to 53%. The same renal behavior occurs in sheep, which increase Na excretion at 40°C, while Europeans rapidly retain Na (MACFARLANE et al., 1958). These osmoregulations derive from differences in dynamics of evaporative cooling. Heated sheep lose water without Na, largely from the respiratory tract, so Na remains in the plasma, then is excreted. Similarly, Aboriginal sweat has less than one third the Na concentration of Europeans. As sweat is evaporated, therefore, there is a relative plasma surfeit of Na in Aboriginals, and this is excreted. Europeans lose sufficient Na in sweat (80-100 mEq/l) to release aldosterone, so that Na is strongly retained.

Lack of Water. When sheep are without water in summer heat, redistributions of water and salt occur (MACFARLANE et al., 1961). After 5 days, body weight was reduced by 23%, PV and ECV by 45%. Plasma Na rose by only 9%, while Cl increased by 28%, and plasma osmolality by 34%, as differential adjustments of ion species took place. Only after 3 days, with 16% loss of weight, was vasopressin detectable in plasma, however.

The rate of loss of water determines the decrement of PV. Cell and gut fluids become more available to plasma, the more slowly dehydration proceeds. At a slow (2.6% daily) rate of water loss, only 4% of the fluid derived from plasma, while rapid (4.7% daily) dehydration took 12.7% of the loss from plasma, and less from cells and gut. The camel without water loses relatively less plasma than sheep or cattle. The low rate of water turnover by camels allows slow dehydration, and this (with time to synthesize more albumin for onchotic pressure) accounts for much of the desert competence of the camel (MACFARLANE et al., 1963). The low energy and water turnover rates of camelids are not due to low turnover of thyroxine. They have very high plasma T_4 levels, but the T_4 secretion rate is the same as that of cattle or horses of the same size. The low metabolism of camels probably derives from the genetically low protein-turnover rate (MACFARLANE, 1976).

Feeding. Ingestion of food reflexly produces saliva which draws water, Na, HCO_3, Cl and some K from the plasma. This is recorded by the buffer system, and shows in the urine. Alkaline, hypertonic saliva is secreted by sheep in large quantities to deal with dry food, so acid urine is produced (KINNE et al., 1961) to balance the buffers. Urine volume falls as vasopressin saves water (STACY and BROOK, 1965), and aldosterone helps reabsorb Na after feeding. When a man or pig eats, however, there is compensatory renal excretion of alkali, and water is retained, since salivary volume is small; but gastric acid secretion reduces both plasma acid and plasma water, so alkaline urine is secreted, and urine volume is reduced.

The microflora of the rumen generates fatty acids and amino acids, and releases plant electrolytes, so that 3 h after a meal, the rumen osmotic pressure may reach 450 mosmol/l. This would attract water from the plasma. The fluids entering and leaving the abomasum are thus nearly iso-osmotic with plasma. Gastrin, secretin and other peptides influence gut osmotic status, as secretions are stimulated.

Many other adjustments of gut, interstitial and cell fluids occur in starvation, lactation, disease, dehydration, or overnutrition. Lactation and starvation are similar to the effects of sweating, being associated with increases of ECV and PV, from retention of water and Na, and resetting of the fluid volume control. Overall, however, aldosterone adjusts the extracellular Na, vasopressin the water content, and cortisol the cell membrane controls. Other hormones add small variations to the general theme.

Summary

Osmoregulation takes place in a water flow system. Hormones take some major and many minor roles in the diverse mechanisms by which water, electrolyte and protein distributions are adjusted.

Water. Vasopressins increase the permeability of collecting ducts through cyclic AMP, opening pores to allow water to return to the interstitial fluid of the kidneys without urea. Adrenalin induces excretion of water without electrolytes probably by altering sensitivity of baroreceptors and reducing release of vasopressin. Thyroxine and cortisol increase water excretion by modifying nephric cell work functions.

Sodium is reabsorbed by renal, sweat, salivary, gut, lachrymal, and mammary gland cells under the influence of aldosterone or deoxycorticosterone, and the Na retained increases ECV. Cortisone, cortisol, and corticosterone also encourage Na reabsorption by the nephron, affecting NaK ATPase. Parathormone increases renal absorption of Na, Cl, PO_4 and Ca. Thyroxine facilitates active transport in gut and kidney, while NaK ATPase activity is increased in kidney, gut and liver, by T_4 or T_3.

Sodium excretion - natriuresis - is enhanced by pituitary and renal peptides, diencephalic small molecules, and prostaglandins PGA_2 and PGE_2.

Potassium. Parathormone and thyroxine raise K excretion rates. In man, pig, rat and dog, aldosterone increases K excretion. In ruminants, little K is lost while aldosterone reabsorbs Na and Cl. Vasopressins increase ruminant K secretion.

Calcium. Parathormone leads to PO_4 loss, while Ca and Mg ions are retained. Calcitonin increases Ca excretion. Thyroxine raises both PO_4 and Ca excretion.

Plasma proteins derive from liver (albumin and globulin) and lymph tissues (γ-globulins) both being influenced by growth hormone and insulin.

Intracellular Osmolality. Membrane NaK ATPase (Mg activated) is involved with pump action on electrolytes. The amount of enzyme and its activity are influenced by cortisol, cortisone and corticosterone, thyroxine and prolactin, which thus help to maintain cell turgor.

Cell protein is under the influence in part of growth hormone, thyroxine, testosterone, oestrogen, insulin, and prolactin.

Transcellular Osmolalities. Gastrin, secretin, and pancreozymin influence the electrolytes and protein of stomach, pancreatic, and intestinal glands. All fluids approximate 300 mosmol/l. Tears, sweat, and milk are electrolyte-containing secretions in which the acinar product is modulated by aldosterone, cortisol, progesterone, and estradiol acting on the duct fluids.

The fluids affected by these hormones have an intrinsic genetic composition that can be changed. Osmoregulatory processes call up endocrine reinforcements when water supplies are depleted, when Na intake is low, and when shifts of fluid between body spaces take place during exercise in the heat, hemorrhage, or chemical damage.

References

BREWER, N.L., MACFARLANE, W.V.: Structure and secretion of the naso-labial glands of cattle. Aust. J. Exp. Biol. Med. Sci. 45, P. 37 (1967)

BLAIR-WEST, J.R., COGHLAN, J.P., DENTON, D.A., WRIGHT, R.D.: Effect of endocrines on salivary glands. In: Handbook of Physiology. Alimentary Canal. Washington, D.C.: Am. Physiol. Soc., 1967, pp. 633-664

BROOKS, F.P., PICKFORD, M.: The effect of posterior pituitary hormones on the excretion of electrolytes in dogs. J. Physiol. 142, 468-493 (1958)

CROSS, R.B., THORNTON, W.M., TWEDDELL, E.D.: The effect of vasopressin on water and electrolyte excretion by the sheep. Aust. J. Exp. Biol. Med. Sci. 41, 629-636 (1963)

DENTON, D.A.: Evolutionary aspects of the emergence of aldosterone secretion and salt appetite. Physiol. Rev. 45, 245-295 (1965)

DOBSON, A., HARROP, C.J.F., PHILLIPSON, A.T.: Osmotic effects of carbon dioxide absorption from the rumen. Federation Proc. 31, 260 (1972)

FERGUSON, D.R., HELLER, H.: Distribution of neurophypophysial hormones in mammals. J. Physiol. 180, 846-863 (1965)

FITZSIMONS, J.T.: The effect on drinking of peptide precursors and of shorter chain peptide fragments on angiotensin II injected into the rats diencephalon. J. Physiol. 214, 295-304 (1971)

GANS, J.H.: Vasopressin-induced saluresis in sheep. Am. J. Vet. Res. 25, 918-923 (1964)

HAINES, H., MACFARLANE, W.V., SETCHELL, C., HOWARD, B.: Water turnover and pulmocutaneous evaporation of Australian desert dasyurids and murids. Am. J. Physiol. 227, 958-963 (1974)

KINNE, R., MACFARLANE, W.V., BUDTZ-OLSEN, O.E.: Hormones and electrolyte excretion in sheep. Nature (London) 192, 1084-1085 (1961)

KLAHR, S., RODRIGUEZ, H.J.: Natriuretic hormone. Nephron 15, 387-408 (1975)

KUHN, E., PEETERS, G.: Influence de l'arginine vasopressine sur l'excretion d'electrolytes chez la brebis. Arch. Int. Pharm. Ther. 168, 14-20 (1967)

KURTZMAN, N.A., BOONJARERN, S.: Physiology of antidiuretic hormone and the interrelationship between the hormone and the kidney. Nephron 15, 167-185 (1975)

KURTZMAN, N.A., ROGERS, P.W.: The diuretic effect of antidiuretic hormone. Clin. Res. 20, 600-612 (1972)

LEE, J.B., ATTALLAH, A.A.: Renal prostaglandins. Nephron 15, 360-369 (1975)

MACFARLANE, W.V.: Endocrine functions in hot environments. In: Environmental Physiology and Psychology in Arid Conditions. Reviews of Research. Paris: UNESCO, 1963, pp. 153-222

MACFARLANE, W.V.: Functions of Aboriginal nomads during summer. In: The Human Biology of Aborigines in Cape York. Kirk, R.L. (ed.). Canberra: Institute of Aboriginal Studies, 1973, pp. 183-194

MACFARLANE, W.V.: Ecophysiological hierarchies. Israel J. Med. Sci. 12, 723-731 (1976)

MACFARLANE, W.V., HOWARD, B.: Comparative water and energy economy of wild and domestic mammals. Symp. Zool. Soc. Lond. 31, 261-294 (1972)

MACFARLANE, W.V., HOWARD, B., SCROGGINS, B., SKINNER, S.L.: Water, electrolytes, hormones and blood pressure of Melanesians in relation to European contact. Proc. Int. Union Physiol. Sci. 7, 274 (1968)

MACFARLANE, W.V., KINNE, R., WALMSLEY, C.M., SIEBERT, B.D., PETER, D.: Vasopressins and the increase of water and electrolyte excretion by sheep, cattle and camels. Nature (London) 214, 979-981 (1967)

MACFARLANE, W.V., MORRIS, R.J.H., HOWARD, B.: Turnover and distribution of water in desert camels, sheep, cattle and kangaroos. Nature (London) 187, 270-271 (1963)

MACFARLANE, W.V., MORRIS, R.J.H., HOWARD, B., MCDONALD, J., BUDTZ-OLSEN, O.E.: Water and electrolyte changes in tropical merino sheep exposed to dehydration during summer. Aust. J. Agr. Res. 12, 889-912 (1961)

MACFARLANE, W.V., ROBINSON, K.W.: Seasonal changes in plasma anti-diuretic activity produced by a standard heat stimulus. J. Physiol. 135, 1-11 (1957)

MACFARLANE, W.V., ROBINSON, K.W., HOWARD, B., KINNE, R.: Heat, salt and hormones in panting and sweating animals. Nature (London) 182, 672 (1958)

MILLS, I.H.: The non-aldosterone hormonal control of sodium. Mem. Soc. Endocrinol. 13, 17-24 (1963)

MUNRO, H.N.: A general survey of mechanisms regulating protein metabolism in mammals. In: Mammalian Protein Metabolism. Munro, H.N. (ed.). New York: Academic Press, 1970, pp. 3-130

ROBINSON, J.R.: Water regulation in mammalian cells. Symp. Soc. Exp. Biol. 19, 237-258 (1965)

ROBINSON, K.W., HOWARD, B., MACFARLANE, W.V.: Observations on seasonal fluctuations of 17-ketosteroid output in the subtropics and tropics. Med. J. Aust. 2, 756-760 (1955)

SCHNEYER, L.H., YOUNG, J.A., SCHNEYER, C.A.: Salivary secretion of electrolytes. Physiol. Rev. 52, 720-777 (1972).

SCHRIER, R.W., BERL, T., HARBOTTLE, J.A., MCDONALD, K.M.: Catecholamines and renal water excretion. Nephron 15, 186-196 (1975)

STACY, B.D., BROOK, A.H.: Antidiuretic hormone activity in sheep after feeding. Quart. J. Exp. Physiol. 50, 65-78 (1965)

WIRZ, H., HARGITAY, B., KUHN, W.: Lokalisation des Konzentrierungsprozesses in der Niere durch direkte Kryoskopie. Helvet. Physiol. Pharmacol. Acta 9, 196-207 (1951)

Chapter IV. Endocrine Responses to Stress

1. Feedback and Facilitation in the Adrenocortical System and the Endocrine Responses to Repeated Stimuli

M. F. DALLMAN and CH. W. WILKINSON

In this paper we limit ourselves to discussion of stress-inducing stimuli and adrenocortical responses to stress in mammals. Emphasis is placed on the modification of these responses by feedback inhibition of glucocorticoids on (CRF and) ACTH secretion and by stress-induced facilitation in the adrenocortical system. Finally we discuss the effects of repeated activation of this system on the responses of other endocrine systems.

Stimuli (stressors) impinge on the adrenocortical system primarily via neural pathways to the hypothalamus where neuronal secretion of CRF into the hypothalamo-hypophysial portal vasculature is stimulated. As a result of the action of CRF on pituitary corticotroph cells, ACTH is released into the systemic circulation and acts on the adrenal cortex to provoke synthesis and secretion of corticosteroids which, in turn, act on most of the tissues of the body. In addition they exert physiologic feedback actions on the hypothalamus and pituitary that limit CRF and ACTH secretion after stimuli of low-to-moderate intensity (SATO et al., 1975; BUCHER et al., 1973; JONES et al., 1972).

The variety of stimuli that excite the activity of this system is bewildering. Some stimuli, such as ether vapors (GREER and ALLEN, 1975), restraint, intraperitoneal injection of saline, and novel environment (DALLMAN, unpublished), that are very successful in provoking adrenocortical activity in conscious animals, are much less effective in the pentobarbital-anesthetized rat. Such "psychic" stimuli probably excite the adrenocortical system in large part through increased activity in associative and limbic regions of the brain that are blocked by the anesthetic from receiving the stimulus or exciting the CRF neuron.

There is evidence supporting the view that there must be an adequate rate of change or absolute intensity of the stimulus presented for activation of the adrenocortical system to occur. For instance, the rate of blood withdrawal has been shown to determine whether an adrenocortical response to hemorrhage will occur in dogs (GANN, 1969). Similarly, acute reduction of ambient temperature to $0^{o}C$ provoked corticosteroid secretion in dogs, whereas slow cooling (over a 45-min period) to the same temperature did not (CHOWERS et al., 1964). Also, MASON (1974) reported increased urinary 17-OH corticosteroids in rhesus monkeys after rapid elevation of ambient temperature to $30^{o}C$, but not when the temperature was increased gradually.

Relationship among Intensity of Stimuli, Adrenal Responses, and Glucocorticoid Feedback

There is a logarithmic relationship between the quantity of hemorrhage and the magnitude of the adrenocortical response (GANN and CRYER, 1973). Similarly, increasing degrees of cold, or doses of histamine or vasopressin given intravenously, or increasing voltage in an electrical shock administered to a hind leg have been shown to provoke increasing adrenocortical responses (FORTIER et al., 1970; DALLMAN and YATES, 1968; DALLMAN and JONES, 1973). Each of these studies determined that there was a maximal adrenal response to a given intensity of stressor, and that increasing the quantity of the stimulus beyond this maximum did not increase its magnitude. However, the conclusion that more steroid was not secreted after still more intense stimuli than those provoking maximal secretion is probably not warranted, since the duration of maximal adrenocortical response was not determined in these experiments. The characteristic adrenocortical response to ACTH is a graded linear response to the log of the dose up to a maximal secretion rate. Further increase in the dose of ACTH prolongs the duration of the maximal secretion rate of the adrenal (GANN et al., 1961; STOCKHAM, 1964). There is no comparable information as to whether the ACTH response is increased in magnitude, extended temporally, or both, with increasing stimulus strength.

The effects of pretreatment with various doses of a potent synthetic glucocorticoid, dexamethasone, on responses to increasing quantities of hemorrhage, vasopressin, or histamine have been determined. The results are in agreement that, in dogs and rats, at low-to-moderate doses of the applied stimuli, inhibition of the adrenocortical response is proportional to the log of the dose of dexamethasone used. With intense stimulation, maximally effective doses of dexamethasone produce no apparent inhibition of the adrenocortical response to the stressor. However, it is likely that inhibition could be measured if sampling were extended in time, since maximally effective quantities of dexamethasone have been shown to attenuate the plasma ACTH response to laparotomy under ether without inhibiting the corticosterone response (SATO et al., 1975).

We have studied the inhibition by dexamethasone of the adrenocortical response to scald of the pentobarbital-anesthetized rat. The logarithmic relationship between the dose of dexamethasone given 2 h before application of this relatively low intensity stimulus and the plasma corticosterone response is shown in Figure 1.

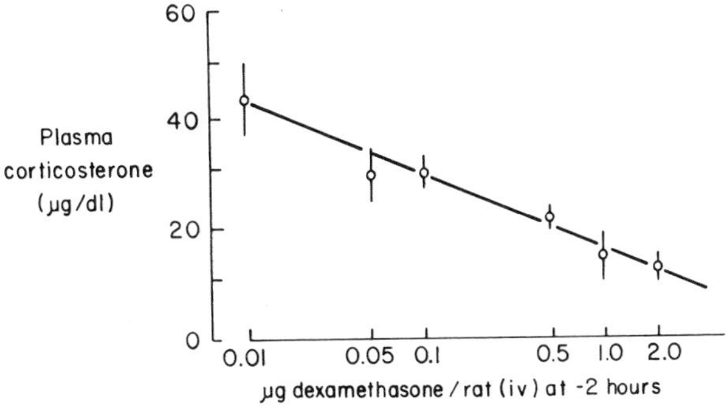

Fig. 1. Plasma corticosterone levels observed 15 min after immersion of a hind foot in water at 70°C for 20 s in female rats under deep pentobarbital anesthesia. Corticosterone levels are decreased in proportion to the log of the dose of dexamethasone administered two hours earlier. Each point represents the mean value ± SEM for 5-12 rats. (From DALLMAN and YATES, 1968)

Because most of the investigations of interactions between ACTH secretion and steroid feedback have been done with either highly potent synthetic glucocorticoids or large doses of naturally occurring steroids, it was of interest to determine whether cortisol infused over the low part of the range of adrenocortical secretion rates reported in the dog could inhibit the high circulating ACTH levels observed in the chronically adrenalectomized dog (taken off steroid maintenance therapy for periods up to 72 h). Dogs were brought to the laboratory, lightly anesthetized with pentobarbital, and either 2% EtOH in 0.9% saline or various concentrations of cortisol in this vehicle were infused at a constant rate for 2 h. As was the case after dexamethasone treatment of the rat, a linear inhibition of ACTH levels was found between 105 and 120 min when plotted as a function of the log of the cortisol infusion rate (DALLMAN et al., 1974b). In summary, either synthetic or naturally secreted glucocorticoids exert a profound effect on ACTH secretion during the period 2-7 h after their administration.

Effect of Prior Stress and Corticosteroid Secretion on the Subsequent Response to Stress

Because of the marked inhibitory effect of corticosteroids on ACTH secretion discussed above, one would predict that stressor-induced secretion of corticosteroids would inhibit the response of the adrenocortical system to subsequently administered stressors. There have been many attempts to demonstrate such an effect, and, with few exceptions, the adrenocortical response to a second stressor presented with 24 h of the first has been shown to be as large or larger than the initial response.

Recently, circulating ACTH and corticosterone levels were measured before and after multiple episodes of 2-min restraint applied to rats, and each repetition provoked responses of similar magnitude in both hormones (VAN LOON, personal communication). Similarly, rats exposed to cold or faradic foot shock for 2 or 10 min at hourly intervals for 24 h, show as high levels of corticosterone in plasma after the last exposure as after the first (FORTIER et al., 1970). HENNESSY et al. (1977) reported that corticosterone levels of mice exposed daily to a novel environment for 10 days were not different from those of animals that had been exposed only once. In female and castrate male mice, corticosteroid responses were greater after the tenth daily treatment with foot shock than after one shock. In agreement with these reports, we have found that after repeated exposures of rats to electrical shock or ether, there appears to be no inhibitory effect of the corticosterone secreted in response to the first stimulus on the responses to subsequent stimuli. Thus, the corticosteroids secreted in response to repeated stimuli with an intervening rest period do not usually result in decreasing adrenocortical responses.

Stressor-Induced Facilitation of Subsequent Stimulus-Induced Responses in the Adrenocortical System

It is difficult to reconcile the two sets of results just presented, high sensitivity to the feedback effects of glucocorticoids, and lack of inhibition of subsequent responses as a result of steroid secreted during the initial response to a stressor. Experiments were designed to test whether stress leaves a facilitatory trace in some element of the adrenocortical system such that the system remains responsive to stimuli even after periods of elevated corticosteroid secretion. Rats were subjected to restraint for a period of 90 min and the plasma corticosterone response to this stimulus was measured over time. In other rats doses of corticosterone or ACTH were found that produced elevations in circulating corticosterone similar to that found after restraint. Three h after restraint, ACTH, corticosterone, or saline control injections were given, rats in all groups were subjected to the stimulus of handling and intraperitoneal injection. Plasma corticosterone levels 15 min later were low in the groups given the steroid or ACTH treatments, compared to the high values observed after prior saline or restraint (Fig. 2). These results suggest strongly that subsequent responses of the adrenocortical system are facilitated by an initial stimulus, so that corticosteroid feedback is counterbalanced.

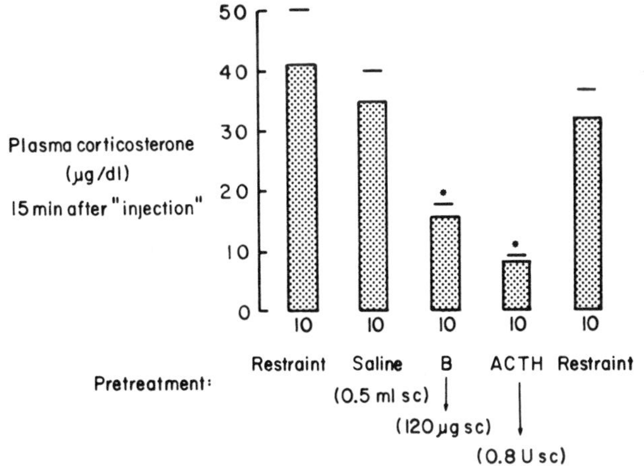

Fig. 2. A facilitatory component of the stress response allows responsiveness of the adrenocortical system to application of a subsequent stimulus despite secretion of a sufficient quantity of corticosterone to inhibit the response. The corticosterone response to 60 min of restraint was matched in other rats either by two injections 40 min apart of 60 μg each corticosterone, or by one injection of 0.8 U ACTH. Control rats were injected with saline. Three h after these treatments all animals were stimulated by "injection", the intraperitoneal insertion and withdrawal of a needle. In the absence of restraint, the quantity of corticosterone was adequate to inhibit the response to injection. (From DALLMAN and JONES, Endocrinol. 92, 1367-1375, 1973)

Recently GANN et al. (1977) have reported both physiologic inhibition and facilitation of the adrenocortical response to the second of two sequential hemorrhages depending upon the magnitude of the first hemorrhage. Stressor-induced facilitation of subsequent adrenocortical responses to stressors may not be limited to periods of one day since DANIELS-SEVERS et al. (1973) have demonstrated a potentiating effect of chronic stressors that lasts up to 8 weeks, and that is not accounted for by an enhanced adrenal responsiveness to ACTH.

If the facilitatory effect of stressors usually balances the inhibitory effects of the secreted corticosteroids on subsequent stimulus-induced ACTH secretion, then what function might this system have, other than to maintain uniform responsiveness in the adrenocortical system in a rather complicated manner? We have suggested previously that the feedback acts to offset the facilitatory effect of repeated application of stressors, thus conserving the modest supplies of pituitary ACTH (DALLMAN and JONES, 1973; DALLMAN et al., 1974a). However, other, more interesting possibilities of the consequences of balanced stress-induced facilitation and corticosteroid-induced inhibition of the responsiveness to repeated stimuli occur when other endocrine responses to stressors are considered.

Endocrine Responses to Hemorrhage, to Insulin-Induced Hypoglycemia, and to "Psychic" Stimuli

Table 1. Some endocrine responses to three stressors (+ = increased activity; - = decreased activity

	Stimuli to the adrenocortical system		
Hormone	Hemorrhage	Insulin-induced hypoglycemia	"Psychic" (restraint, mild electric shock, novelty)
Epinephrine	+ (1)	+ (5)	+ (10)
ADH (vasopressin)	+ (2)		+ (11)
Renin (PRA)	+ (3)	+ (6)	+ (12)
Growth hormone	+ (4)	+ (7)	+ (primate) - (rat) (13)
Prolactin		+ (8)	+ (14)
Insulin			
Glucagon		+ (9)	

(1) dog (HUME: Federation Proc. 20, Suppl. 9, 75-98 1961)
(2) dog (WEINSTEIN et al.: Endocrinology 66, 712-718, 1960)
(3) dog (NANNI et al.: Surgery in Italy 4, 198-204, 1974)
rabbit (WEBER et al.: Kidney Int. 7, 331-341, 1975)
(4) rhesus monkey (MEYER and KNOBIL: Endocrinology 80, 163-171, 1967)
(5) dog (MÜLLER et al.: Metabolism 25, 1077-1086, 1976)
man (BRANDSBORG et al.: Gastroentereology 68, 455-460, 1975)
(6) man (HATA et al.: J. Clin. Endocrinol. Metab. 43, 173-177, 1976)
(7) man (COPINSCHI et al.: C.R. Acad. Sci. (Paris) 275, 1419-1421, 1972)
(8) man (COPINSCHI et al.: C.R. Acad. Sci. (Paris) 275, 1419-1421, 1972; OSTERMAN et al.: Acta Endocrinol. (Kbh) 84, 237-245, 1977)
(9) dog (MÜLLER et al.: Metabolism 25, 1077-1086, 1976)
rat (PEREZ et al.: Diabetologia 12, 414, 1976)
(10) rat (KVETNANSKY et al.: Endocrinology 89, 46-49, 1971)
(11) adrenalectomized dog (TRAVIS and SHARE: Endocrinology 89, 246-253, 1971)
dog (O'CONNOR and VERNEY: Quart. J. Exp. Physiol. 31, 393-408, 1942)
(12) baboon (BLAIR et al.: Am. J. Physiol. 231, 772-776, 1976)
(13) rhesus monkey (MEYER and KNOBIL: Endocrinology 80, 163-171, 1967)
rat (KRULICH et al.: Neuroendocrinology 16, 293-311, 1974)
(14) rat (MATTHEIJ and VAN PIJKEREN: Acta Endocrinol. (Kbh) 84, 51-61, 1977; KRULICH et al.: Neuroendocrinology 16, 293-311, 1974)

Table 1 provides a partial list of the endocrine responses to three stimuli to the adrenocortical system. The humoral responses to the three different stimuli, all of which result in ACTH and corticosteroid secretion, have in common increased secretion of epinephrine, renin, probably prolactin, and ADH (vasopressin). After the application of stressors, growth hormone secretion falls in the rat, but rises in primates. Glucose concentrations are reported to increase in all cases, and glucagon and insulin concentrations may or may not increase.

If one proposes that the facilitatory effect of stressors is specific to some component of the adrenocortical system, and does not affect the controlling elements in other endocrine systems, then the constancy of corticosteroid secretory responses after repeated exposures to a stressor could have real consequences on the profile of the subsequent responses to stressors in other hormonal systems.

Table 2. Hormonal systems sensitive to the actions of glucocorticoids (+ = increased activity; - = decreased activity)

Epinephrine	+	rat	(WURTMAN, AXELROD: J. Biol. Chem. 241, 2301-2305, 1966)
ADH (vasopressin)	-	man	(DINGMAN et al.: J. Clin. Invest. 44, 1041, 1965)
Renin	+	dog	(REID et al.: Endocrinology 93, 107-114, 1973; REID et al.: Endocrinology 95, 1482-1485, 1974)
Growth hormone	-	man	(FRANTZ, RABKIN: N. Engl. J. Med. 271, 1375-1381, 1964)
Prolactin	-	man	(OSTERMAN et al.: Acta Endocrinol. (Kbh) 84, 237-245, 1977)
Insulin	+	man	(PERLEY, KIPNIS: N. Engl. J. Med. 274, 1237-1241, 1966)
Glucagon	+	man	(MARCO et al.: N. Engl. J. Med. 288, 128-131, 1973)

Table 2 lists some of the reported effects of treatment with either synthetic or natural glucocorticoids on the responses of seven hormones. Treatment with corticosteroids inhibits the secretion of ADH, prolactin, and growth hormone in response to provocative stimuli. By contrast, treatment with corticosteroids, or elevated rates of corticosteroid secretion, augment the secretion of epinephrine, glucagon, and insulin as well as increasing plasma renin activity by increasing angiotensinogen production.

Thus, although the consequences of previous stimulus-induced corticosteroid secretion may not be apparent in the subsequent responses of the adrenocortical system to stressors, the results of corticosteroid secretion may affect the subsequent levels of responses in other endocrine systems. The secretion of epinephrine in response to repeated bouts of restraint in rats provides evidence to support this contention. KVETŇANSKÝ et al. have demonstrated the increase in the adrenal medullary enzymes responsible for epinephrine synthesis, as well as the increase in urinary epinephrine excretion that occur with time in rats that are repeatedly restrained. The increase in the activity of both dopamine-B-hydroxylase and phenylethanolamine-N-methyl transferase is dependent on the presence of the pituitary and increased ACTH secretion (KVETŇANSKÝ et al., 1970, 1971). MIKULAJ et al. (1976) also report that adrenal and plasma corticosterone levels during the period of restraint may be of similar magnitude during the first and 40th bout of the stimulus.

Additional evidence that corticosteroids secreted in response to an initial stressor may affect other endocrine responses to repetition of the stimulus are provided by SACHS et al. The ADH response to a second hemorrhage applied to dogs 90 min after the first, and 60 min after reinfusion of the shed blood is markedly smaller than the first response (SACHS et al., 1967). Yet, using the same conditions of timing,

GANN et al. (1977) found that the cortisol responses were of similar magnitude. Although the two groups did not use hemorrhages of similar magnitude, it is very likely that the hemorrhage applied by Sachs' group provoked more cortisol secretion than that applied by GANN (GANN and CRYER, 1973). In vitro studies indicated that the diminished ADH response to a second stimulus was not due to decreased capacity to secrete ADH, nor did the ADH released inhibit its further secretion. The posterior lobe in vitro was shown to be capable of ADH secretion of equal magnitude when stimulated electrically at periods 90 min apart (SACHS and HALLER, 1968).

The evidence that glucocorticoids secreted in response to stressors will alter subsequent responses in other endocrine systems is still scant. However, experiments can readily be designed to pursue this line of investigation. It seems likely that repeated applications of stressors would result in decreased responses by those hormones that may be "stimulus-specific", such as growth hormone, prolactin and ADH, a glucocorticoid response of normal magnitude, and increased responses in renin, epinephrine and glucagon secretion. The latter responses would act to increase vascular tone and volume, and the synthesis and mobilization of glucose. These responses are those most generally associated with the flight or fight response to stressors.

Acknowledgment. This work was supported in part by USPHS grants AM06704, AM05613, NS00072 and NASA-Ames University interchange NCA2-OR665-502.

References

BUCHER, B., KOCH, B., MIALHE, C.: Sur l'existence d'un mécanisme de "feedback rapide" ACTH-corticostérone. J. Physiol. (Paris) 66, 199-209 (1973)

CHOWERS, I., HAMMEL, H.T., STROMME, S.B., MCCANN, S.M.: Comparison of effect of environmental and preoptic cooling on plasma cortisol levels. Am. J. Physiol. 207, 577-582 (1964)

DALLMAN, M.F., DEMANINCOR, D., SHINSAKO, J.: Diminishing corticotrope capacity to release ACTH during sustained stimulation: The twenty-four hours after bilateral adrenalectomy in the rat. Endocrinology 95, 65-73 (1974a)

DALLMAN, M.F., JONES, M.T.: Corticosteroid feedback control of stress-induced ACTH secretion. In: Brain-Pituitary-Adrenal Interrelationships. Brodish, A., Redgate, E.S. (eds.). Basel: Karger, 1973, pp. 176-196

DALLMAN, M.F., SHACKELFORD, R.L., MORGAN, G.S., SHINSAKO, J.: Feedback regulation of ACTH secretion: Cortisol (F) infused over the physiological range results in a concentration-dependent decrease in plasma ACTH in the dog. Federation Proc. 33, 205 (1974b)

DALLMAN, M.F., YATES, F.E.: Anatomical and functional mapping of central neural input and feedback pathways of the adrenocortical system. Mem. Soc. Endocrinol. 17, 39-72 (1968)

DANIELS-SEVERS, A., GOODWIN, A., KEIL, L.C., VERNIKOS-DANELLIS, J.: Effect of chronic crowding and cold on the pituitary-adrenal system: Responsiveness to an acute stimulus during chronic stress. Pharmacology 9, 348-356 (1973)

FORTIER, C., DELGADO, A., DUCOMMUN, P., DUCOMMUN, S., DUPONT, A., JOBIN, M., KRAICER, J., MACINTOSH-HARDT, B., MARCEAU, H., MIALHE, P., MIALHE-VOLOSS, C., RERUP, C., VAN REES, G.P.: Functional interrelationships between the adenohypophysis, thyroid, adrenal cortex and gonads. C.M.A. Journal 103, 864-874 (1970)

GANN, D.S.: Parameters of the stimulus initiating the adrenocortical response to hemorrhage. Ann. N.Y. Acad. Sci. 156, 740-755 (1969)

GANN, D.S., CRYER, G.L.: Feedback control of ACTH secretion by cortisol. In: Brain-Pituitary-Adrenal Interrelationships. Brodish, A., Redgate, E.S. (eds.). Basel: Karger, 1973, pp. 197-223

GANN, D.S., CRYER, G.L., PIRKLE, J.C., Jr.: Physiological inhibition and facilitation of adrenocortical response to hemorrhage. Am. J. Physiol. 232, R5-R9 (1977)

GANN, D.S., KINGSBURY, B., DRUCKER, W.R., TRAVIS, R.H.: Diminished adrenal corticoid response to burn and ACTH in the nephrectomized dog. Proc. Soc. Exp. Biol. Med. 108, 99-103 (1961)

GREER, M.A., ALLEN, C.F.: The effect of pentobarbital on basal and ether-stimulated ACTH secretion in intact and adrenalectomized rats. Neuroendocrinology 17, 258-264 (1975)

HENNESSY, J.W., LEVIN, R., LEVINE, S.: Influence of experiential factors and gonadal hormones on pituitary-adrenal responses of the mouse to novelty and electric shock. J. Comp. Physiol. Psych. 91, 770-777 (1977)

JONES, M.T., BRUSH, F.R., NEAME, R.L.B.: Characteristics of fast feedback control of corticotrophin release by corticosteroids. J. Endocrinol. 55, 489-497 (1972)

KVETŇANSKÝ, R., GEWIRTZ, G.P., WEISE, V.K., KOPIN, I.J.: Effect of hypophysectomy on immobilization-induced elevation of tyrosine hydroxylase and phenylethanolamine-N-methyl transferase in the rat adrenal. Endocrinology 87, 1323-1329 (1970)

KVETŇANSKÝ, R., WEISE, V.K., GEWIRTZ, G.P., KOPIN, I.J.: Synthesis of adrenal catecholamines in rats during and after immobilization stress. Endocrinology 89, 46-49 (1971)

MASON, J.W.: Specificity in the organization of neuroendocrine response profiles. In: Frontiers in Neurology and Neuroscience Research 1974. Seeman, P., Brown, G. M. (eds.). Toronto: Univ. of Toronto Press, 1974, pp. 68-80

MIKULAJ, L., KVETŇANSKÝ, R., MURGÁS, K., PAŘÍZKOVÁ, J., VENCEL, P.: Catecholamines and corticosteroids in acute and repeated stress. In: Catecholamines and Stress. Usden, E., Kvetňanský, R., Kopin, I.J. (eds.). Oxford: Pergamon, 1976, pp. 445-452

SACHS, H., HALLER, E.W.: Further studies on the capacity of the neurohypophysis to release vasopressin. Endocrinology 83, 251-262 (1968)

SACHS, H., SHARE, L., OSINCHAK, J., CARPI, A.: Capacity of the neurohypophysis to release vasopressin. Endocrinology 81, 755-770 (1967)

SATO, T., SATO, M., SHINSAKO, J., DALLMAN, M.F.: Corticosterone-induced changes in hypothalamic corticotropin-releasing factor (CRF) content after stress. Endocrinology 97, 265-274 (1975)

STOCKHAM, M.A.: Changes of plasma and adrenal corticosterone levels in the rat after repeated stimuli. J. Physiol. 173, 149-159 (1964)

2. Is Posterior-Hypophysial Corticotropin Involved in Neurogenic Stress?

C. Mialhe, B. Briaud, and B. Koch

By disconnecting the pituitary from the central nervous system (CNS), FORTIER (1951) distinguished between two categories of stress : neurogenic and systemic, according to whether they act at the hypothalamo-pituitary level through the CNS, or through the circulatory system. Neurogenic stress may be characterized by: (1) the necessity of an intact neural input to the hypothalamus, (2) a fast ACTH response and, (3) a great sensitivity to the circulating corticosteroid levels (cf. review by MIALHE and BRIAUD, 1977).

We have shown the existence of an ACTH activity at the posterior pituitary level (MIALHE-VOLOSS, 1958). KRAICER et al. (1973) showed that the ACTH of the neurointermediate lobe (NIL) is, in fact, present in the intermediate lobe (IL), and SCOTT et al. (1973) demonstrated that the molecular structure of NIL ACTH appears to be similar to the ACTH molecule extracted from the anterior pituitary (AP).

The results obtained with a bioassay utilizing dispersed adrenal cells showed that the AP contains 50 to 60 mU of ACTH, and the NIL 2 to 3 mU. This observation means that some ACTH could be released from NIL during stress. Indeed, when hypophysectomized rats are used, the intravenous injection of 300 µU is sufficient to produce a plasma corticosterone level similar to those obtained after systemic or neurogenic stimuli. This means that 300 µU of ACTH may be secreted during stress. This quantity represents 11% to 16% of the ACTH content of the NIL or 0.5 to 0.6% of that of the AP.

Several authors (cf. review by MIALHE and BRIAUD, 1977) showed that, during neurogenic stress, a decrease in the NIL ACTH level is observed. The ACTH content in the AP seems unaffected. Under these conditions, it can be suggested that the ACTH of NIL plays a physiologic rôle, particularly in the response to neurogenic stimuli. However it has never yet been possible to find in vivo a functional ACTH activity after anterior lobectomy.

The arguments for and against a physiologic rôle of NIL ACTH may be thus summarized. (1) The decrease in the ACTH level of NIL during neurogenic stress may result from the release of the hormone into the blood, or be the consequence of an in situ cleavage of the ACTH molecule into CLIP and MSH (SCOTT et al., 1973). However, in this case the reason for this cleavage during neurogenic stress should be explained. Moreover, the apparent lack of decrease in the AP ACTH may be due to the fact that only 0.5% of the AP ACTH content is released, and is thus indetectable. (2) Total or partial inhibition of the response after posterior lobectomy (SMELIK et al., 1962) may be the consequence of the suppression of NIL ACTH or of the section of the hypothalamo-hypophysial pathway incident to the operation. (3) In a superfusion system, like the AP, NIL releases ACTH. This release may be increased when a median eminence extract is added to the superfusion medium. Contrary, however, to AP, neurotransmitters such as serotonine (KRAICER and MORRIS, 1976) or acetylcholine (FISCHER and MORIARTY, 1977) stimulate the in vitro release of ACTH from NIL. The amounts needed may be considered as physiologic, since they are compatible with the quantities of neurotransmitters found in the hypothalamic area of the brain (BROWNSTEIN et al., 1976). Moreover, contrary to the effect on AP, the corticosterone added to the perfusion medium does not inhibit the stimulating effect of a median eminence extract. This may explain why corticosterone inhibits differently the response to these two types of stimuli. Contrary to what is seen in vitro, NIL ACTH disappears in vivo in the absence of AP, and the adrenal of the totally hypophysectomized rat does not differ from the adenohypophysectomized animal (GREER et al., 1975).

In conclusion, in the present stage of our knowledge, and because we are unable to ascertain whether blood ACTH is of AP or NIL origin, we can only conclude that NIL ACTH may possibly be involved in the response to neurogenic stimuli.

References

BROWNSTEIN, M.J., PALKOVITZ, M., SAAVEDRA, J.M., KIZER, J.S.: Distribution of hypothalamic hormones and neurotransmitters within the diencephalon. In: Frontiers in Neuroendocrinology. Martini, L., Gannong, W.F. (eds.). New York: Raven Press, 1976, pp. 1-23

FISCHER, J.L., MORIARTY, C.M.: Control of bioactive corticotropin release from the neuro-intermediate lobe of the rat pituitary in vitro. Endocrinology 100, 1047-1054 (1977)

FORTIER, C.: Dual control of adrenocorticotrophin release. Endocrinology 49, 782-788 (1951)

GREER, M.A., ALLEN, C.F., PATON, P., ALLEN, J.P.: Evidence that the pars intermedia and pars nervosa of the pituitary do not secrete functionally significant quantities of ACTH. Endocrinology 96, 718-724 (1975)

KRAICER, J., GOSBEE, J.L., BENCOSME, S.A.: Pars intermedia and pars distalis: two sites of ACTH production in the rat hypophysis. Neuroendocrinology 11, 156-176 (1973)

KRAICER, J., MORRIS, A.R.: In vitro release of ACTH from dispersed rat pars intermedia cells: effect of secretagogues. Neuroendocrinology 20, 79-96 (1976)

MIALHE, C., BRIAUD, B.: Possible involvement of pars intermedia of the rat pituitary in neurogenic stress. In: Frontiers of Hormone Research. Van Wimersma Greindanus (ed.). Basel: Karger, 1977, pp. 193-199

MIALHE-VOLOSS, C.: Posthypophyse et activité corticotrope. Acta Endocrinol. Copenh. 35, Suppl. pp. 1-96 (1958)

SCOTT, A.P., RATCLIFFE, J.G., REES, L.H., LANDON, J., BENNETT, H.P., LOWRY, P.J., MCMARTIN, C.: Pituitary peptide. Nature (New Biol.) 244, 65-67 (1973)

SMELIK, P.G., GAARENSTROOM, J.H., KONIJNENDIJK, W., DE WIED, D.: Evaluation of the rôle of the posterior lobe of the hypophysis in the reflex secretion of corticotrophin. Acta Physiol. Pharmacol. Neerl. 11, 20-33 (1962)

3. Endocrine Responses to Acoustic Stresses

B. METZ, G. BRANDENBERGER, and M. FOLLENIUS

The progress of technical civilization and urbanization is paralleled by continuous intensification of noise. It is becoming increasingly apparent that prolonged exposures to environmental noise may contribute to the development in man of pathologic states such as coronary vascular disease, gastrointestinal disorders and hypertension. Workers exposed to noise, and residents annoyed by aircraft noises appear to suffer more neurologic disorders than the rest of the population.

Few investigators have attempted to correlate these medical disorders with neuroendocrine disturbances in men exposed to environmental noise. Many more investigations have been concerned with separate assessments of adreno-cortico-medullary hormones to see if noise may be included among other physical and physiochemical stresses that induce a pattern of endocrinologic responses associated with the general adaptation syndrome (SELYE, 1946, 1976). In this respect, the most commonly cited nonauditory effect of noise is adrenocortical activation via the hypothalamo-pituitary axis; a second channel for stress response consists of release of catecholamines under the influence of discharge of acetylcholine at autonomic nerve endings, especially in the adrenal medulla.

In man, information on hormone levels in the blood is scarce; most investigations have evaluated the adrenocortico-medullary hormones in the urine; it is then assumed that an increase in adrenal secretion is followed by an increase in urinary output of its hormone metabolites.

It has generally been reported that exposure to noise causes significant increases in adrenaline excretion, whereas noradrenaline excretion is less strongly affected. LEVI (1961) reported an increased output of both catecholamines in men exposed to "disagreeable industrial noise" at 97-104 dBA. HAWEL and STARLINGER (1967) examined students who were exposed to noise (90 dBA, 1 h) and found a significant increase in urinary adrenaline, but no such increase in noradrenaline. Even moderate noise (80 dBA) caused a significant increase in adrenaline excretion, in so far that students exposed to noise did not show the afternoon decrease observed under quiet control conditions. A similar effect, albeit less marked, was found for noradrenaline excretion, whereas no effect could be detected on corticosteroids (SLOB et al., 1973).

Along with these studies emphasizing the role of the adrenal medulla in man under laboratory conditions, there are also field studies on changes in the catecholamine excretion of workers exposed to less well-defined noise levels. ANITESCO et al. (1973) examined 100 employees exposed to noise and industrial vibrations (97-127 dB, 40-100 Hz). After 4 h of work, the group had significantly higher urinary adrenaline and noradrenaline than the group of 20 controls. Marked increases in catecholamine excretion, blood pressure and pulse rate were reported in 72% of the workers from an aircraft factory exposed to turbine noise for 3 h (ORTIZ et al., 1974). Similarly, in workers exposed to vibrations and industrial noise, an increase in urinary vanilic-mandelic acid (VMA) indicates a strong stress response (MORELLI et al., 1973).

Little is known of the effect of noise on the adrenocortical function in man. The lack of specifity in analytic methods and the influence of renal and hepatic functions mean that the urinary corticosteroid level is a poor index to adrenal function under stress. Discrepant results appear in investigations on the effects of exposure to noise on urinary 17-ketosteroid excretion; both increased (ARGUELLES et al., 1962; SERRA et al., 1964) and decreased (ANITESCO and CONTULESCO, 1972; ATHERLY et al., 1970) outputs have been observed. It should be kept in mind that urinary 17-ketosteroids are derived not only from cortisol, but also from androgens secreted by the adrenal gland in both sexes, and from testicular secretion in the male. So changes in 17-ketosteroids urinary excretion may not depend only on changes in adrenal cortex activity.

Very few investigations have examined the effects of exposure to noise on urinary 17-OH-CS. Significant increases due to exposure to pure-frequency sounds have been reported by ARGUELLES et al. (1962) and at least constant levels by SLOB et al. (1973) will moderate noise exposure (80 dB). Since the same exposure caused a significant increase in adrenaline excretion, the authors concluded that "the strongest reaction to noise as a stressor is shown by adrenaline excretion."

An important and often neglected factor that complicates every study on the effects of experimental noise in man is the individual psychologic reaction to the sound. In the studies mentioned above, stimulus characteristics are generally well defined; but the reaction patterns may be partially conditioned by the specific attitudinal or physiologic characteristics of the individual.

A clue to the importance of such a modulation is provided by the experiments of ATHERLY et al. (1970) who showed that exposure to noises of "high subjective importance" (aircraft and typewriter) caused a marked decrease in 24-h urinary 17-ketosteroid and eosinophils, and an increase in total cell-count in lymphocytes and in neutrophils, whereas noise of "low subjective importance" (white noise) produced no significant changes from control levels. It seems that the effect of rather high noise levels (up to 94 dB for 6 h) may have been counteracted by such psychologic factors as "the familiarity of the noise and the generally positive attitudes of the subjects to the job" as stated by CARLESTAM et al. (1973) in their study on IBM operators at their usual work. The authors reported nonsignificant changes in adrenaline and noradrenaline excretion from control to noise periods and concluded that, under some favorable circumstances, intense noise may not act as a stressor.

Further evidence that the reaction of the individual to noise is particularly important comes from the experiments of ARGUELLES et al. (1970). Comparing the adrenal hormone reactions to noise of healthy controls with those of patients with cardiovascular diseases or schizophrenia, they found higher increases in adrenaline and noradrenaline excretion in both patient groups. The authors suggested that heart patients and schizophrenics react to audiogenic stress because of a "more active psychologic personality."

Thus, although many aspects of the interrelation between susceptibility to noise and measurable endocrinologic changes have not yet been investigated, it seems clear that emotional or psychologic factors associated with noise play a highly significant role.

Similar conclusions may be drawn from the studies of BRANDENBERGER et al. (1977), who demonstrated that exposure to broad- and narrow-band pink noises of different sound-pressure levels, frequencies, and

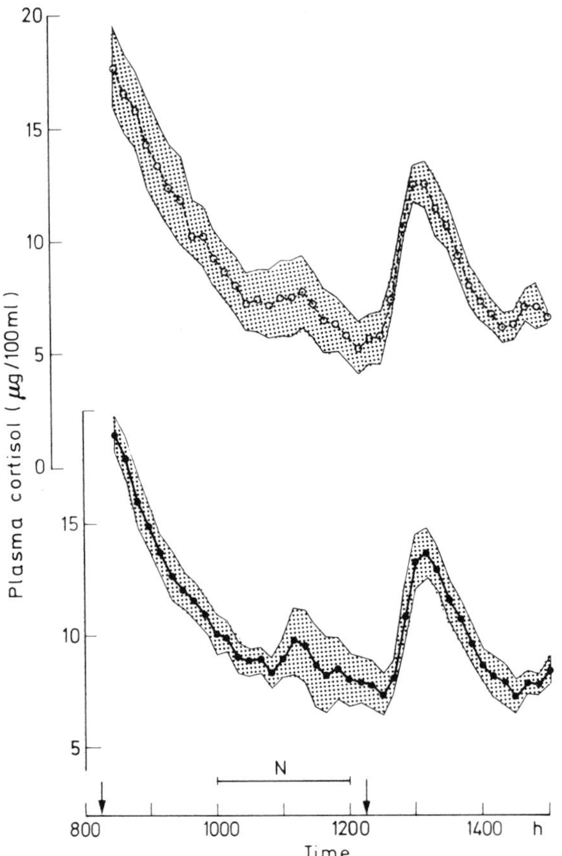

Fig. 1. Mean and standard deviation of plasma cortisol concentration in five subjects during control days (above) and during days with exposure to pink noise (N) of 120 min duration and 96 dB (A) intensity. Arrows indicate meals. (From BRANDENBERGER et al., 1977)

durations did not produce any appreciable modification in the temporal pattern of plasma cortisol levels in man. This study takes into account the continuously variable pattern of circulating cortisol throughout the day, due to episodic secretion. Under stable physiologic conditions, a fairly constant pattern with an early morning decline and meal-related peaks was observed on control days; however, some subjects did show small, apparently haphazard, fluctuations; slight additional increases during noise exposure may be difficult to characterize, especially if individual results are considered. However, there are no significant differences between the mean patterns for control days and noise-exposure days (Fig. 1). Thus, it appears that noise doses safe for conservation of human hearing induce no significant increase in plasma cortisol concentration in subjects fully informed of the experimental design, although these exposures induced auditory fatigue and annoyance, revealed by deterioration of their sensory-motor performances, and by their subjective assessments. The authors concluded that noise itself, when not associated with other potentially agressive stimuli, does not stimulate the hypophysio-adrenocortical axis.

Other data on the effect of exposure to noise on blood corticosteroid levels are still scanty, but lead to similar conclusion. ARGUELLES et al. (1962), with wide-interval blood sampling, observed "substantial" increases in plasma 17-OH-CS due to exposure to pure frequency sounds. Only at the highest frequency (10,000 Hz) and intensity (93 dB) were these increases statistically significant. FAVINO et al. (1973) investigated, in the laboratory, the effects of 5 h of continuous industrial noise on circulating hormone levels, by simultaneous radioimmunoassays of cortisol, growth hormone (GH), luteinizing hormone (LH) and thyroxine. They found no appreciable modifications in plasma cortisol, except for a transient initial increase and irregular increases of GH, and no significant changes in LH and thyroxine.

These results differ from those observed in animals, that do not remain indifferent to noise, but generally react with hostility or fright. The responses in animals may be related to a more general stressing situation. Noise has therefore been considered as a typical neurogenic stress known to activate the hypothalamo-hypophysial axis. Animal studies enabled investigations of the interaction between the activating neuronal systems and the inhibitory systems, which determines the level of peripheral modifications. Furthermore, attempts have been made to outline the role of brain neurotransmitters in controlling several central nervous system functions in response to auditory stimulations.

It is well established that stressful agents increase the secretion of corticotropin (ACTH) from the adenohypophysis, and that the resulting increase in plasma concentration of ACTH causes in increased secretion of adrenal corticosteroids. HENKIN and KNIGGE (1963) studied the changes in adrenal secretion of corticosterone in rats exposed to a continuous high intensity pure tone (130 dB, 220 Hz). The pattern of adrenocortical response consists of an initial high rate of hormone secretion, followed by a depression of corticosterone output to normal or subnormal levels if the stimulus is continued for a period of 12 h. This sudden suppression of adrenal corticosteroid secretion has been attributed to an inhibition of ACTH release.

Inhibitory mechanisms induced by repeated sound stimulation were studied by BRIAUD et al. (1971) who exposed rats to continuous sounds of different frequencies at 100 dB for 15 min, and found that adrenocortical response increased concomitantly with frequency. Their results showed that higher plasma corticosterone level inhibited subsequent stimulation by sound, but did not affect the response to an ether stress. Further comparisons between the inhibition of the adrenal response to neurogenic or systemic stress (BRIAUD, 1973) showed that the minimum amount of exogenous corticosterone needed to inhibit the response to a systemic stress was twice as large as the amount necessary to inhibit the response to a neurogenic stress. The time-lag in inhibition is also greater for systemic stress than for neurogenic stress. These results lead to the conclusion that different neurohumoral mechanisms are involved in the two types of stress.

MIALHE-VOLOSS (1955, 1958) demonstrated the presence of ACTH in the intermediate lobe of the rat pituitary, and showed that the corticotropic cells intervene in the response to sound used as a neurogenic stress, whereas a systemic stimulation leads to the depletion of ACTH in the adenohypophysis. These results have beeen confirmed more recently by MORIARTY et al. (1975), who found marked ultrastructural and immuno cytochemical changes in intermediate lobe cells after 30 min of neurogenic stress, whereas no cytologic changes were observed following systemic stimulation. Some investigators (KRAICER et al., 1973; MORIARTY et al., 1975; MIALHE and BRIAUD, 1976) sought a possible functional relationship between neuro-intermediate corticotropic activity and circulating adrenocorticosteroids, but found no evidence for it. That the intermediate lobe does play a role in the neurogenic stress response was borne out recently by experiments of BERAUD et al. (1976). In rats subjected to continuous noise of 90 dB, they noted an increased plasma corticosterone level and, in the neurointermediate lobe, significantly increased ACTH and α-MSH levels with parallel patterns, whereas anterior lobe ACTH was depleted.

The neurogenic stressor effect of noise has also been related to other hypophysial hormones. MIALHE and LUTZ (1969) measured the plasma levels of antidiuretic hormone (ADH) and ACTH and found a simultaneous increase of both hormones in noise-exposed rats, whereas ADH liberation precedes that of ACTH in the case of systemic stimulation. BROWN et al. (1971) suggested that the plasma GH level may increase in squirrel monkeys exposed to an intermittent-sound stimulus of 120 dB produced by a high range automobile horn. However, the evidence for auditory stimulation is meager, and the response seems rather to be elicited by other psychogenic stressors. BLOOM et al. (1973), found in rhesus monkeys that plasma glucagon rose rapidly when they were alarmed by a load noise of fluctuating frequency and amplitude, or by banging on a metal sheet. This increase was followed by a rise in blood glucose, but not in insulin. They conclude that the rapid increase in glucagon seems to be caused by α-cell secretion either under direct neural control, or, indirectly, by catecholamine release mediated by the nervous system.

Several studies suggest that catecholamines may control some important central functions. Their level in the organism can indicate the magnitude of stress, as well as the reactivity of the sympathetic nervous system. Many authors have found increased urinary excretion of catecholamines due to noise of high intensity. OGLE and LOCKETT (1968) reported an increased urinary adrenaline output in rats exposed to a noise of 20 kHz and 98-100 dB, and stated that it would "prevent an emotional release of antidiuretic hormone." MARKIEWICZ (1973), in experiments on rats subjected to long-lasting acoustic stimulation, measured catecholamines in tissues, blood and urine. He concluded that metabolic disturbances of catecholamines and serotonin, consisting of an increase in catecholamines in the urine, and also at high concentrations in blood and brain during the initial phase occurred, while further stimulation led to changes in synthesis and degradation of biogenic amines.

Thus, the role of brain neurotransmitters in controlling various functions of the central nervous system has been demonstrated; research has been mainly concentrated on noradrenaline, dopamine and serotonin. Catecholaminergic and serotoninergic pathways have been mapped out since the development of histochemical fluorescence methods. Very few studies have so far been published on the relationship between biogenic amines and auditory functions. Since the level of brain catecholamines represents a dynamic equilibrium between synthesis and efflux, stress-induced changes in the turnover of brain catecholamines have generally been evaluated. VASSOUT (1977) exposed rats to sonic booms of variable characteristics. He reported a significant increase in the noradrenaline turnover rate, whereas no systematic variations in the dopamine turnover rate were observed (Fig. 2). These results tally with those of SMOOKLER and BUCKLEY (1969), who demonstrated significant variations in brain norepinephrine. CALOGERO and VETRANO (1973) attempted to determine whether changes in the monoamine content of specific areas of the brain were related to specific auditory stimulation rather than to a general stressing situation. They used two different types of stimulus, and observed that the most important changes were those of serotonin and 5-hydroxyindolacetic acid, which were correlated with changes

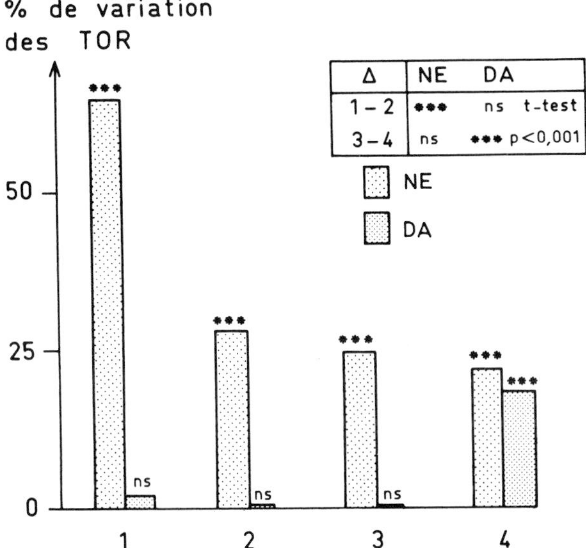

Fig. 2. Effect of sonic booms on turnover rate of brain norepinephrine (NE) and dopamine (DA).

Sonic boom type	1	2	3	4
Total duration (ms)	84	18	76	56
Rise time (ms)	7	7	3	3

Peak levels: 3.5 mb.
(From VASSOUT, 1977)

in the auditory transmission. Adrenocortical stimulation and decrease in brain noradrenaline were only observed with intense and stressing auditory impulses, while serotonin seemed to be involved in the control of the auditory transmission. The author concluded that serotonin might inhibit auditory-stressing stimulation in the brain areas containing the auditory pathways. Other transmitters, such as γ-amino-butyric acid (GABA) have been studied (VASSOUT, 1977), but no significant changes of its concentration in brain could be established.

The activation of central noradrenergic sites has been shown to play an important role in the hypertensive effects of auditory stimulations (SMOOKLER et al., 1973). Paradoxically, LOCKETT and MARWOOD (1973) described "sound-deprival hypertension" involving changes in hypophysial secretion in rats transferred from the stock room to a sound-proofed room. These findings may well stimulate further research on the endocrinologic changes induced by sound deprivation, and thus give a clearer overall picture of the effects of noise or its absence.

References

ANITESCO, C., BUBUIANU, E., CONTULESCO, A.: Interaction des catécholamines et des électrolytes dans le traumatisme sonore vibratoire industriel. Arch. Malad. Prof. Paris 34, 503-510 (1973)

ANITESCO, C., CONTULESCO, A.: Etude de l'influence du bruit et des vibrations sur le comportement des catécholamines dansl l'agression sonore vibratoire industrielle. Arch. Malad. Prof. Paris 33, 365-372 (1972)

ARGUELLES, A.E., IBEAS, D., OTTONE, J.P., CHEKHERDEMAN, M.: Pituitary-adrenal stimulation by sound of different frequencies. J. Clin. Endocr. 22, 846-852 (1962)
ARGUELLES, A.E., MARTINEZ, M.A., PUCCIARELLI, E., DISISTO, M.V.: Endocrine and metabolic effects of noise in normal, hypertensive and psychotic subjects. In: Physiological Effects of Noise. Welch, B.L., Welch, A.S. (eds.). New York-London: Plenum Press, 1970, pp. 43-55
ATHERLY, G.R.C., GIBBONS, S.L., POWELL, J.A.: Moderate acoustic stimuli: the interrelation of subjective importance and certain physiologic changes. Ergonomics 13, 536-545 (1970)
BERAUD, G., KRAICER, J., LYWOOD, D.W.: ACTH et α-MSH hypophysaires après un stress neurotrope. J. Physiol. 72, 35A (1976)
BLOOM, S.R., DANIEL, P.M., JOHNSTON, D.I., OGAWER, O., PRATT, O.E.: Release of glucagon, induced by stress. Quart. J. Exp. Physiol. 58, 99-108 (1973)
BRANDENBERGER, G., FOLLENIUS, M., TRÉMOLIÈRES, C.: Failure of noise exposure to modify temporal patterns of plasma cortisol in man. Eur. J. Appl. Physiol. 36, 239-246 (1977)
BRIAUD, B.: Réponse corticosurrénalienne aux agressions neurotrope et systémique après injection de corticostéroides. J. Physiol. 66, 259-270 (1973)
BRIAUD, B., LUTZ, B., MIALHE, C.: Réponse corticosurrénalienne à une agression neurotrope: influence de la fréquence et de la répétition du stimulus. C.R. Soc. Biol. 165, 1435-1440 (1971)
BROWN, G.M., SCHALCH, D.S., REICHLIN, S.: Patterns of growth hormone and cortisol responses to psychological stress in the squirrel monkey. Endocrinology 88, 956-963 (1971)
CALOGERO, B., VETRANO, G.: Variations of the biogenics amines content in some different areas of the brain of rats subjected to physiological auditory stimulation and acoustic trauma. Rev. Laryng. 94, 429-443 (1973)
CARLESTAM, G., KARLSSON, C.G., LEVI, L.: Stress and disease in response to exposure to noise. A review. Proceedings of the international congress on noise as a public health problem. Dubrovnik, Yugoslavia pp. 479-486 (1973)
FAVINO, A., MAUGERI, V., KAUCHTSCHISCHVILI, G., ROBUSTELLI DELLA CUNA, G., NAPPI, G.: Radioimmunoassay measurements of serum cortisol, thyroxine, growth hormone and luteinizing hormone with simultaneous electroencephalographic changes during continuous noise in man. J. Nucl. Biol. Med. 17, 119-122 (1973)
HAWEL, W., STARLINGER, H.: Einfluß von wiederholten vierstündigen, intermittierenden, sogenannten rosa Rauschen auf Catecholaminausscheidung und Pulsfrequenz. Int. Z. Angew. Physiol. Einschl. Arbeitsphysiol. 24, 351-362 (1967)
HENKIN, R.I., KNIGGE, K.M.: Effect of sound on the hypothalamic-pituitary adrenal axis. Am. J. Physiol. 204, 710-714 (1963)
KRAICER, J., GOSBEE, J.L., BENCOSME, S.A.: Pars intermedia and pars distalis: two sites of ACTH production in the rat hypophysis. Neuroendocrinology 11, 156-176 (1973)
LEVI, L.: A new stress tolerance test with simultaneous study of physiological and psychological variables. Acta Endocrinol. (Kbh) 37, 38 (1961)
LOCKETT, M.F., MARWOOD, J.F.: Sound deprivation causes hypertension in rats. Federation Proc. 32, 2111-2114 (1973)
MARKIEWICZ, L.: Some data on the influence of noise on neurohumoral substances in tissues and body fluids. Proc. Int. Cong. on Noise as a Public Health Problem. Dubrovnik, Yugoslavia pp. 473-478 (1973)
MIALHE, C., BRIAUD, B.: L'ACTH du lobe intermédiaire de l'hypophyse. J. Physiol. 72, 261-276 (1976)
MIALHE, C., LUTZ, B.: Libération des hormones antidurétique et corticotrope au cours de différents types d'agressions. Neuroendocrinologie. Paris: CNRS (ed.), 1969, pp. 163-171
MIALHE-VOLOSS, C.: Variations des teneurs en hormone corticotrope des lobes antérieur et postérieur de l'hypophyse du rat soumis à différents types d'agressions. C.R. Acad. Sci. 241, 105-107 (1955)
MIALHE-VOLOSS, C.: Posthypophyse et activité corticotrope. Acta Endocrinol. Suppl. 35, 1-96 (1958)
MORELLI, G., BELOTTI, C., PERRELA, F.: Stress' vibratorio nell' uomo: aspetti etiopatogenetici e lavorativi. Nuovo Arch. Ital. Otol. 1, 94-1P1 (1973)

MORIARTY, G.C., HALMI, N.S., MORIARTY, C.M.: The effect of stress on the cytology and immunocytochemistry of pars intermedia cells in the rat pituitary. Endocrinology 96, 1426-1436 (1975)

OGLE, C.W., LOCKETT, M.F.: The urinary changes induced in rats by high pitched sound (20 kcyc./sec). J. Endocrinol. 42, 253-260 (1968)

ORTIZ, G.A., ARGUELLES, A.E., CRESPIN, H.A., SPOSARI, G., VILLAFANE, C.T.: Modifications of epinephrine, norepinephrine, blood lipid fractions and the cardiovascular system produced by noise in an industrial medium. Horm. Res. 5, 57-64 (1974)

SELYE, H.: The general adaptation syndrome and the diseases of adaptation. J. Clin. Endocrinol. 6, 117-230 (1946)

SELYE, H.: Stress in Health and Disease. Boston-London: Butterworths, 1976

SERRA, C., BARONE, A., DEVITA, C., LAURINI, F.: Riposta neuroumorali alla stimulazione acustica intermittente. Acta Neurologica 19, 1018-1035 (1964)

SLOB, A., WINK, A., RADDER, J.J.: The effect of acute noise exposure on the excretion of corticosteroids, adrenaline and noradrenaline in man. Int. Arch. Arbeitsmed. 31, 225-235 (1973)

SMOOKLER, H.H., BUCKLEY, J.P.: Relationships between brain catecholamine synthesis, pituitary adrenal function and the production of hypertension during prolonged experimental stress. J. Neuropharmacol. 8, 33-41 (1969)

SMOOKLER, H.H., GOEBEL, K.H., SIEGEL, M.I., CLARKE, D.E.: Hypertensive effects of prolonged auditory visual and motion stimulation. Federation Proc. 32, 2105-2110 (1973)

VASSOUT, P.: Action du bang sonique sur divers métabolites sanguins et cérébraux. Thèse 3e cycle, Univ. Louis Pasteur, Strasbourg (1977)

4. Concentrations of Certain Hormones in the Blood of Human Males Subjected to Steady-State Noise

A. FAVINO

Audiogenic stress although well established in rodents, has not been demonstrated as occurring in humans exposed to steady-state noise within the range of current industrial standards for hearing protection (FAVINO et al., 1973; this vol., Ch. IV,3). To learn more about the short-term effects of noise on endocrine function in man, blood samples were drawn from human males while they were subjected to noise. These samples were analyzed for different hormones.

Methods

Six normal males, 20-35 years old, were seated in a room with a noise level of 40-50 dBA from 15.00 to 17.00, two subjects at a time. Blood samples were removed with a catheter placed in an antecubital vein every 10 min for 40 min, before, during, and after administration of 100 dBA steady-state noise of the same frequency spectrum as used earlier by FAVINO et al. (1973). The noise was administered either continuously, or was interrupted every 10 min for 10 min.

Assays were performed with commercially available assay kits (Table 1a).

Table 1a. Details of assays employed

Hormone	Source of kit	Type	Variation within assay %	Variation between assays %
Thyroid-stimulating hormone	CIS	Double antibody	13	15
Growth hormone	CIS	Double antibody	10.7	12.5
Prolactin	Biodata	Single antibody	10.5	14.3
ACTH	CIS	Single antibody	15.8	23.7
Effective thyroxine ratio (ETR)	Mallinckrodt	Competitive protein binding	3.5	3.8
Corticoids	CIS	Competitive protein binding	15.7	21.25

Results and Discussion

From Table 1 it is clear that high noise levels, within the limits required for protection, do not induce conspicuous changes in hormones

Table 1. Endocrine responses of human males to noise

	Type	Time after beginning of the experiment (min)											
	of	Before noise				During noise				After noise			
Hormone	noise	10	20	30	40	50	60	70	80	90	100	110	120
ACTH	C	61.1 (17.7)	32.1 (9.4)	44.6 (11.5)	72.2 (40.8)	51.0 (12.9)	38.5 (12.2)	42.0 (12.6)	31.7 (7.1)	18.4 (4.2)	16.9 (17.0)	12.7 (6.6)	21.6 (11.3)
	I	76.1 (20.1)	68.5 (23.3)	69.4 (14.9)	68.7 (22.0)	56.3 (8.2)	41.6 (7.8)	45.4 (6.8)	60.1 (8.3)	56.3 (19.9)	16.6 (7.6)	61.3 (13.2)	51.8 (31.1)
Prolactin	C	17.7 (5.4)	16.0 (4.2)	16.5 (4.2)	15.4 (4.8)	18.9 (5.1)	16.2 (4.3)	14.5 (3.7)	12.9 (2.8)	13.2 (2.8)	10.3 (2.7)	11.7 (2.8)	20.9 (9.2)
ng/ml	I	17.6 (5.3)	17.3 (3.9)	14.7 (3.7)	13.3 (2.5)	12.9 (2.2)	12.9 (2.5)	12.4 (1.5)	11.7 (1.2)	10.8 (1.1)	11.1 (1.7)	12.7 (2.4)	12.5 (2.2)
TSH	C	2.0 (0.6)	1.9 (0.5)	2.5 (0.5)	2.0 (0.6)	2.3 (0.3)	2.1 (0.4)	2.6 (0.4)	2.4 (0.5)	2.4 (0.6)	2.6 (0.4)	2.8 (0.7)	2.4 (0.6)
ng/ml	I	2.4 (0.5)	2.2 (0.5)	2.2 (0.6)	2.4 (0.5)	2.6 (0.6)	2.5 (0.4)	2.3 (0.7)	3.1 (0.7)	3.0 (0.8)	3.4 (0.9)	3.4 (0.9)	3.4 (0.8)
GH	C	0.9 (0.8)	1.3 (1.0)	1.9 (1.5)	2.5 (1.7)	2.8 (1.6)	2.3 (1.3)	2.0 (1.0)	2.1 (1.3)	1.5 (1.0)	1.3 (0.9)	0.9 (0.5)	0.7 (0.3)
ng/ml	I	1.8 (1.3)	2.7 (1.8)	3.7 (2.2)	3.0 (1.8)	2.8 (1.7)	2.5 (1.3)	2.0 (1.1)	1.9 (0.9)	1.6 (0.9)	1.8 (0.9)	1.3 (0.8)	1.0 (0.5)
Corticoid	C	6.1 (2.9)	5.7 (2.4)	5.3 (2.3)	5.6 (1.6)	3.8 (0.6)	5.6 (1.1)	5.2 (1.9)	3.9 (1.2)	5.6 (2.3)	5.3 (1.8)	5.2 (2.5)	3.1 (1.3)
µg/100 ml	I	4.8 (1.2)	9.6 (2.5)	11.9 (6.6)	8.4 (3.8)	8.3 (3.5)	9.3 (4.3)	8.7 (4.1)	8.2 (2.8)	4.5 (1.9)	6.0 (2.5)	5.9 (3.5)	5.2 (1.9)
ETR effective	C	0.98 (0.01)	0.97 (0.01)	0.98 (0.01)	0.95 (0.02)	0.97 (0.01)	0.98 (0.02)	0.96 (0.02)	0.96 (0.01)	1.00 (0.02)	0.97 (0.01)	0.94 (0.03)	0.97 (0.03)
thyroxine ratio	I	0.92 (0.03)	0.92 (0.02)	0.92 (0.02)	0.92 (0.02)	0.92 (0.02)	0.92 (0.03)	0.94 (0.01)	0.92 (0.02)	0.95 (0.02)	0.91 (0.02)	0.91 (0.02)	0.90 (0.03)

ACTH, PRL, GH, corticoids and effective thyroxine ratio (ETR) as well as serum TSH levels at 10 min intervals between 15.00 and 17.00, before, during, and after administration of 100 dbA steady-state continuous (C) and intermittent (I) noise. Mean values ± SE (in parenthesis in six subjects. TSH 1 ng = 5 µU MRC 68/38; corticoid: mainly cortisol, but cross reactions also with corticosterone and deoxycortisol not significantly present in normals.

over the course of 2 h. The continuous decreases in ACTH and corticoids can be at least partially attributed to the persistance of the circadian rhythm for both hormones. On the other hand, a variance analysis of the data (Table 2) shows a slight but significant increase in TSH during and after intermittent noise. A significant augmentation was also demonstrated for GH during continuous noise, which conforms to the changes previously reported with more stressful noise (FAVINO et al., 1973). After exposure to both types of noise, the GH levels were significantly decreased. Finally, continuous noise decreased the concentrations in prolactin.

Table 2. Results of variance analysis of the data

Hormone	Type of noise	Mean values of data within blocks					
		Before noise (B)		During noise (R)		After noise (S)	
ACTH pg/ml	C	52.60	o	40.79	+	17.38	o,+
	I	70.67	o,+	50.38	+	46.68	o
Prolactin ng/ml	C	16.39	o	15.65	=	14.00	o,=
TSH ng/ml	I	2.30	o,	2.59	●	3.27	o,●
GH ng/ml	C	1.65	+,‡	2.29	+,o	1.09	o,‡
	I	2.79	o	2.30	●	1.41	o,●
Corticoid µg/100 ml	C	5.67	=,‡	4.62	=	4.77	‡
	I	8.66	+,[+]	8.61	+	5.41	[+]

Significantly different terms of the comparisons are labeled with the same symbol:
o, ● for $p < 0.001$
+, [+] for $p < 0.01$
=, ‡, [=] for $p < 0.05$
Each of the values reported is the mean of four samples at 10-min interval (block) in six subjects (see Table 1). Variance analysis for randomized blocks B, R, S, showed in fact that the variance was due to difference between subjects, and not to difference between time intervals within each block, except for prolactin with intermittent noise (I) and TSH with continuous noise (C). Further analysis of the variance was then performed, using a split-plot design for prolactin (I) and TSH (C), which showed that all the variance was due to differences between subjects. The application of t Tukey's test for the comparisons between blocks with replication in all other experimental groups led to the conclusions reported on Table 2.

These changes are tentatively attributable to a hypothetical decrease of serotonin levels, similar to that occurring in the mouse brain at nonstressing noise levels (CALOGERO, 1971), and in view of the demonstration that serotonin in man stimulates release of ACTH and prolactin (IMURA et al., 1973), and suppresses release of TSH (MAC INDOE and TURKINGTON, 1973).

References

CALOGERO, B.: Sul ruolo della serotonina nella trasmissione centrale del messagio sonoro. La Clin. ORL 5-6, 291-302 (1971)

FAVINO, A., MAUGERI, U., KAUCHTSCHISCHVILI, G., ROBUSTELLI DELLA CUNA, G., NAPPI, G.: Radioimmunoassay measurements of serum cortisol, thyroxine, GH, LH with simultaneous EEG changes during continuous noise in man. J. Nucl. Biol. Med. 17, 119-122 (1973)

IMURA, H., NAKAI, Y., YOSHIMI, T.: Effect of 5-hydroxytryptophan (5-HTP) on growth hormone and ACTH release in man. J. Clin. Endoc. Metab. 36, 204-206 (1973)

MACINDOE, J.H., TURKINGTON, R.W.: Stimulation of human prolactin secretion by intravenous infusion of l-tryptophan. J. Clin. Invest. 52, 1971-1978 (1973)

Chapter V. Endocrine Responses to Hyperbaria and Hypobaria

1. Endocrine Responses to Elevated Ambient Pressure

A. C. WEIHL

Introduction

The hyperbaric environment represents an extraordinary situation, in which essentially all environmental parameters are artificially changed. Exposure to hyperbaric conditions exposes an organism to an environment in which all parameters are different from those encountered in the normal atmospheric surroundings, and even those parameters that are nominally maintained at the same levels encountered under normal atmospheric conditions are altered in physiologic terms. Such features must always be kept in mind in evaluating physiologic effects observed under hyperbaric conditions, and great caution must be exercised in attributing an observed effect to a change in a specific environmental parameter.

Hyperbaric Environment

To understand the factors involved, one must dissect the hyperbaric environment into its many components, recognizing that alterations in two components may have synergistic or antagonistic physiologic effects. In addition to the essential feature of ambient pressure above one atmosphere absolute (ATA), the hyperbaric environment encompasses alterations in the type and partial pressures of the inert gases present, changes in oxygen partial pressure, alterations in the thermal properties of the gas mixtures, changes in gas density, and the additional variable of water immersion versus dry hyperbaric exposures (Table 1).

Table 1. Components in hyperbaric environment

1.	Hydrostatic pressure	4.	Thermal conductivity
2.	Inert gas	5.	Gas density
3.	Oxygen partial pressure	6.	Immersion

Even this list of variables is incomplete, in that it neglects other parameters, such as humidity, alterations in light-dark cycles, and alterations in speech and sound characteristics. The range of potential alterations is great, as men have been exposed to pressures as great as 61 ATA, and animals to hundreds of atmospheres of pressure. The range of relative density of gases covers a span of 20:1, thermal conductivity a span of 10:1, and sound velocity a range of 4:1. Each of these parameters may be altered, some quite independently, and then magnified by an increase in pressure.

Additional consideration must be given to the fact that exposure to a hyperbaric environment must be carried out in a progressive, stepwise fashion. Due to a number of physiologic factors, one cannot enter or leave a hyperbaric atmosphere rapidly. As exposure to greater pressures occurs, the rate of increase in pressure must be reduced, such that many hours, or even days, may be spent reaching a pressure of 40 to 50 ATA. Likewise, the rate of pressure reduction must be even more gradual than the rate of pressure increase. As seen in Figure 1, the rate of reduction in pressure from 50 ATA to one ATA may require weeks to achieve safely. Thus, any hyperbaric exposure consists of three distinct phases: (1) a compression or descent phase, (2) a period of constant elevated pressure, and (3) a decompression or ascent phase.

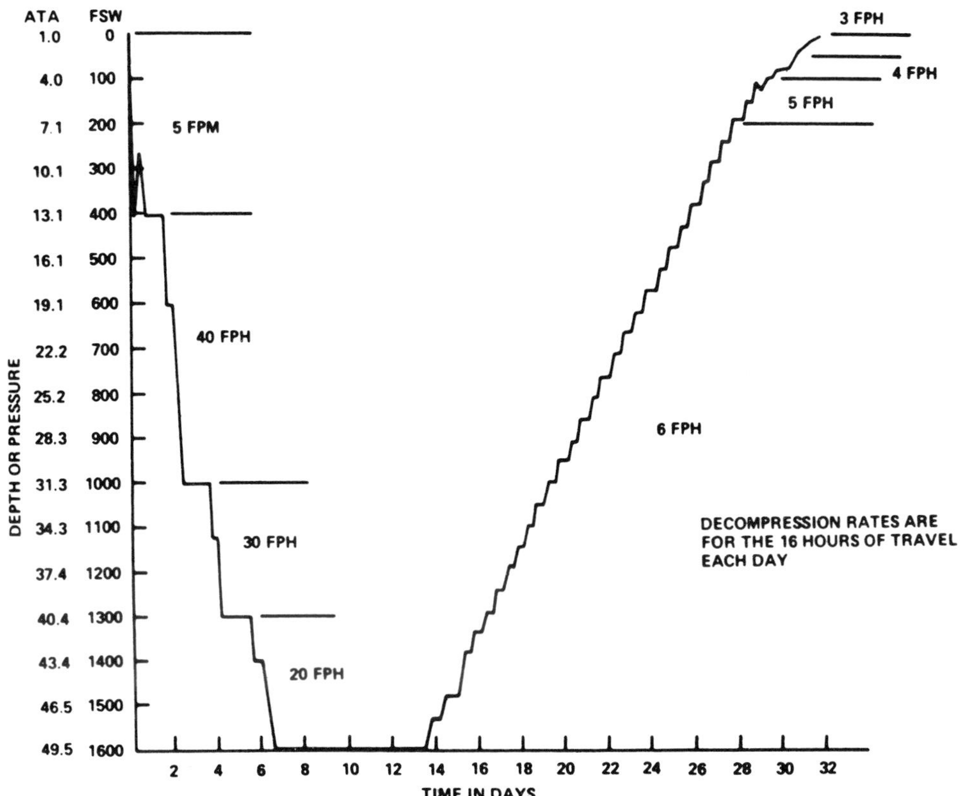

Fig. 1. Dive profile for U.S. Navy 1600 foot dive. Decompression rates are for the 16 h of travel each day

Saturation Exposure

During this discussion, attention will be focused primarily on long-term or saturation exposures to elevated ambient pressures, in which the organism reaches an equilibrium state from the standpoint of the amount of inert gas dissolved in body tissues. For practical purposes, a state of saturation exposure is achieved during exposure to a constant hyperbaric pressure for a period of approximately 12 h in a helium-oxygen environment, and approximately 24 h in a nitrogen-oxygen environment. After these lengths of time, further exposure at a constant pressure does not alter the requirements for decompression at the end of the exposure.

The last decade has brought a great increase in interest in saturation exposures. As the need arises to work at greater depths in the ocean, saturation exposures become increasingly important, since the time required for decompression remains a constant, independent of the duration of exposure. A team of men can remain at a constant pressure and work for weeks, without spending any time in decompression until the end of the task. Conventional diving techniques, in which a diver returns to a one-atmosphere environment at the end of each task, require enormous amounts of time for decompression compared to actual time spent working, especially when work is carried out at great depth.

In recent years, man has been able to work routinely at depths as great as 200 m in the open sea, and open sea dives to depths of almost 400 m have been made. Additionally, in the last 5 years, dry-chamber dives have been made to depths of 400 to 610 m in France, Great Britain, and the United States. The record depth for human exposure has been attained twice in France at a depth of 610 m or 61 ATA, without serious short- or long-term adverse effects (ROSTAIN et al., 1977).

Atmospheric Analysis

Thus, man is being exposed increasingly to hyperbaric environments for prolonged periods of time. These environments are almost without exception synthetic, meaning that the partial pressures of the constituent gases are set at levels different from atmospheric air. Even in the situation in which nitrogen-oxygen atmospheres are used, the fractional concentration of oxygen is below the normal of 0.21. If atmospheric air is used, at any pressure greater than 2 ATA or 10 m of sea-water, the partial pressure of oxygen exceeds 0.4 ATA and oxygen toxicity occurs.

However, the predominant atmosphere used in prolonged hyperbaric exposures is a helium-oxygen (heliox) mixture, with the percentage of oxygen varying according to depth. Nitrogen is avoided as the inert gas for two main reasons. First, at pressures greater than 6 to 8 ATA, nitrogen has a significant narcotic effect, progressing to anesthesia and eventual death at great depths. Second, nitrogen-oxygen mixtures impose high respiratory loads at depth due to increased density. Helium, in contrast, has no apparent narcotic effects, and is one-seventh as dense as nitrogen. Thus, helium at 7 ATA has the same density as air at one atmosphere, and helium at 60 ATA or 600 m possesses a density roughly equivalent to air at 9 ATA (Table 2).

Table 2. Molecular weight, density and thermal conductivity of helium, nitrogen and oxygen

	Helium	Nitrogen	Oxygen
Molecular weight	4	28	32
Density (g/l)	0.1784	1.251	1.429
Thermal conductivity × 10^5 (cal per $^{o}C\ cm^{-2}s^{-1}$)	34	5.66	5.83

An additional significant feature of a helium-oxygen atmosphere is the partial pressure of oxygen maintained. As mentioned previously, an upper limit on oxygen partial pressure, in the range of 0.4 to 0.5 ATA, must be maintained to avoid long-term oxygen toxicity that affects the lungs. However, studies have shown that maintainance of a so-called normal oxygen partial pressure of 0.21 ATA leads to physiologic abnormalities that are completely reversed when its partial pressure is raised to 0.3 to 0.4 ATA (CHOUTEAU, 1969). The precise explanation for this phenomenon is unclear, but an apparent hypoxia has been reproducibly observed in high-pressure exposures utilizing an oxygen partial pressure of 0.21 ATA, with dramatic improvement in the well-being of the experimental subjects brought about through increase in the oxygen partial pressure to 0.3 to 0.4 ATA.

No systematic study has been performed to investigate the endocrine and metabolic abnormalities produced by exposure to so-called "normal" oxygen partial pressures during prolonged high-pressure exposures. Nor have detailed studies fully examined the possible short- and long-term consequences of exposure to elevated oxygen partial pressures.

It is important to point out at this juncture that an oxygen partial pressure of 0.3 to 0.4 ATA often constitutes only 0.5 to 2% of the total hyperbaric atmosphere, with the vast bulk of the remainder made up by helium. Thus, in a 50 ATA exposure, the atmosphere will consist of 0.3 to 0.4 ATA of oxygen, approximately 0.5 to 1 ATA of nitrogen, and 48 to 49 ATA or 96% to 98% helium. From the standpoint of the physical properties of the hyperbaric atmosphere, virtually all the properties represent those of helium.

Thermal Properties

The markedly increased thermal conductivity of helium plays a major role in hyperbaric exposure (Table 2). It is significant that the comfort, or neutral, ambient temperature in a high-pressure helium environment approaches the neutral temperature for water immersion, approximately 33°C. Perturbations in ambient temperature in a helium environment which might seem to be insignificant may produce noticeable physiologic changes due to cold or heat stress. Human subjects at 50 ATA are able to sense changes in ambient temperature as small as 0.3°C (RAYMOND et al., 1975a). Many hyperbaric exposures have been plagued by inability to maintain an adequate ambient temperature for thermal comfort. Consequently, a number of reported endocrine and metabolic changes have been due at least in part to cold stress.

To summarize the significant environmental parameters of hyperbaric exposure, the following features must be kept in mind:

1. elevated absolute pressure
2. predominant use of helium as the inert gas
3. elevated partial pressure of oxygen
4. significantly increased thermal conductivity
5. elevation of absolute density.

Scope of Studies - Man

Endocrine and metabolic studies in hyperbaric environments have used man as the primary experimental subject. A variety of reasons account for this fact. First, it is difficult to maintain adequate, long-term life support for animals in hyperbaric chambers, and second, even where it is possible to maintain animals in hyperbaric chambers for prolonged periods of time, difficulties are encountered with sample collection. Human intervention is usually required for sample collection, and it is not feasible to expose an investigator to high pressure for a brief period due to the limitations previously discussed.

Further impetus for human hyperbaric experimentation has been produced by the need actually to utilize men in high-pressure environments to perform necessary tasks. This need has led naval and industrial sponsors to support human research with a readily identifiable goal of allowing men to work safely under high-pressure conditions.

Other factors to consider are the extreme expenses involved in hyperbaric operations, often reaching tens of thousands of dollars per day. This has limited the number of experiments performed. The total experience is small, with fewer than ten separate human research projects having been carried out at depths greater than 300 m. Consequently, many observations have not been repeated or confirmed, and conflicting data have been collected in other areas.

Endocrine Responses

Two areas of investigation have received the greatest attention in the past. Interest has focused on adrenal responses, both cortical and medullary, and on alterations in hormones involved in body fluid balance.

A variety of different hyperbaric exposures, both human and animal, have consistently revealed elevations in daily catechol excretion, measured as total catechols, or fractionated into epinephrine and norepinephrine components (RAYMOND et al., 1975b; LEACH et al., 1973; MATSUDA et al., 1975; WALDVOGEL and BUHLMAN, 1968; BUHLMAN et al., 1970). The causative factors for these elevations in catechol levels are multiple. The possibility of stress reaction or response to hypothermia must be considered, in addition to reaction to hyperbaric exposure.

Adrenal cortical responses to high-pressure helium environments have been consistently elevated (ROSTAIN et al., 1977; BENNETT and GRAY, 1971; HAMILTON et al., 1966). Additionally, reports have documented shifts in diurnal rhythms of cortisteroid excretion, with both shifts in timing of peak output and prolongation of the diurnal cycle being reported (ROSTAIN et al., 1977).

Some of the most significant observations made during hyperbaric exposure have related to body weight and body fluid balance. Multiple exposures under different conditions of pressure, time, and temperature have consistently resulted in decreases in body weight (RAYMOND et al., 1975b). Although some studies have detected a decrease in actual tissue weight, the majority have reported a diuresis accompanied by a decrease in total body fluid volume (MATSUDA et al., 1975; RAYMOND et al., 1975b).

Various mechanisms for this diuresis have been proposed, involving changes in ADH levels, or alterations in renal responsiveness to ADH. One principal theory involves increase in intra-thoracic blood volume as a result of cold stress and breathing of dense gas, leading to a reduction in ADH. Supporting this theory are the observations of MATSUDA et al. (1975) that diuresis under pressure varied inversely with ambient temperature.

Another report of hyperbaric diuresis describes an increase in urine flow in spite of an ambient temperature of 31°C in an 18.6 ATA exposure. ADH decreased significantly, and was accompanied by significant increases in plasma and urine aldosterone. The theory was proposed that increased urine output and ADH suppression were both due to marked reductions in insensible water loss.

In contrast, analysis of data collected during exposure to 50 ATA maximum pressure with ambient temperature maintained at 30° to 32°C revealed a 5% loss in initial body weight due to water loss. In this study, urinary ADH was found to increase, as did urinary aldosterone, accompanied by a reduction in urinary osmolality (RAYMOND et al., 1975b).

Clearly, detailed further studies are needed of the inter-relationships of body weight, fluid balance, urine osmolality, and ADH and aldosterone excretion. The effect of changes in fluid balance is significant, with a potential to alter performance under hyperbaric conditions, and perhaps to increase susceptibility to other problems, such as decompression sickness. Current data are conflicting, and further carefully controlled studies are most necessary.

Immersion

Another major environmental parameter to consider is that of immersion in water. Although hyperbaric exposures are performed in dry habitats for the majority of the time, it is important to recognize that the basic intent of these exposures is to permit man to work in an immersed state. Therefore, the interaction of immersion effects with those already discussed must be considered.

Immersion has been shown to increase urinary sodium and water excretion significantly. Immersion studies in man have revealed marked reduction in plasma renin, urinary and plasma aldosterone, and antidiuretic hormone (EPSTEIN et al., 1976). Return to the nonimmersed state leads to a gradual decline of natriuresis, suggesting the presence of a humoral natriuretic factor (EPSTEIN et al., 1976). Additional studies have shown that the suppression of aldosterone and plasma renin by immersion occurs without decreases in 17-hydroxy-corticosteroids.

The observed effects of immersion are most important when combined with the additional effect of hyperbaric exposure and cold, inducing diuresis. The immersed diver will be exposed to all three factors simultaneously, immersion, cold, and hyperbaria, leading to a potentially disabling diuresis.

Implications and Summary

Man's exposure to hyperbaric conditions represents exposure to alterations in virtually all environmental parameters. The hyperbaric environment presents many hazardous and potentially disabling conditions from which man cannot be isolated if he is to function underwater.

Human responses to the hyperbaric environment include responses to elevated pressure, altered inert gas and oxygen pressures, cold exposure and increased gas density. Some responses are primarily stress responses and may be considered adaptive. Other responses, such as those concerning body weight and fluid balance, may lead to hazardous long-term consequences. Such responses are indicative of a need for extensive further investigations as the need to extend the depth and duration of man's exposure to high-pressure environments becomes increasingly great.

References

BENNETT, P.B., GRAY, S.P.: Changes in human urine and blood chemistry during a simulated oxygen-helium dive to 1500 feet. Aerosp. Med. 42, 868-874 (1971)

BUHLMAN, A.A., MATTHYS, H., OVERRATH, G., BENNETT, P.B., ELLIOTT, D.H., GRAY, S.P.: Saturation exposures at 31 ATA in an oxygen-helium atmosphere with excursions to 36 ATA. Aerosp. Med. 41, 394-402 (1970)

CHOUTEAU, J.: Saturation diving: The Conshelf experiments. In: The Physiology and Medicine of Diving and Compressed Air Work. Bennett, P.B., Elliott, D.H. (eds.). London: Bailliere, Tindall and Cassell, 1969

EPSTEIN, M., LEVINSON, R., LOUTZENHISER, R.: Effects of water immersion on renal hemodynamics in normal man. J. Appl. Physiol. 41, 230-233 (1976)

HAMILTON, R.W., MACINNIS, J.B., NOBLE, A.D., SCHREINER, H.R.: Saturation diving to 650 feet. Oceans Systems, Inc., Technical Memorandum B-411, 116-123 (1966)

HONG, S.K.: Body fluid balance during saturation diving. In: Int. Symp. Man in the Sea. Hong, S.K. (ed.). Bethesda, Md.: Undersea Med. Soc. 1975, pp. IV-127 - IV-140

LEACH, C.S., ALEXANDER, W.C., FISHER, C.L., LAMBERTSEN, C.J., JOHNSON, P.C.: Endocrine studies during a 14-day continuous exposure to 5.2% O_2 in N_2 at pressure equivalent to 100 fsw (4 ATA). Aerosp. Med. 44, 855-859 (1973)

MACINNIS, J.B., BOND, G.F.: Saturation diving: man-in-sea and Sealab. In: The Physiology and Medicine of Diving and Compressed Air Work. Bennett, P.B., Elliott, D.H. (eds.). London: Bailliere, Tindal and Cassell, 1969, pp. 505-523

MATSUDA, M., NAKAYAMA, H., KURATA, F.K., CLAYBAUGH, J.R., HONG, S.K.: Physiology of man during a 10-day dry heliox saturation dive (SEATOPIA) at 7 ATA. II. Urinary water, electrolytes, ADH, and aldosterone. Undersea Biomed. Res. 2, 119-131 (1975)

PHILP, R.B.: A review of blood changes associated with compression-decompression: relationship to decompression sickness. Undersea Biomed. Res. 1, 117-150 (1974)

RAYMOND, L.W., SODE, J., LEACH, C.S.: Vasopressin, aldosterone and catecholamines during weight loss in diver breathing helium-oxygen at 1-50 atmospheres. Clin. Res. 23, 602A (1975b)

RAYMOND, L.W., THALMANN, E., LINDGREN, G., et al.: Thermal homeostasis of resting man in helium-oxygen at 1-50 atmospheres absolute. Undersea Biomed. Res. 2, 51-67 (1975a)

ROSTAIN, J.C., FRUCTUS, X., GHATA, J., et al.: Changes in physiological circadian rhythms during helium-oxygen saturation dives to 500 M and 610 M. Undersea Biomed. Res. 4, A46 (1977)

WALDVOGEL, W., BUHLMANN, A.A.: Man's reaction to long-lasting overpressure exposure. Examination of the saturated organism at a helium pressure of 21-22 ATA. Helv. Med. Acta 34, 130-150 (1968)

2. High Altitude Hypoxia and Adrenal Development in the Rat: Enzymes for Biogenic Amines

A. VACCARI, J. CIMINO, S. BROTMAN, and P. S. TIMIRAS

Exposure to a hypoxic environment may be regarded as a form of stress capable of stimulating the sympathoadrenal system; the type and magnitude of the response to hypoxia, however, appear to vary depending on the duration of the exposure and its severity.

Earlier reports (CUNNINGHAM et al., 1965; CANTU et al., 1966) were concerned primarily with the effects of short-term hypoxia on adrenal monoaminergic systems; yet little is known of the effects of more prolonged exposure. More current research shows that an initial decrease in adrenal epinephrine levels occurs after a few hours of exposure, but when exposure is prolonged up to 60 h, it is followed by normalization (STEINSLAND et al., 1970; RAAB, 1973; KOOB and ANNAU, 1974). Additionally, an example of the differential response of the adrenal medulla to the degree of hypoxia is represented by dopamine levels that increase with severe, but decrease with moderate hypoxia (SNIDER et al., 1974).

It is quite possible that the synthesizing and catabolizing pathways of monoamines are more directly affected by oxygen deficiency than the monoamine levels by themselves, in view of the oxygen dependency of some of the enzymes involved in monoamine metabolism. However, no data are yet available on the effects of hypoxia on the monoamine enzymes in the adrenals - a lack of information that is quite surprising in view of the importance of the adrenocortical and adrenomedullary interrelationships in maintaining homeostasis in response to various stressors (WURTMAN et al., 1972). We may take as indirect evidence of a hypoxia-induced activation of tyrosine hydroxylase the work of SNIDER et al. (1974).

The purpose of the investigation described here was to study the development of the enzymes for biogenic amines in the adrenals of rats chronically exposed to moderate hypoxia (natural high altitude) from conception until adulthood, and to correlate changes in enzymes activity with adrenocortical function.

Adult Long-Evans rats were acclimatized for one month before breeding at the Barcroft Laboratory of the White Mountain Research Station (3.800 m; 480 mm Hg; 12.8% O_2 in inspired air). The animals of the first generation (F_1) born at high altitude (HA) and the sea level (SL) controls of the same age were divided by sex and killed at 1, 7, 12, 20, and 60 days of age. SL controls were maintained on the Berkeley campus (76 m; 766 mm Hg; 20% O_2 in inspired air) under housing conditions (temperature, humidity) similar to those at HA. Glands from one or more litters grouped by age, sex and environmental conditions were pooled; 6-12 assays (3-6 males + 3-6 females) were conducted per age.

Enzyme Assays. The procedures for the enzyme assays (tyrosine-hydroxylase, TH; tryptophan-hydroxylase, TPH; DOPA- and 5-HTP-decarboxylase, DOPAdC, 5-HTPdC; catechol-O-methyl transferase, COMT; monoamine oxidase, MAO) have been described elsewhere (VACCARI et al., 1977).

Other Measurements

Corticosterone. Plasma and adrenal corticosterone levels were assayed by the fluorimetric method of JAMES et al. (1971).

Tyrosine and Tryptophan. The levels of adrenal tyrosine (WAALKES and UDENFRIEND, 1957), and tryptophan (DENCKLA and DEWEY, 1967) were measured by fluorimetric methods.

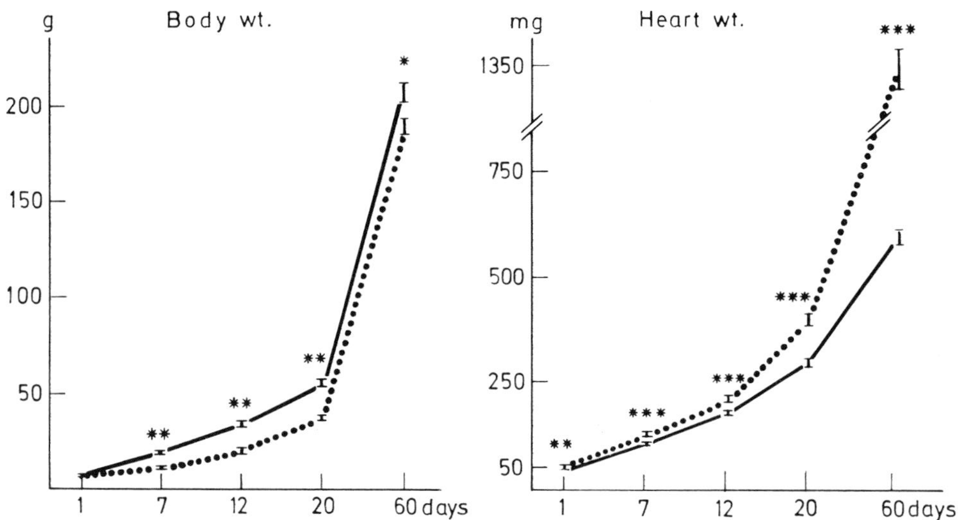

Fig. 1. High-altitude induced impairment of body weight (left figure), and cardiac hypertrophy (right figure) during development of F_1 rats. (·——·) Sea level, SL; (····) high altitude, HA. Number of rats ranged from 50 to 85. * $p < 0.05$; ** $p < 0.02$; *** $p < 0.001$

All HA animals were restless, aggressive toward the handler, and displayed frequent tremors, clearly observable from the 12th postnatal day. A mortality of 45% occurred in the HA rats, during the preweaning period, as compared to 2% at SL. Whole-body growth was markedly impaired throughout the experimental period, and a marked, persistent cardiac hypertrophy was present as early as at 1 day of age (Fig. 1). The adrenals were moderately enlarged in HA rats only at 7 days after birth, 4.0 ± 0.1 mg/pair glands (n = 80) as compared with 2.7 ± 0.1, in SL rats (n = 70).

Effects of High Altitude Hypoxia on Enzyme Activities

Enzyme activity was expressed as units per g wet wt, rather than as units per pair adrenals inasmuch as, at the early ages, pooled tissue samples had to be used. The total activity essentially resembled the specific activity (units g protein^{-1}); the only exceptions were MAO (6.8 ± 0.3 SL; 8.4 ± 0.2 HA, μmol h^{-1} g protein^{-1}) and COMT (1.31 ± 0.05 SL; 1.67 ± 0.04 HA μmol h^{-1} g protein^{-1}), which were significantly

(p < 0.001) more active at HA at one day only. The specific activity, however, did follow the same trend as total activity at later ages.

The effects of HA on the development of the two catecholamine-synthesizing enzymes TH and DOPAdC are shown in Figure 2. TH activity was

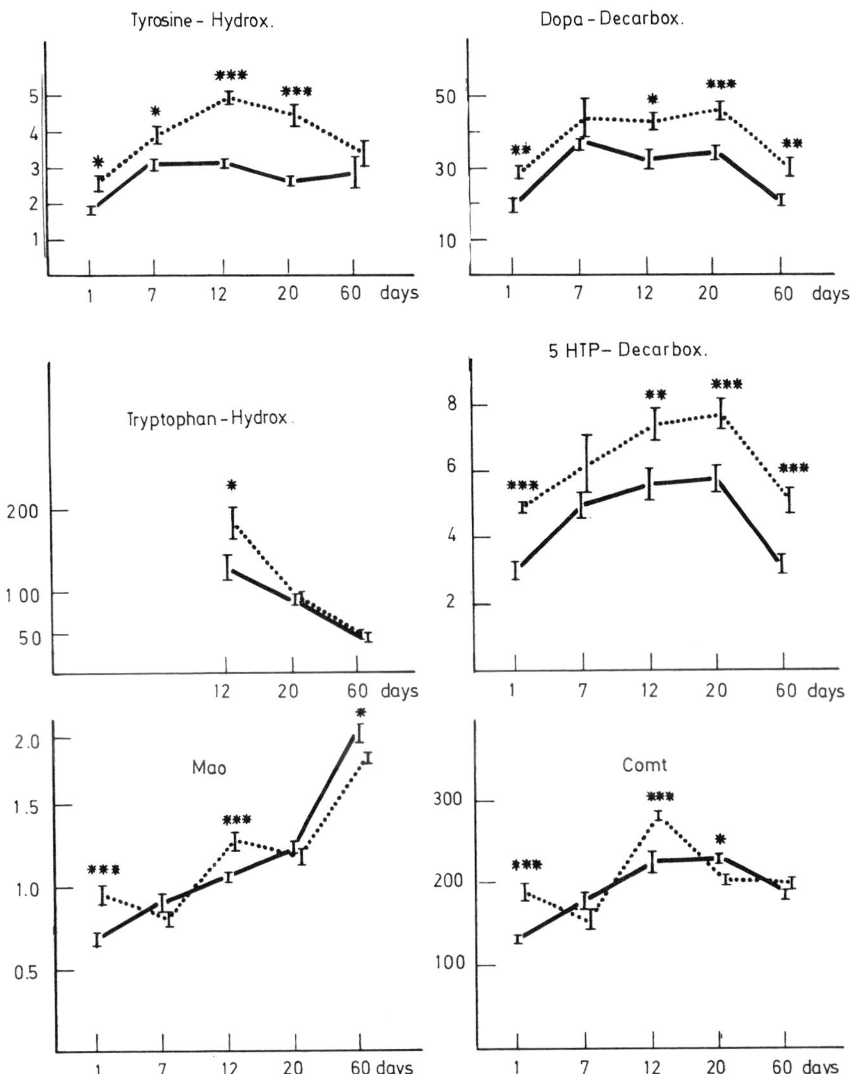

Fig. 2. Effects of high altitude (·····; 3.800 m; 466 mm Hg; 12.8% P_{O_2}) on the development of the activity of Tyrosine-hydroxylase and DOPA-decarboxylase (μmol h^{-1} g wet wt^{-1} ± SEM; top figures), Tryptophan-hydroxylase (pmol h^{-1} g wet wt^{-1} ± SEM) and 5-HTP-decarboxylase (μmol h^{-1} g wet wt^{-1} ± SEM) (middle figures), Catechol-O-methyltransferase (nmol h^{-1} g wet wt^{-1} ± SEM) and monoamine oxidase (μmol h^{-1} g wet wt^{-1} ± SEM) (lower figures), as compared to the sea level, F_1 rats (·——·). Number of experiments was 6-12; * p < 0.05; ** p < 0.02 or < 0.01; *** p < 0.001

markedly and persistently stimulated throughout the two months of exposure to HA. The mean increase from 1 to 20 days was 53%; at 60 days, although the difference was not statistically significant, the activity remained 20% higher in HA than in SL rats. DOPAdC activity followed the same trend as TH and was dramatically higher at HA at all ages considered, 36% higher on the average from day 1 to 20, and 42% higher on day 60. TPH activity was 41% higher in the adrenals of HA animals at 12 days, but was unchanged at the other two ages (Fig. 2); 5-HTPdC at HA showed an average increase of 38% from 1 to 20 days, and of 62% at 60 days (Fig. 2). COMT activity was stimulated by HA at 1 and 12 days of age with an average increase of 28%; however, at day 20, the HA effects were reversed and COMT activity was decreased significantly by 11%. At 60 days the activity was similar in HA and SL rats (Fig. 2). MAO activity showed essentially the same pattern as COMT; it was markedly increased after HA exposure at days 1 and 12 (23% average increase); at 20 days it had decreased, and activity was still depressed at 60 days (Fig. 2).

<u>Corticosterone Levels.</u> Plasma levels of corticosterone in HA rats were dramatically increased as early as 1 day of age and remained elevated until 60 days of age. The average increase during the 2 months of the experiment was of 141%, the maximum (449%) was reached at 7 days, and the minimum (24% at 60 days (Fig. 3). Adrenal corticosterone concen-

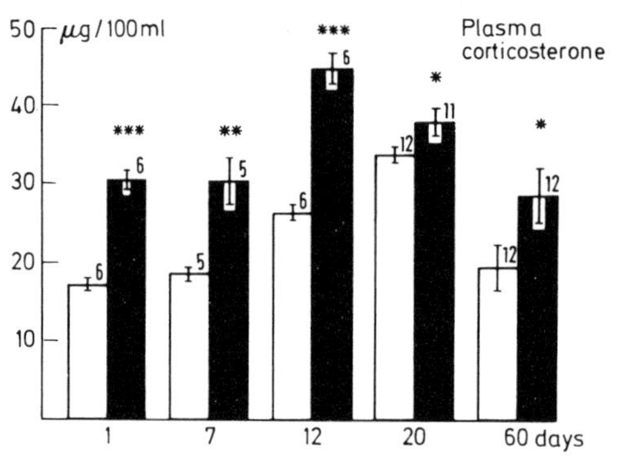

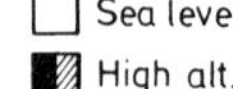

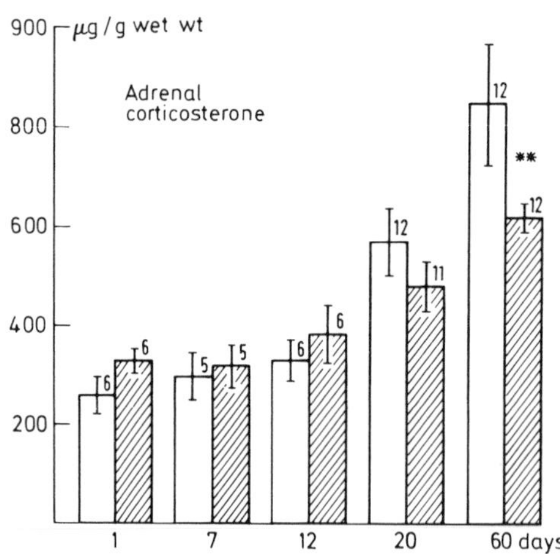

Fig. 3. Effects of high altitude on the levels of plasma (μg/100 ml) (top figure), and of adrenal (μg g wet wt^{-1} ± SEM) corticosterone (lower figure). Number of experiments is indicated at top of barograms. * $p < 0.05$; ** $p < 0.01$; *** $p < 0.001$

trations were not significantly altered by exposure to HA except on day 60 when a 37% decrease was observed in the HA rats (Fig. 3).

Tyrosine and Tryptophan Concentrations. The concentrations of tyrosine and tryptophan, the respective amino acid precursors for the synthesis of catecholamines and 5-HT were measured in the adrenals at 60 days only. Tyrosine levels were unaffected, but tryptophan levels were slightly (13%) but significantly ($p < 0.02$) increased by HA.

Tissue Proteins. Development at HA affected significantly the adrenal concentration of proteins during the first 20 days of life, when an average increase of 15% was observed; differences were no longer evident at 60 days.

Discussion

The relatively high activity of most enzymes in the adrenals on the first postnatal day was comparable to adult levels. Exposure to HA markedly and continuously altered all activities. These long-term effects of HA are distinct from the transitory enzymatic changes occurring in adult animals after acute or sub-acute exposure to hypoxia, in which altered catecholamine levels rapidly return to normal, suggesting also a transient effect on the relative enzymes (STEINSLAND et al., 1970; KOOB and ANNAU, 1974; SNIDER et al., 1974). The activity of the synthesizing enzymes at HA appears to be stimulated continuously, while that of the catabolizing enzymes undergoes a diphasic change (an increase followed by a decrease). The observation as early as the first postnatal day that both synthesizing and catabolizing enzymes are induced by HA may be interpreted as an exceptionally rapid induction of these enzymes in the neonatal period or as a prenatal phenomenon involving a deficiency in the placental protection of the fetus from environmental hypoxia (PETROPOULOS and TIMIRAS, 1974).

The assumption that hypoxia represents the primary stimulus at HA is supported by several studies from our and other laboratories in which the effects of natural HA on endocrine development and maturation of the central nervous system was duplicated in decompression chambers (TIMIRAS and WOOLLEY, 1966). Malnutrition prior to weaning cannot, however, be completely excluded. In our experiments, blood-oxygen saturation was not measured. However, evidence shows that there is a direct relation between ambient oxygen concentration and organ and blood O_2 (SAWIN, 1970). The increased activity of oxygen-dependent enzymes, such as TH and TPH, resulting from relatively moderate hypoxia is surprising, since inhibition of their activity would be expected. Possibly other factors, such as stress-induced hyperfunction of the adrenal cortex during early development, cause a nonspecific induction of enzyme activity which overcomes the direct influence of oxygen deficiency on enzyme molecules. Indeed, we know that the release of adrenocortical hormones is stimulated by exposure to hypoxia, but the consequent hypersecretion of glucocorticoids in humans (HORBEIN, 1962) and in adult rats (LAU and TIMIRAS, 1972) is usually temporary and ceases as soon as adaptation has been achieved. On the other hand, when rats are exposed to HA during their early development, adaptation does not occur or, if it does, it is incomplete as evidenced by impaired growth (e.g., reduced body weight), and delayed development (e.g., retarded brain maturation) (TIMIRAS and WOOLLEY, 1966), as well as continuing high levels of circulating adrenocortical hormones. In addition, the finding that plasma levels of corticosterone are high at birth suggests that the hypothalamo-hypophysio-adrenocortical axis is already competent and capable of responding to stress at a very early age, contrary to the belief that the first postnatal days represent a "stress nonresponsive" period (BUTTE et al., 1973). It is possible that exposure to HA has a chronic effect on those inhibitory circuits in the brain that regulate hypothalamo-hypophysial negative feedbacks and thereby continuously stimulates adrenocortical function as long as the hypoxic stress persists (MAROTTA and GARCY, 1975).

The increase in adrenocortical seçretion at HA also correlates with the stimulating influence of glucocorticoids on enzymes of neurotransmitters such as TH (see PLETSCHER, 1972) and TPH (SZE et al., 1976) by induction of new enzyme proteins (WURTMAN et al., 1972) and/or increased uptake of tryptophan (NECKERS and ŞZE, 1975). Conversely, COMT activity is depressed by stress (KVETŇANSKÝ et al., 1975) and both COMT and MAO activity are decreased by hypophysectomy and returned to normal by ACTH administration (WURTMAN et al., 1972). On the other hand, according to PARVEZ and PARVEZ (1973), high levels of plasma glucocorticoids inhibit, and low levels stimulate MAO and COMT activity. Thus, enhanced enzymatic activity may be related to increased protein content of the adrenals in HA animals.

The diphasic effects of HA and MAO and COMT are difficult to interpret. Other factors than the secretion of ACTH or glucocorticoids may be involved in the regulation of these enzymes. With respect to the possible implication of the precursor amino acids in enzymatic activity, our results show unchanged tyrosine levels, but significantly increased tryptophan levels at 60 days of age. Not having measured tryptophan levels prior to 60 days, at ages when TPH was stimulated by HA, we cannot conclude that hypoxia induces TPH activity through an increase of tryptophan levels in the adrenals. However, this possibility cannot be excluded.

In conclusion, continuous exposure to moderate hypoxia induces long-lasting changes in the development of adrenal neurotransmitter systems, as suggested by permanent changes in the activity of monoaminergic metabolic enzymes. These changes are represented by an increase in the activity of the synthesizing enzymes from birth to adulthood and a biphasic pattern in the catabolizing enzymes which are increased during early development and then decreased. Inasmuch as the increase in synthetic activity predominates, it is proposed that these enzymatic changes are responsible for an increased availability of catecholamines and perhaps 5-HT in the adrenal glands. Such an increase could be interpreted as a compensatory response to prenatal alterations or as an adaptive response to postnatal hypoxia and may contribute to the maintenance of homeostasis.

Acknowledgments. This investigation was supported by NIH grant NS-08989, training grant 5-T01-GM01021 to S.B., and a University of California Regents Fellowship to J.C.

References

BUTTE, J.D., KAKIHANA, R., FARNHAM, M.L., NOBLE, E.P.: The relationship between brain and plasma corticosterone stress response in developing rats. Endocrinology 92, 1775-1779 (1973)

CANTU, R.C., NAHAS, G.G., MANGER, W.M.: Effects of hypercapnic acidosis and of hypoxia on adrenal catecholamine output of the spinal dog. Proc. Soc. Exp. Biol. Med. 122, 424-427 (1966)

CUNNINGHAM, W.L., BECKER, E.J., KREUZER, F.: Catecholamines in plasma and urine at high altitude. J. Appl. Physiol. 20, 607-610 (1965)
DENCKLA, W.D., DEWEY, H.K.: The determination of tryptophan in plasma, liver and urine. J. Lab. Clin. Med. 69, 160-169 (1967)
HORBEIN, T.F.: Adrenal cortical response to chronic hypoxia. J. Appl. Physiol. 17, 246-248 (1962)
JAMES, V.H.T., MATTINGLY, D., DALY, J.R.: Recommended method for the determination of plasma corticosteroids. Brit. Med. J. 2, 310-313 (1971)
KOOB, G.F., ANNAU, Z.: Behavioral and neurochemical alterations induced by hypoxia in rats. Am. J. Physiol. 227, 73-78 (1974)
KVETŇANSKÝ, R., TORDA, T., JAHNOVA, E., SALEH, N.: Activity of catecholamine degrading enzymes in rat adrenal medulla and cortex after acute and repeated stress. Endocrinol. Exp. 9, 79-86 (1975)
LAU, C., TIMIRAS, P.S.: Adrenocortical function in hypothalamic deafferent rats maintained at high altitude. Am. J. Physiol. 222, 1040-1042 (1972)
MAROTTA, S.F., GARCY, A.M.: Effects of altering monoamine metabolism on the adrenocortical response to hypoxia. Aviat. Space. Env. Med. 46, 1368-1372 (1975)
NECKERS, S.L., SZE, P.Y.: Regulation of 5-hydroxytryptamine metabolism in mouse brain by adrenal glucocorticoids. Brain Res. 93, 123-132 (1975)
PARVEZ, H., PARVEZ, S.: The effects of metopirone and adrenalectomy on the regulation of enzymes monoamine oxydase and catechol-O-methyltransferase in different brain regions. J. Neurochem. 20, 1011-1020 (1973)
PETROPOULOS, E.A., TIMIRAS, P.S.: Effects of hypoxic environment on prenatal brain development: recent evidence versus earlier dogma. In: Drugs and the Developing Brain. Vernadakis, A., Weiner, N. (eds.). New York: Plenum Press, 1974, pp. 429-449
PLETSCHER, A.: Regulation of catecholamine turnover by variations of enzyme levels. Pharmacol. Rev. 24, 225-232 (1972)
RAAB, W.Z.: Medullary hormone content of the adrenals of white rats subjected to low atmospheric pressure. J. Aviat. Med. 14, 284-288 (1973)
SAWIN, C.F.: Hemathology of sea level and high altitude native Sonoran deer mice. Am. J. Physiol. 218, 701-703 (1970)
SNIDER, S.R., BROWN, R.M., CARLSSON, A.: Changes in biogenic amine synthesis and turnover induced by hypoxia and/or foot shock stress. I. The adrenal medulla. J. Neural Transm. 35, 283-291 (1974)
STEINSLAND, O.S., PASSO, S.S., NAHAS, G.G.: Biphasic effect of hypoxia on adrenal catecholamine content. Am. J. Physiol. 218, 995-998 (1970)
SZE, P.Y., NECKERS, L., TOWLE, A.C.: Glucocorticoids as a regulatory factor for brain tryptophan hydroxylase. J. Neurochem. 26, 169-173 (1976)
TIMIRAS, P.S., WOOLLEY, D.E.: Functional and morphologic development of brain and other organs of rats at high altitude. Federation Proc. 25, 1312-1320 (1966)
VACCARI, A., BROTMAN, S., CIMINO, J., TIMIRAS, P.S.: Sex differentiation of neurotransmitter enzymes in central and peripheral nervous systems. Brain Res. 132, 176-185 (1977)
WAALKES, T.P., UDENFRIEND, S.: A fluorometric method for the estimation of tyrosine in plasma and tissues. J. Lab. Clin. Med. 50, 733-736 (1957)
WURTMAN, R.J., POHORECKY, L.A., BALIGA, B.S.: Adrenocortical control of the biosynthesis of epinephrine and proteins in the adrenal medulla. Pharmacol. Rev. 24, 411-426 (1972)

3. Endocrine Responses to Chronic High Altitude Exposure

M. L. Nelson

Exposure of animals to hypobaric hypoxia throughout development is a stress that results in a variety of endocrine-related changes. In the rat, neonatal mortality is common at high altitude (HA) with losses as high as 80% by weaning age (CHIODI, 1964; KELLEY and PACE, 1968; NELSON and CONS, 1975). Altered activity of several endocrine organs has been reported in those rats which survive.

Rats born and raised either at an altitude of 3800 m, or at equivalent simulated altitude conditions, are stunted in their growth when compared with sea-level controls (MOORE and PRICE, 1948; TIMIRAS and WOOLLEY, 1966; NELSON and CONS, 1975). This has partially been attributed to an impairment of the growth-promoting activities of the adenohypophysis, since female HA rats at 40 days of age have a reduced pituitary content of growth hormone compared with controls at sea level (NELSON and CONS, 1975).

Thyroid activity of adult rats exposed to natural or simulated HA for short periods (GORDON et al., 1943; VAN MIDDLESWORTH and BERRY, 1951; SURKS, 1966), and of immature rats born and raised at HA (NELSON, 1971), is also impaired. A reduction in the thyroidal uptake of iodine and plasma PBI, as well as decreased follicular cell heights, have been reported. No differences from sea level controls were found in either pituitary or plasma TSH levels in young female rats raised at simulated HA (NELSON and CONS, 1975), but similar rats at natural HA had decreased pituitary content of TSH compared to controls (NELSON et al., 1968). An increased percentage of basophils and a degranulation of acidophils has also been observed in the adenohypophyses of HA rats (NELSON, 1973).

Reproductive function in the female rat is significantly impaired by exposure to hypobaric hypoxia throughout development. Elevated pituitary content of gonadotropins, reduced ovarian and uterine weights, and delayed vaginal opening were found in HA female rats at 40 days of age as compared with sea-level controls (NELSON and CONS, 1975). Consequently, the onset of puberty appears to be somewhat delayed in female rats at high altitude. In addition, adult first-generation HA rats have irregular estrous cycles with long periods of diestrus, a high incidence of infertile matings and a reduction in litter size (NELSON and SREBNIK, 1970). Fertility is rare in second-generation HA rats. Delayed onset of puberty and infertility have also been reported in human populations native to high altitudes (DONAYRE, 1966; ABELSON, 1976; PAWSON, 1976) although socio-economic conditions must be considered in these studies and the degree of endocrine involvement is not known. Clearly, much more data are needed on the effects of high altitude on the developing organism particularly with reference to the endocrine system and its target organs.

References

ABELSON, A.E.: Altitude and fertility. Human Biol. 48, 83-91 (1976)

CHIODI, H.: Action of high altitude chronic hypoxia on newborn animals. In: The Physiological Effects of High Altitude. Weihe, W.H. (ed.). New York: Macmillan, 1964, pp. 97-112

DONAYRE, J.: Population growth and fertility at high altitude. In: Life at High Altitudes. Hurtado, A. (ed.). Washington, D.C.: Pan Am. Health Org., 1966, pp. 74-79

GORDON, A.S., TORNETTA, F.J., D'ANGELO, S.A., CHARIPPER, H.A.: Effects of low atmospheric pressures on the activity of the thyroid, reproductive system and anterior lobe of the pituitary in the rat. Endocrinology 33, 366-383 (1943)

KELLEY, F.C., PACE, N.: Etiological considerations in neonatal mortality among rats at moderate high altitude (3,800 m). Am. J. Physiol. 214, 1168-1175 (1968)

MIDDLESWORTH, L. VAN, BERRY, M.M.: Iodide metabolism during anoxia, nephrectomy, trauma, avitaminoses and starvation in the rat. Am. J. Physiol. 167, 576-580 (1951)

MOORE, C.R., PRICE, D.: A study at high altitude of reproduction, growth, sexual maturity, and organ weights. J. Exp. Zool. 108, 171-216 (1948)

NELSON, M.L.: Thyroid function in immature rats developing at high altitude. Environ. Physiol. Biochem. 1, 96-103 (1971)

NELSON, M.L.: Microscopic appearance of the anterior pituitary gland in rats born and raised at high altitude (3800 m). Pacific Regional Conf. Gen. Comp. Endocrinol. Abstracts 39 (1973)

NELSON, M.L., CONS, J.M.: Pituitary hormones and growth retardation in rats raised at simulated high altitude (3800 m). Environ. Physiol. Biochem. 5, 273-282 (1975)

NELSON, M.L., SREBNIK, H.H.: Comparison of the reproductive performance of rats at high altitude (3800 m) and at sea level. Int. J. Biometeorol. 14, 187-193 (1970)

NELSON, M.L., SREBNIK, H.H., TIMIRAS, P.S.: Reduction in pituitary growth hormone and thyroid-stimulating hormone at high altitude. Excerpta Med. Int. Cong. Ser. 157, 196 (1968)

PAWSON, I.G.: Growth and development in high altitude populations: a review of Ethiopian, Peruvian and Nepalese studies. Proc. R. Soc. Lond. (Biol.) 194, 83-98 (1976)

SURKS, M.I.: Effect of hypoxia and high altitude on thyroidal iodine metabolism. Endocrinology 78, 307-315 (1966)

TIMIRAS, P.S., WOOLLEY, D.E.: Functional and morphologic development of brain and other organs of rats at high altitude. Federation Proc. 25, 1312-1320 (1966)

Chapter VI. Endocrine Responses to Ambient Temperature

1. The Endocrine Component of Human Adaptation to Cold and Heat

K. J. COLLINS

Introduction

Climatic physiologists recognize different levels of adaptation to environmental temperature. In the acute stage of exposure to heat or cold, neural and neuro-endocrine processes act synergistically to maintain homeostasis. Through its sensory input from the environment and control of physical, chemical, and behavioral thermoregulation, the nervous system plays the primary role in integrating these adjustments. Not surprisingly, the immediate response has come to be regarded as a stress reaction, and in some respects the initial endocrine involvement closely resembles that induced by nonspecific stress stimuli. In common with other stressors, it is usually difficult to eliminate or control the psychologic influences on the endocrine response to temperature.

Adaptation following repeated exposure to thermal stress develops over weeks or months, and leads to reversible acquired functional modifications. The change in function produced by environmental temperature alone, as in most laboratory studies, is described as temperature acclimation, and when a complex of environmental factors is present, e.g., with seasonal climatic changes, the adaptive response is described as acclimatization. Eventually, in the long term, adaptation to the environment becomes a more permanent feature with the acquisition of characteristics which favor survival in a particular climate. The study of human ecosystems requires the multidisciplinary approach pioneered by the International Biological Programme (COLLINS and WEINER, 1977) but at present there is scant information on a population basis of the effects of climatic temperature alone. Such evidence is difficult to obtain, for in tropical and polar indigenes one not infrequently finds that the temperature stimulation is inadequate to produce full acclimatization. The reason for this is that man, in adapting to climatic extremes, successfully avoids temperature stress by behavioral and insulative adjustments to his surroundings.

The endocrine responses clearly become more difficult to assess in proceeding from short-term to long-term adaptation, and there is often a tendency to try to predict the acquired pattern from the immediate responses to temperature change. This may not, however, be justified, for when adaptation has occurred, exposure to the given temperature is no longer stressful, unless there is reversion to the unadapted condition again. HAMMEL (1964) reasons that an adaptive response produced by a cause not directly related to the actual stress is probably more readily sustained, and yields a more lasting advantage than one produced as a direct result of the stress.

Endocrine Responses to Temperature Change in Man

In thermoregulation two main components of the neuro-endocrine system are involved. First the hypothalamo-hypophysial axes that control thyroid, growth, and adrenocortical hormones, act together with the sympathico-adrenomedullary system by a dual response (a) to the stress of a change in environmental temperature and (b) to the increased metabolic requirements in cold, and reduced metabolism in hot conditions. As body temperature rises outside the thermal neutral zone in extreme heat, metabolism becomes subject to the Arrhenius Van't Hoff effect, thereby increasing rather than decreasing calorigenesis. A second principal component assumes importance when sweating becomes a predominant mechanism of heat loss, and major cardiovascular and body fluid adjustments take place. In this the hypophysio-adrenal, the renin-angiotensin-aldosterone system and posterior pituitary hormones all play a part in re-establishing salt and water balance. An analysis of the participation of these components in different stages of climatic adaptation in man has been made through studies of hormone excretory patterns and the levels and turn-over rates in blood (COLLINS and WEINER, 1968; CHAFFEE and ROBERTS, 1971; GALE, 1973). Recent work has indicated that physiologic changes induced by heat and cold, particularly in the nonsteady state, can lead to misleading conceptions of the endocrine involvement, unless careful interpretation is made of the in vivo hormone dynamics. Intrinsically, investigations in man have experimental limitations that may sometimes be overcome by studies in other mammalian homeotherms. There are, however, important species differences in the comparative biochemistry and endocrinology of temperature acclimation.

Endocrine Control of Energy Metabolism in the Cold

Exposure to cold induces a decrease in skin temperature, the onset of shivering, and an increase in metabolic heat production. In many animals acclimated by repeated exposure to cold, shivering and peripheral vasoconstriction decline, while heat production remains high. In cold-acclimation the development of nonshivering thermogenesis involves the "metabolic" hormones of the thyroid, adrenal cortex and medulla (SMITH and HOIJER, 1962). The conversion from shivering to nonshivering thermogenesis with adaptation to cold stems mainly from an increased sensitivity of brown adipose and other tissues to the effects of noradrenaline.

Primarily, both shivering and nonshivering aspects of cold-acclimation depend on an increased secretion of noradrenaline and adrenaline from adrenergic terminals and from the adrenal medulla, but the contribution of nonshivering thermogenesis differs from species to species. Whereas in the laboratory rat the increased secretion rate of noradrenaline declines after 4 weeks in the cold, and reaches a baseline again at 8 weeks, a different pattern occurs in the baboon. The baboon shivers very little at 6°C air temperature, and there is a prompt increase in nonshivering thermogenesis without hypertrophy of brown adipose tissue. In this species, maintenance of nonshivering thermogenesis is presumed to require continued secretion of noradrenaline. The miniature pig lacks brown adipose tissue and nonshivering thermogenesis, but develops its capacity for shivering thermogenesis (BRÜCK et al., 1969). In man the metabolic contribution of brown adipose tissue likewise appears to be small (CHAFFEE and ROBERTS, 1971). Many of these species differences in the development of cold adaptation might be explained by the ability of different animals to replace costly mechanisms of energy utilization by more stable long-term changes, such as an increase in insulation by growth of pelage.

In the short term, cold stimulates the release of TRF, TSH, and thyroid hormones, and it was formerly believed that in both acute and chronic exposure to cold the increase in metabolic rate is a function of an increased rate of secretion and utilization of thyroid hormones. Recently, more emphasis has been placed on the diet-dependency of thyroid-hormone turnover in cold conditions. HÉROUX and BRAUER (1965) critically examined thyroid secretion rates in cold-adapted rats (see Fig. 1)

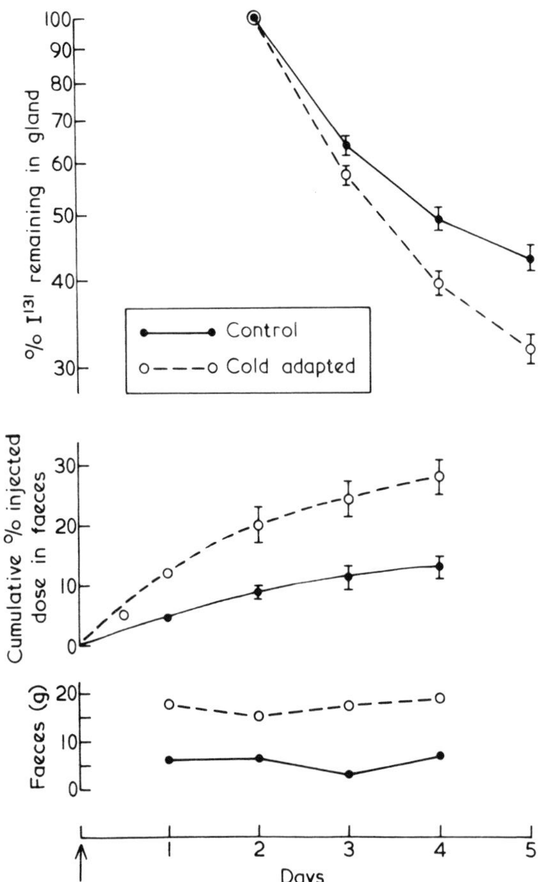

Fig. 1. Release of thyroid hormone and fecal excretion of I^{131} (injected at day 0) in cold-acclimated (6°C) and control (23°C) rats (data from HÉROUX and BRAUER, 1965)

and suggested that the greater requirement for thyroxine in cold-adapted animals was at least partly due to greater fecal loss of the hormone. Increased fecal bulk resulting from a significantly greater food intake in the cold thus enhances the enterohepatic clearance of thyroxine. The augmented turnover of T4 may therefore lead to an increased release of TRH and TSH, and a rise in T4 secretion. In fact, when the intake of non-nutritive bulk is adjusted so that both cold-acclimated and control animals excrete the same amount of feces, the difference between the fecal excretion of T4 is largely reduced (HILLIER, 1968). The whole question of the influence of ambient temperature and food intake on thyroxine utilization is, however, not a simple one. It has recently been suggested that the energy content of the diet is the dominant factor, rather than dietary bulk (INGRAM and KACIUBA-USCILKO, 1977). Whether increased entero-hepatic clearance of T4 may be balanced by preferential secretion of the more calorigenically potent T3, and thus still lead to a net increase in metabolic stimulation, is a question yet to be resolved. GALE (1973) suggests that the evidence points to a synergistic and permissive role of thyroid and glucocorticoids in the calorigenic action of catecholamines during cold exposure.

Cold Adaptation in Man

In the Ama divers of Japan, who become cold-adapted by repeated water immersion, BMR is generally higher in winter than in summer (ITOH, 1974). It is recognized, however, that this annual periodicity can be largely accounted for by the increased energy content of the diet in winter. Elevation of metabolic rate in man during continuous exposure has also been shown to depend on physical conditioning rather than cold exposure per se. Different patterns of natural acclimatization to cold have been described in various primitive populations (HAMMEL, 1964), involving increased resting metabolism (in the Alacaluf Indian of Tierra del Fuego), predominantly increased surface insulation by vasoconstriction (in the Australian Aborigine) or a combination of these mechanisms (in the Alaskan Eskimo and Andean Indian), but again these differences could be largely accounted for by differences in natural diet, physical training, and behavior.

As in animals, acute exposure to cold results in increased urinary excretion of noradrenaline, and an increased oxygen uptake. After 29 weeks' residence in Antarctica, BUDD and WARHAFT (1970) found that human excretion rates of catecholamines did not differ from the pre-exposure condition, though there was evidence of cold acclimatization from the changes in cardiovascular responses, and an increased calorigenic response to noradrenaline. It has also been claimed that the well-adapted Japanese Ainu, whose metabolic response is particularly sensitive to exogenous noradrenaline (ITOH, 1974), provide further evidence of nonshivering thermogenesis in man. However, as noted by BRÜCK (1976), exogenous noradrenaline increases oxygen uptake in some species by a reaction which is not elicited by cold exposure, and thus the noradrenaline test alone does not convincingly demonstrate cold-induced nonshivering thermogenesis. Tissue sensitization to catecholamines is a cold-adaptive mechanism, that in the long term may result in an irreversible change in target organ response. Another example of a change in sensitivity of effector organs has been described in the African Pygmy in which peripheral sensitivity to growth hormone is low although the hormone is present in normal amount in plasma (RIMOIN et al., 1969).

In other investigations of men during prolonged exposure to cold in Antarctica, significant increases in circulating T4 and T3 have been reported (EASTMAN et al., 1974). There were also individual variations in serum cortisol concentration that were thought to reflect the degree of general stress rather than cold stress per se. The secretion rate, metabolic clearance rate, dietary intake, the level of hormone-binding protein and hemoconcentration in the cold are all important parameters that need to be measured in order to make a meaningful assessment of the serum hormone changes. Evidence is not available to show that increased amounts of thyroid or glucocorticoid hormones are secreted and utilized to maintain thermal homeostasis in cold-adapted man. From comparative studies there does not appear to be a relationship between thyroxine turnover and metabolic rate in different animals; thyroxine secretion rate is shown to be a direct function of food intake and inversely related to body mass in any species (MACFARLANE, 1976). By analogy with animal studies, and assuming that nonshivering thermogenesis develops in cold-adapted man, tissues of high metabolic activity may be sensitized to the calorigenic action of catecholamines which act synergistically in the presence of constant levels of thyroid and adrenocortical hormones.

Energy Metabolism in Heat

Abrupt exposure of animals and man to high temperatures may result in an increase in deep body temperature, and an increase in metabolism. In man, the increased metabolic response to a rapidly rising body temperature is shown by higher oxygen consumption, increased secretion of glucocorticoids (COLLINS et al., 1969) and growth hormone (FEW and WORSLEY, 1975), and increased sympatho-adrenal activity (HARRISON, 1975). Information on the thyroid response in man under these conditions is lacking. The reaction to a given high-temperature stress is less easily evoked following heat acclimation, because improved physical channels of heat loss limit the level of increase of deep body temperature.

There have been few investigations of the "metabolic" endocrine response to heat acclimation in man. In an experiment in which 14 young adults were artificially acclimated to heat over a period of 2 weeks, it was found that there were no significant differences in resting metabolic rate, cumulative excretion of I^{131}, 17-OH corticosteroid excretion, or cortisol secretion rate before and after acclimation (COLLINS and FEW, unpublished). With prolonged exposure to heat, the endocrine adjustment of energy metabolism is likely to be the converse of that of cold adaptation, the suppression of calorigenesis being partly accounted for by reduced energy intake. This is confirmed by experiments in rats shown to have reduced thyroid activity when kept at $34^{o}C$ compared with controls at $28^{o}C$ (YOUSEF and JOHNSON, 1968). When the food intake of the controls was restricted to the levels of the rats fed ad libitum in the heat, the differences in thyroid activity mostly disappeared.

Many species of small mammals native to hot climates have a low metabolic rate relative to that predicted on the basis of body weight, and this is accompanied by a reduction in size of internal heat-producing organs, and in the activity of oxidative enzymes (CHAFFEE and ROBERTS, 1971). Chemical thermosuppression of metabolism can clearly be regarded as a beneficial adaptive response to hot conditions to complement an increased rate of heat loss. Several investigators have reported a lower BMR in people living in hot climates, as compared with those in temperate regions, though this is not undisputed. If adequate allowance is made for subjects to familiarize themselves with the test equipment, and the daily procedure is standardized, the depression of metabolism in the tropics is smaller than is usually reported, and of the order of 5% (COLLINS and WEINER, 1968). Taken together with factors of diet, body size and individual variability (MASON and JACOB, 1972), the evidence of ethnic differences in BMR related to climatic temperature is slight.

Regulation of Salt and Water Balance

Changes in ambient temperature bring about changes in urine flow and salt retention in man. There is a large body of evidence that shows that increased aldosterone and vasopressin secretion promote restoration of water and salt balance (COLLINS and WEINER, 1968). The endocrine component of these adjustments is often judged by the degree to which the plasma concentration of hormones is altered. Some of the errors in this assumption may be shown by the experiment illustrated in Figure 2, in which the core temperature of a resting man was raised from an

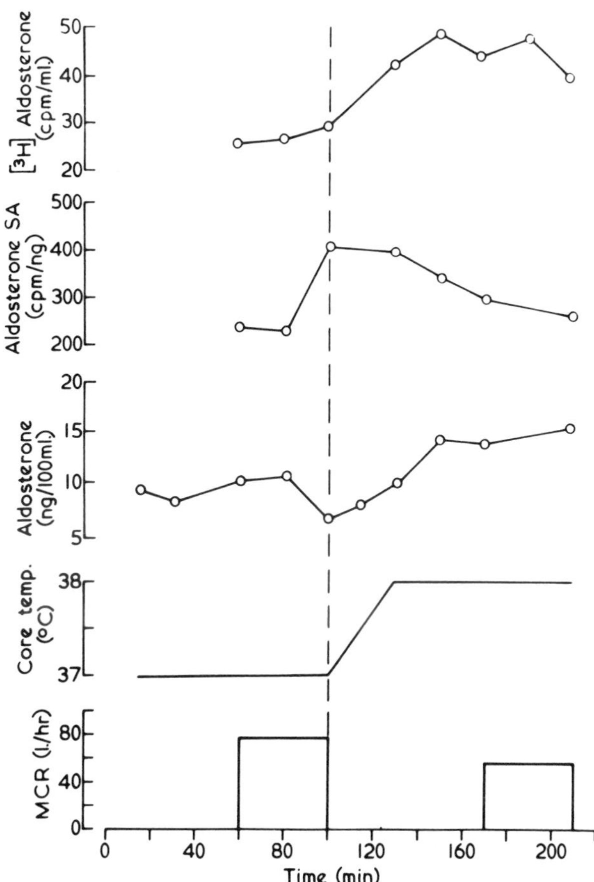

Fig. 2. Metabolic clearance rate (MCR), plasma concentration and specific activity (SA) of aldosterone during continuous infusion of [1, 2, 6, 7^3 H] aldosterone in a resting subject with normal and raised core temperature. (Data from COLLINS et al., 1977)

equilibrium level at 37°C to a second equilibrium at 38°C during continuous infusion of tracer quantities of labeled aldosterone (COLLINS et al., 1977). It is evident that the increased levels of aldosterone during heating may arise not only from increased adrenocortical secretion, as shown by a fall in specific activity of plasma aldosterone, but also from a decrease in the metabolic clearance rate (MCR). During heat exposure there is a redistribution of cardiac output resulting in enhanced blood flow in the skin at the expense of splanchnic and renal flow. Reduction in hepatic clearance rate can be demonstrated by a significant increase in the half-life of injected indocyanine green. Although the MCR of aldosterone was significantly smaller (in six experiments) there was no change in cortisol MCR, and this reveals another factor affecting plasma aldosterone concentration levels. The higher binding affinity of plasma proteins for cortisol can increase displacement of aldosterone from carrier proteins (ZAGER et al., 1976), and in stressful conditions raised plasma cortisol concentrations will facilitate aldosterone MCR. The MCR is a resultant of these factors, and of the efficiency of hepatic cellular function. Thus, in acute heat exposure the effect of a lower splanchnic blood flow appears to predominate in producing the reduction in aldosterone MCR.

With the development of heat acclimation leading to restoration of fluid and electrolyte balance and expansion of blood volume, it may be expected that the drive to increased aldosterone secretion is removed. This appears to be the case as demonstrated by laboratory studies of heat acclimation (BONNER et al., 1976) and of unacclimatized and naturally acclimatized residents of a semi-desert climate (FINBERG et al., 1974). The contribution to aldosterone turnover made by changes in hepatic clearance during acclimation has not been elucidated. The expectation would be that the smaller rise in internal temperature with heat exposure following acclimation should diminish the vasoconstriction in visceral organs, and restore hepatic clearance rate.

There are few studies of hormone functions in indigenous tropical populations, and these are, on the whole, cross-sectional and, as already mentioned, provide little opportunity for a comparative analysis of the effects of high temperature alone. The importance of the dietary factor is well demonstrated by MACFARLANE et al. (1968). In remote, essentially herbivorous people of New Guinea, potassium levels are found to be high and sodium low in body fluids. Although dynamic studies of steroid turnover were not possible, plasma aldosterone and renin concentrations were found to be abnormally high in this population group, while in coastal New Guinea people exposed to varying degrees of European economy and sodium availability, plasma aldosterone levels were lower, and reflected in a reciprocal way the degree of acculturation.

Summary

The immediate endocrine responses to temperature stress become modified and diminished during adaptation. "Metabolic" hormones increase heat production in acute cold or heat stress, but with adaptation to cold, costly increases in energy utilization may be replaced by more stable long-term changes in which the endocrine system plays only a permissive role. Changes in hormone activity may represent the response to non-equilibrium conditions, or incomplete adaptation to environmental change. In man there is little evidence at present of an adaptational effect of temperature alone in establishing new equilibria of hormone secretion and utilization. Further understanding of the adaptive changes leading to sensitization of effector organs and of the cellular basis of adjustment to temperature extremes is needed.

References

BONNER, R.M., HARRISON, M.H., HALL, C.J., EDWARDS, R.J.: Effect of heat acclimatization on intravascular responses to acute heat stress in man. J. Appl. Physiol. 41, 708-713 (1976)

BRÜCK, K.: Temperature regulation and catecholamines. Isr. J. Med. Sci. 12, 924-933 (1976)

BRÜCK, K., WUNNERBERG, W., ZEISBERGER, E.: Comparison of cold-adaptive metabolic modifications in different species, with special reference to the miniature pig. Federation Proc. 28, 1035-1041 (1969)

BUDD, G.M., WARHAFT, N.: Urinary excretion of adrenal steroids, catecholamines and electrolytes in man, before and after acclimatization to cold in Antarctica. J. Physiol. 210, 799-806 (1970)

CHAFFEE, R.R.J., ROBERTS, J.C.: Temperature acclimation in birds and mammals. Ann. Rev. Physiol. 33, 155-202 (1971)

COLLINS, K.J., FEW, J.D., FINBERG, J.P.M.: Metabolic clearance rate of cortisol and aldosterone during controlled hyperthermia in man. J. Physiol. 268, 7-8P (1977)

COLLINS, K.J., FEW, J.D., FORWARD, T.J., GIEC, L.A.: Stimulation of adrenal glucocorticoid secretion in man by raising the body temperature. J. Physiol. 202, 645-660 (1969)

COLLINS, K.J., WEINER, J.S.: Endocrinological aspects of exposure to high environmental temperatures. Physiol. Rev. 48, 785-839 (1968)

COLLINS, K.J., WEINER, J.S.: Human Adaptability. A History and Compendium of Research in the International Biological Programme. London: Taylor and Francis, 1977

EASTMAN, C.J., EKINS, R.P., LEITH, I.M., WILLIAMS, E.S.: Thyroid hormone response to prolonged cold exposure in man. J. Physiol. 241, 175-181 (1974)

FEW, J.D., WORSLEY, D.E.: Human pituitary-adrenal response to hyperthermia. J. Endocrinol. 66, 141-142 (1975)

FINBERG, J.P.M., KATZ, M., GAZIT, H., BERLYNE, G.M.: Plasma renin activity after acute heat exposure in nonacclimatized and naturally acclimatized man. J. Appl. Physiol. 36, 519-523 (1974)

GALE, C.C.: Neuroendocrine aspects of thermoregulation. Ann. Rev. Physiol. 35, 391-430 (1973)

HAMMEL, H.T.: Terrestrial animals in cold: recent studies on primitive man. In: Handbook of Physiology, Section 4, Adaptation to the Environment. Dill, D.B., Adolph, E.F., Willson, C.G. (eds.). Washington, D.C.: Am. Physiol. Soc., 1964, pp. 413-434

HARRISON, M.H.: Metabolic effects of a short exposure to a hot environment in man. Ann. Hum. Biol. 2, 41-48 (1975)

HÉROUX, O., BRAUER, R.: Critical studies on determination of thyroid secretion rate in cold-adapted animals. J. Appl. Physiol. 20, 597-606 (1965)

HILLIER, A.P.: The biliary-faecal excretion of thyroxine during cold exposure in the rat. J. Physiol. 197, 123-124 (1968)

INGRAM, D.L., KACIUBA-USCILKO, H.: The influence of food intake and ambient temperature on the rate of thyroxine utilization. J. Physiol. 270, 431-438 (1977)

ITOH, S.: Physiology of Cold-Adapted Man. Sapporo, Japan: Hokkaido Univ. School of Medicine, 1974, p. 2

MACFARLANE, W.V.: Ecophysiological hierarchies. Isr. J. Med. Sci. 12, 723-731 (1976)

MACFARLANE, W.V., HOWARD, B., SCROGGINS, B., SKINNER, S.L.: Water, electrolytes, hormones and blood pressure of Melanesians in relation to European contact. Proc. 24th Int. Congr. Physiol. Sci. Vol. VII, No. 822, 1968, p. 274

MASON, E.D., JACOB, M.: Variation in basal metabolic rate responses to changes between tropical and temperate climates. Hum. Biol. 44, 141-172 (1972)

RIMOIN, D.L., MERIMEE, T.J., RABINOWITZ, D.: Peripheral subresponsiveness to human growth hormone in the African Pygmies. New Engl. J. Med. 281, 1383-1388 (1969)

SMITH, R.E., HOIJER, D.J.: Metabolism and cellular function in cold acclimation. Physiol. Rev. 42, 60-142 (1962)

YOUSEF, M.K., JOHNSON, H.D.: Effects of heat and feed restriction during growth on thyroxine secretion rate of male rats. Endocrinology 82, 353-358 (1968)

ZAGER, P.G., BURTIS, W.J., LEUTSCHER, J.A., DOWDY, A.J., SOOD, S.: Increased plasma protein binding and lower metabolic clearance rate of aldosterone in plasma of low cortisol concentration. J. Clin. Endocrinol. Metab. 42, 207-213 (1976)

2. Human Growth Hormone Secretion in Responses to Cold and Heat

Y. OKADA and Y. KUMAHARA

Secretion of growth hormone (hGH) in response to cold and heat has been studied in normal adult subjects aged 21 to 38 years (2 males and 4 females) exposed to $4^{\circ}C$ for 1 or 2 h. Body temperature decreased to less than $34^{\circ}C$ in all cases. The serum level of cortisol increased from 18.4 to 23.8 μg/100 ml in one subject, but changed little in the others. FFA increased progressively to 113%, 136%, 226%, and 268% of the initial value in four of the subjects. Levels of hGH did not change or decrease during cooling, but increased from less than 1.1 ng/ml to more than 4.2 ng/ml (7.48 ± 4.13 ng/ml) on rewarming. Figure 1 shows a typical

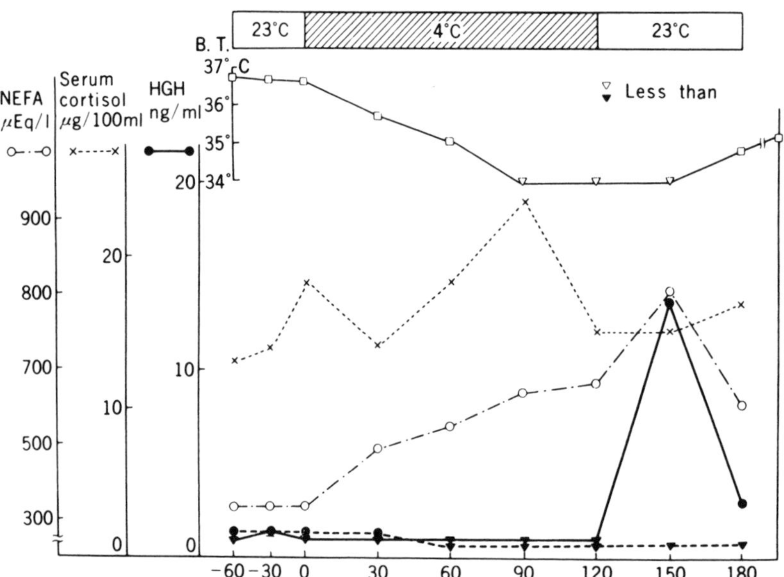

Fig. 1. Effect of 2-h exposure to cold on the serum levels of hGH, NEFA, and cortisol in a normal adult subject. The hGH level did not change during the cold exposure but increased from 0.8 to 13.5 ng/ml on rewarming (●——●). Control study at room temperature showed no significant change in hGH level (o---o)

pattern of hGH secretion during and after cold exposure. An insulin tolerance test at a dose of 0.05 U/kg of body weight was performed on the two male subjects during cold exposure. hGH values reached maxima of 32 and 7 ng/ml in the two subjects. Two female subjects were given 20 mg of propranolol orally and then exposed to cold air for 1 h. FFA changed little throughout the test. Levels of hGH did not increase during cooling, but increased from 1.7 and 2.2 to 9.5 and 6.8 ng/ml, respectively, on rewarming. There were no significant changes in hGH levels in control subjects held at room temperature (OKADA et al., 1970).

Four nonobese and one moderately obese subjects were exposed to heat in a Sauna bath (48°C) for the period of 1 h. In the four nonobese subjects, hGH levels increased from less than 1.6 ng/ml to maximum ranging from 6.2 to 30 ng/ml at 60 min after the onset of heat exposure. In the obese subject, hGH increased from 2.0 to 3.5 ng/ml at 60 min (Fig. 2). Control studies at room temperature showed no increase in

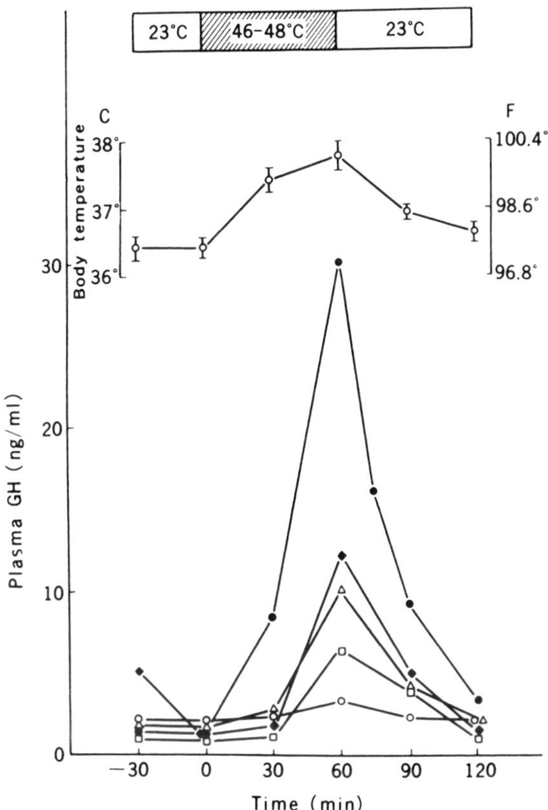

Fig. 2. Change of body temperature and plasma hGH levels before and after exposure to hot air (46°-48°C) in a Sauna bath for 1 h in four normal and one obese male subjects. Levels of hGH increased from less than 1.6 ng/ml to maximum ranging from 6.2-30 ng/ml at 60 min in four normal male subjects, but from 2.0 to 3.5 ng/ml in one obese subject

hGH levels in any of the normal subjects. FFA increased to the maxima ranging from 146.3% to 187.5% of the initial values in four of five subjects, but did not change in one subject. Cortisol levels changed little during heat exposure, but increased by 9.3 and 10.4 μg/100 ml after the test in two of five subjects. Blood glucose, hematocrit, and serum thyroxine levels did not change significantly. Secretion of hGH in response to heat was eliminated completely by oral pre-administration of glucose (100 g) in two subjects (OKADA et al., 1972).

All blood samples obtained during cold and heat exposure were analyzed for TSH and thyroxine, but the results revealed no significant changes. The mechanism of the hGH responses to cold and heat is not known.

References

OKADA, Y., MIYAI, K., IWATSUBO, H., KUMAHARA, Y.: Human growth hormone secretion before and after cold exposure in normal adult subjects. J. Clin. Endocrinol. Metab. 30, 393-395 (1970)

OKADA, Y., MATSUOKA, T., KUMAHARA, Y.: Human growth hormone secretion during exposure to hot air in normal adult male subjects. J. Clin. Endocrinol. Metab. 34, 759-763 (1972)

Chapter VII. Endocrine Responses to Malnutrition

1. Neuroendocrine Aspects of Reproduction in Experimental Malnutrition

H. H. SREBNIK, W. H. FLETCHER, and G. A. CAMPBELL

Introduction

It is now abundantly clear that diets qualitatively or quantitatively deficient in essential nutrients interfere with normal reproductive function. The degree to which these diets are detrimental varies with the type, severity, and duration of dietary manipulation, as well as with the age, strain, and sex of the animal under investigation. A broad consensus has been reached that nutritional deficiencies modify the gonadotrophic function of the adenohypophysis, and evidence has been adduced to implicate the central nervous system in the etiology of reproductive disturbances of function or behavior. Both morphologic and physiologic studies have served to establish the effects of malnutrition as breakdowns in neuro-endocrine mechanisms.

Effects of Malnutrition on Male Animals

The effects of malnutrition have included one or more of the following: delay in onset of puberty, gonadal atrophy, involution of accessory reproductive organs, and infertility - conditions that generally have been attributed to inadequacies of circulating gondadotrophic hormones. With the availability of radioimmunoassays we have recently tested these assumptions in young male rats, averaging 150 g in weight. They were placed on diets containing either optimal amounts of protein (20%), or no protein at all (SREBNIK et al., 1961), and groups of deficient and well-nourished animals were exsanguinated under ether anesthesia at various times after onset of the experiment to obtain plasma for radioimmunoassay (RIA) of FSH, LH, and testosterone.

Table 1 summarizes the autopsy data for a typical experimental series. Protein-deficient (PFD) rats lost weight from onset, and, after 4 weeks on the diet, had one-third the body mass of control (CD) rats. Testes of deficient rats did not change in weight for the first 10 days, but they were significantly less by day 21 ($p < 0.05$). The involution of the adenohypophysis gland was even more marked, and weights of ventral prostate glands declined until they reached near-castrate values.

Testosterone concentrations of protein-deficient animals were barely detectable after the first 10 days of the experiment; by day 29, three of the four animals had values below the range of sensitivity of the method. These data are consistent with published reports of markedly depressed testosterone titers in malnourished rats (GREVAL et al., 1971; HOWLAND, 1975).

FSH concentrations, after an initial delay, declined steadily in the absence of dietary protein. LH values were stable for the first 10 days of protein deprivation, but then fell sharply; at the end of the experiment, LH was undetectable in two of the four samples. These re-

Table 1. Body and organ weights (mean values for 4 or more animals), and serum testosterone, FSH, and LH concentrations of male Long-Evans rats, approximately 40 days at onset, and maintained on protein-free (PFD) or control diet (CD). Androgen in extracted serum was measured by RIA employing an antiserum co-specific for testosterone and dihydrotestosterone; protein hormone levels were determined by double antibody RIA according to NIH-NIAMDD. Serum values are means ± standard errors of the mean for animals (usually 3 or more) whose hormone concentrations were in the sensitivity range of the assay

Diet fed	Days on diet	Final body weight (g)	Testes (mg)	Ventral prostate (mg)	Anterior pituitary (mg)	Serum concentrations (ng/ml)		
						Testosterone	FSH	LH
	Onset Controls	152	1643	75.3	4.8	4.9 ± 0.1	972.2 ± 142.0	87.0 ± 14.1
PFD	4	140	1953	83.0	4.5	-	962.5 ± 123.6	111.8 ± 43.8
PFD	7	128	2105	58.1	4.2	-	587.8 ± 123.6	93.3 ± 15.9
PFD	10	117	1880	50.8	3.5	0.6 ± 0.1	323.9 ± 49.6	69.7 ± 32.4
PFD	21	91	1015	22.2	2.4	0.4 ± 0.1	190.1 ± 18.1	27.2 ± 3.0
PFD	29	81	626	17.8	2.4	0.3	166.1 ± 16.3	25.0 ± 0.2
CD	29	249	2918	191.8	5.4	3.6 ± 0.7	692.7 ± 121.1	166.3 ± 45.6

sults indicate that circulating levels of both FSH and LH become attenuated in the course of severe malnutrition, thereby accounting for the gonadal atrophy and sequelae that accompany this condition. As might be expected, total food deprivation has similar consequences (ROOT and RUSS, 1972; HOWLAND and SKINNER, 1973; CAMPBELL et al., 1977b). Taken together with observations of reduced bioassayable pituitary FSH and LH in male rats after 7 days of total starvation (NEGRO-VILAR et al., 1971), or one month of protein deprivation (SREBNIK and FLETCHER, 1972), the data suggest that gonadotrophin synthesis is impaired under conditions of severe malnutrition. Radioimmunoassays failed to demonstrate significant differences in pituitary gonadotrophin concentrations between acutely starved and well-nourished male rats (ROOT and RUSS, 1972; HOWLAND and SKINNER, 1973) and, therefore, did not correlate well with the bioassay measurements. A similar discrepancy exists with respect to determinations of hypothalamic-releasing factor activity of starved male rats, it being reduced when measured by bioassay (NEGRO-VILAR et al., 1971), but unchanged from control values on the basis of RIA (ROOT et al., 1975).

Effects of Malnutrition on Female Animals

Pituitary and serum gonadotrophin concentrations have also been determined for female rats subjected to 50% caloric restriction (PIACSEK and MEITES, 1967; HOWLAND, 1971, 1972; NAKANISHI et al., 1976) or protein deprivation (SREBNIK et al., 1961). Both bioassay and RIA data are in essential agreement that pituitary FSH concentration is elevated in undernourished female rats when compared to ad libitum-fed, diet controls. Serum FSH levels, as measured by radioimmunoassay, were unchanged after 3 to 4 weeks of undernutrition (HOWLAND, 1971; NAKANISHI et al., 1976), but LH concentrations appeared to be diminished by this treatment (HOWLAND, 1971, 1972).

The increase in pituitary FSH in female rats maintained on nutritionally deficient diets has been surmised to indicate failure of hormone release from the gland secondary to insufficiency of hypothalamic releasing factor (PIACSEK and MEITES, 1967). We decided to investigate this relationship further by measuring gonadotrophin-releasing factor (Gn-RF) in hypothalami of protein-deficient rats and attempted to correlate the bioassay data with an electron microscopic examination of the median eminence. Also, in consideration of preliminary reports (LEMMING and KRAUSE, 1963; FLETCHER and SREBNIK, 1971) that administration of estradiol re-established normal pituitary FSH values in undernourished rats, we studied the effects of estradiol benzoate (EB) on hypothalamic content of Gn-RF and ultrastructure of protein-depleted animals.

Table 2 presents autopsy data for protein-deficient and control rats that served as donors of hypothalamic material. PFD rats had lost approximately one-third of their initial body weight by the end of the 5-week deficiency period, and weighed only one-half as much as terminal diet controls. Uterine weights and microanatomy of vehicle-injected, deficient animals were markedly subnormal; most had been anestrous for 3 weeks or more. Their ovaries also were small and characterized by absence of follicular development and atrophic interstitial tissue. Daily injections of small amounts of EB for 10 days preceding autopsy stimulated uterine growth, maintained ovarian weights and histology - possibly by inducing FSH release - and caused vaginal cornification in all animals, including diet controls.

Table 2. Body and organ weights (mean values for 16 or more animals), and pituitary FSH content of female Long-Evans rats, approximately 80 days of age and 200 g at onset, fed protein-free (PFD) or control diet (CD) and injected for 10 days preceding autopsy with estradiol benzoate (EB). FSH content of anterior lobes, pooled by treatment group, was determined by the ovarian weight-augmentation test and expressed as NIH-FSH-S8 equivalents (mean values for 6 or more test rats). Data presented in tables were subjected to computer program analysis for statistical validation. ns = not significant

Diet fed	Weeks on diet	Treatment (day × 10 days)	Final body weight (g)	Uterus (mg)	Ovaries (mg)	Anterior pituitary weight (mg)	Anterior pituitary FSH content (µg)	*p*
PFD	Injection onset controls		150	138	37.8	5.2	130	130 vs. 65: < 0.01
PFD	5	Sesame oil	128	118	29.0	5.6	118	118 vs. 67: < 0.01
PFD	5	0.1 µg EB	123	228	36.8	6.0	65	65 vs. 67: ns
CD	5	Sesame oil	255	400	84.1	12.3	67	
CD	5	0.3 µg EB	254	534	82.3	13.1	52	

Pituitary FSH content of deficient rats 5 weeks after being placed on the protein-free diet was 118 µg, whereas FSH content of animals maintained on the control diet for the same length of time - and killed in estrus - was 67 µg. As pituitary glands of PFD females were smaller than control rat glands, FSH potency was even greater when expressed as µg per mg of tissue. Significantly, physiologic amounts of estradiol benzoate reduced adenohypophyseal FSH of deficient animals from preinjection values of 130 µg to 65 µg. This treatment, therefore, restored FSH content to levels found in normal controls, in which 0.3 µg of steroid was without any effect.

Extracts of stalk-median eminence (SME) from the different treatment groups were evaluated for their ability to deplete pituitary FSH stores in vivo. Intact male rats, which served as assay animals, received each by intravenous injection either the equivalent of two stalk-median eminence fragments, or cerebral cortex of comparable weight. Exactly 45 min later, the recipient rats were killed, so that residual FSH content in their pituitary glands could be determined.

Assay rats given 34 mg of neocortex, or injected with 2 SME from diet controls in estrus - even when treated with 0.3 µg of estradiol benzoate - had similar hypophyseal FSH contents. Recipients of hypothalamic extracts from PFD donors differed, however, in that the same test dose caused a significant (20%) depletion of their FSH stores from this base line level ($p < 0.01$), indicating that hypothalamic Gn-RF, as well as adenohypophyseal FSH, accumulate in female rats deprived of dietary protein for 5 weeks. Contrariwise, hypothalamic extracts of PFD donors treated with 0.1 µg of estradiol benzoate failed to deplete FSH from glands of recipient animals, and this observation suggests that estrogen treatment had lowered the hypothalamic Gn-RF content of PFD rats, even as the steroid had reduced their pituitary FSH content.

Electron microscopic evaluation of the external median eminence region correlated well with our Gn-RF potency estimates: axon terminals of oil-injected PFD rats contained many more small, dense-core, neurosecretory granules than did nerve endings of well-fed females, whereas axon profiles of hormone-treated PFD animals could not be distinguished from those of diet controls on the basis of dense-core inclusions. Marked differences existed also in the fine structure of neuronal cell bodies forming the arcuate nuclei of rats from the various treatment groups. By morphologic indices of cell activity, arcuate neurons of oil-injected PFD rats - unlike those of diet controls - had only limited capacities for either protein synthesis or production of dense-core granules; however, organelle composition and development were greatly improved in protein-depleted animals given EB, pointing to re-activation of the synthesizing and condensation-packaging machineries in response to steroid treatment.

Effects of Malnutrition on Prolactin Secretion

The third adenohypophyseal hormone that influences reproductive function in the rat is prolactin, but the status of this hormone in severely malnourished animals has not been thoroughly studied. It is known that pituitary prolactin is decreased in acutely starved or chronically underfed female rats (MEITES and REED, 1949; NAKANISHI et al., 1976); though, apparently, starvation does not affect pituitary prolactin content of male rats (AKIKUSA, 1971). Circulating hormone appears to be reduced in starved males (SIREK et al., 1976; CAMPBELL et al., 1977b), but not in female rats restricted in their dietary intake to 50% of a stock diet (NAKANISHI et al., 1976).

We have recently studied the effects of protein deprivation on pituitary and plasma prolactin levels of female rats, similar in all respects to those already described. At the end of 5 weeks on their respective diets, PFD and CD animals that were to serve as donors for pituitary assays were killed by decapitation; all others were exsanguinated under nembutal anesthesia. Prolactin content of anterior lobes was determined by both bioassay (deciduoma test) and polyacrylamide gel electrophoresis (NICOLL et al., 1969). Plasma levels of the hormone were measured by double antibody RIA. As determined by chemical assay, anterior pituitaries of PFD rats contained only about one-third as much hormone as glands of control rats killed in diestrus (114 ± 16 ug), and biologic assay gave similar estimates of pituitary prolactin. Plasma concentration of immunoreactive prolactin from animals on the protein-free diet also was reduced to one-third of the control values (24 ± 4 ng/ml). Such parallel decline is in accord with the view that hormone production, rather than release, is adversely affected by protein deprivation. In separate experiments, prolactin-inhibiting activity of hypothalamic extract from protein-deficient and fully fed donors was compared in vitro (NICOLL et al., 1969) and found not to differ.

Conclusion

Taken as a whole, the experiments reported here offer further proof that malnutrition depresses the activity of the hypothalamo-hypophysial axis; but the questions remain: where is the primary locus of breakdown, and what is its nature? The adenohypophysis, male or female, retains its sensitivity to Gn-RF under a variety of nutritional deficiency states, as has been demonstrated repeatedly, both in vivo and in vitro (ROOT and DUCKETT, 1973; HOWLAND, 1976; CAMPBELL et al., 1977b). In fact, the secretory response of the adenohypophysis to injection of a synthetic factor was frequently greater in deficient animals than diet controls.

Other procedures have shown that the hypothalamo-hypophysial unit is able to respond to physiologic stimulus: continuous illumination re-initiated gonadotrophin release in underfed female rats (PIACSEK and MEITES, 1967), and gonadectomy has long been known to bring about over-production and hypersecretion of FSH and LH, even under conditions of complete starvation (MEITES and REED, 1949; ROOT and RUSS, 1972; HOWLAND and SKINNER, 1973; ROOT and DUCKETT, 1973) or total protein deprivation (LEATHEM, 1958; SREBNIK et al., 1961; SREBNIK, 1970). Furthermore, there is now evidence that low doses of estrogen can reduce the postcastration increase in LH more effectively in underfed rats than in ovariectomized rats fed full rations (HOWLAND and IBRAHIM, 1973; CAMPBELL et al., 1977a). These observations collectively imply that the hypothalamus may not only have suffered no loss in sensitivity, but may indeed be more sensitive to the negative feedback action of sex steroids (STEWART et al., 1975). If hypersensitivity of the "gonadostat" under those conditions is confirmed, it may provide an explanation for the puzzling lack of castration changes in intact, malnourished rats with extreme sex steroid deficiencies.

There is presumptive evidence that the positive feedback loop is intact as well, for estrogen and progesterone injected sequentially into ovariectomized rats on a low plane of nutrition raised serum FSH and LH concentrations significantly above pre-injection values (HOWLAND, 1976). Our own results with estrogen-treated, intact, protein-deficient females tend to support this proposition.

Perhaps, then, malnutrition acts first to disrupt ovarian and testicular steroidogenesis, in which case failure of gonadotrophin secretion may follow rather than precede steroid hormone disappearance. Such a peripherally directed mode of action would be compatible with the presence of a functionally competent hypothalamo-hypophysial complex. It would be consistent also with the recorded rapid onset of accessory organ atrophy and delayed pituitary reaction of male protein-deficient rats, but experimental verification of this concept requires serial and simultaneous measurements of circulating gonadotrophic and steroid hormones to judge more precisely the time course of their decline.

Acknowledgments. Our experiments were supported by grants from the National Science Foundation and from the Committee on Research, University of California, Berkeley. Radioimmunoassay kits and standard preparations of pituitary hormones were generously supplied by Dr. A.F. PARLOW and The NIAMDD Rat Pituitary Hormone Distribution Program. We are also indepted to Mrs. JACQUELINE M. EHLERT and Mr. RICHARD F. LAHERTY for skillful technical assistance, and to Dr. PAUL LICHT for help with testosterone radioimmunoassays.

References

AKIKUSA, Y.: Effect of starvation on synthesis and release of growth hormone and prolactin in the rat anterior pituitary. Endocrinol. Jap. 18, 411-416 (1971)

CAMPBELL, G.A., HODSON, C.A., MIODUSZEWSKI, R., MEITES, J.: Increased estrogen suppression of LH in starved, ovariectomized rats. Program of Endocr. Soc., p. 193 (1977a)

CAMPBELL, G.A., KURCZ, M., MARSHALL, S., MEITES, J.: Effects of starvation in rats on serum levels of follicle stimulating hormone, luteinizing hormone, thyrotropin, growth hormone and prolactin; response to LH-releasing hormone and thyrotropin-releasing hormone. Endocrinology 100, 580-587 (1977b)

FLETCHER, W.H., SREBNIK, H.H.: Reduction in pituitary FSH content of female protein-deficient rats induced by estradiol benzoate. Anat. Rec. 169, 317 (1971)
GREVAL, T., MICHELSEN, D., HAFS, H.D.: Androgen secretion and spermatogenesis in rats following semistarvation. Proc. Soc. Exp. Biol. Med. 138, 723-727 (1971)
HOWLAND, B.E.: Gonadotrophin levels in female rats subjected to restricted feed intake. J. Reprod. Fert. 27, 467-470 (1971)
HOWLAND, B.E.: Effects of restricted feed intake on LH levels in female rats. J. Anim. Sci. 34, 445-447 (1972)
HOWLAND, B.E.: The influence of feed restriction and subsequent re-feeding on gonadotrophin secretion and serum testosterone levels in male rats. J. Reprod. Fert. 44, 429-436 (1975)
HOWLAND, B.E.: Gonadotrophin release induced by Gn-RH or progesterone in female rats maintained on high or low levels of feed intake. J. Reprod. Fert. 47, 137-139 (1976)
HOWLAND, B.E., IBRAHIM, E.A.: Increased LH-suppressing effect of oestrogen in ovariectomized rats as a result of underfeeding. J. Reprod. Fert. 35, 545-548 (1973)
HOWLAND, B.E., SKINNER, K.R.: Effect of starvation on gonadotrophin secretion in intact and castrated male rats. Can. J. Physiol. Pharmacol. 51, 759-762 (1973)
LAMMING, G.E., KRAUSE, J.B.: The effect of a low plane of nutrition and the endocrine glands of the female rat. In: Nutrition. Mills, C.F., Passmore, R. (eds.). Edinburgh: Livingstone, 1963, p. 633
LEATHEM, J.H.: Hormones and protein nutrition. Rec. Progr. Horm. Res. 14, 141-182 (1958)
MEITES, J., REED, J.O.: Effects of restricted feed intake in intact and ovariectomized rats on pituitary lactogen and gonadotrophin. Proc. Soc. Exp. Biol. Med. 70, 513-516 (1949)
NAKANISHI, Y., MORI, J., NAGASAWA, H.: Recovery of pituitary secretion of gonadotrophins and prolactin during re-feeding after chronic restricted feeding in female rats. J. Endocrinol. 69, 329-339 (1976)
NEGRO-VILAR, A., DICKERMAN, E., MEITES, J.: Effects of starvation on hypothalamic FSH-RF and pituitary FSH in male rats. Endocrinology 88, 1246-1249 (1971)
NICOLL, C.S., PARSONS, J.A., FIORINDO, R.P., NICHOLS, C.W.: Estimation of prolactin and growth hormone levels by polyacrylamide disc electrophoresis. J. Endocrinol. 45, 183-196 (1969)
PIACSEK, B.E., MEITES, J.: Reinitiation of gonadotropin release in underfed rats by constant light or epinephrine. Endocrinology 81, 535-541 (1967)
ROOT, A.W., DUCKETT, G.E.: In vivo and in vitro effects of synthetic luteinizing hormone-releasing hormone (LH-RH) upon the secretion of luteinizing hormone (LH) and follicle stimulating hormone (FSH) in intact and castrated, fed and starved adult male rats. Proc. Soc. Exp. Biol. Med. 144, 30-33 (1973)
ROOT, A.W., REITER, E.O., DUCKETT, G.E., SWEETLAND, M.L.: Effect of short-term castration and starvation upon hypothalamic content of luteinizing hormone-releasing hormone in adult male rats. Proc. Soc. Exp. Biol. Med. 150, 602-605 (1975)
ROOT, A.W., RUSS, R.D.: Short-term effects of castration and starvation upon pituitary and serum levels of luteinizing hormone and follicle stimulating hormone in male rats. Acta Endocrinol. 70, 665-675 (1972)
SIREK, A.M.T., HORVATH, E., EZRIN, C., KOVACS, K.: Effects of starvation on pituitary growth hormone cells and blood growth hormone and prolactin levels in the rat. Nutr. Metabol. 20, 67-75 (1976)
SREBNIK, H.H.: FSH and ICSH in pituitary and plasma of castrate protein-deficient rats. Biol. Reprod. 3, 96-104 (1970)
SREBNIK, H.H., FLETCHER, W.H.: Pituitary FSH increase in male protein-deficient rats induced by testosterone propionate. Proc. Soc. Exp. Biol. Med. 141, 85-88 (1972)
SREBNIK, H.H., NELSON, M.M.: Anterior pituitary function in male rats deprived of dietary protein. Endocrinology 70, 723-730 (1962)
SREBNIK, H.H., NELSON, M.M., SIMPSON, M.E.: Follicle stimulating hormone (FSH) and interstitial-cell-stimulating hormone (ICSH) in pituitary and plasma of intact and ovariectomized protein-deficient rats. Endocrinology 68, 317-326 (1961)
STEWART, S.F., KOPIA, S., GAWLAK, D.L.: Effects of underfeeding, hemigonadectomy, sex and cyproterone acetate on serum FSH levels in immature rats. J. Reprod. Fert. 45, 173-176 (1975)

2. Endocrine Responses to Malnutrition in Animals with Special Reference to Metabolic Hormones

J. LEATHEM

An interdependence exists between the endocrine glands and nutrition, for not only does nutrition influence the synthesis and release of hormones, but hormones, in turn, through their regulation of metabolism, influence nutrition. Thus dietary deficiencies may create endocrine imbalances, may modify protein binding in transport, may alter metabolic clearance rate, and may influence tissue responsivity possibly through changes in hormone receptors. Hormones, on the other hand, influence the appetite and the absorption, utilization, and excretion of food. Furthermore, hormones can accentuate the effects of a poor diet.

The clinical aspects of malnutrition in infancy and childhood emphasize protein-calorie malnutrition (PCM), as in kwashiorkor and marasmus, or a combination of the two. Thus animal models have been sought, and clinical features of human PCM have been reported (ANTHONY and EDOZIEN, 1975). Furthermore, it should be recalled that MULINOS and POMERANTZ in 1940 suggested that malnutrition in adult rats induced a "pseudo-hypophysectomy". Then too, in normal growth, the rat pituitary increased from 2.6 mg to 7.0 mg between 25 and 60 days of age. An increase in protein and RNA accompanied the growth. An increase in cell number (DNA) and cell size (P/DNA) was associated with the development to day 50, but thereafter only cell size increased. If a protein-free diet was fed initially for 10 days, all protein and nucleic acid changes were prevented. Refeeding 20% casein resulted in a restoration of protein content in 30 days. However, the pattern of growth differed by favoring a continued increase in cell number with a subnormal increase in cell size.

Biochemical analysis may reveal subtle differences, and thus 200 g male rats were examined 28 days after hypophysectomy while fed 18% casein ad libitum for comparison with normal rats pair-fed 0% and 18% casein. The livers from hypophysectomized rats were significantly smaller than those fed 0% casein, but protein content per cell was less in the protein-deprived, possibly due to fatty infiltration. Both hypophysectomy and 0% casein prevented the normal increase in polyploidy as expressed on the basis of DNA/nucleus basis. Incorporation rates and protein-synthetic competence of ribosomes were studied using ^{14}C-l-leucine. In support of prior studies, the membrane-bound ribosomes exhibited greater incorporating capability than did the free ribosomes. However, protein-synthetic competence of the free ribosomes was significantly less after hypophysectomy than after protein deprivation, and both were well below the levels of the rat fed 18% casein. Both hypophysectomy and protein deprivation caused a marked decrease in essential and nonessential free amino acids in liver, with the greater change associated with hypophysectomy. These data reveal comparable directional compositional changes in liver following hypophysectomy and protein-free feeding (Table 1). The meaningfulness of the subtle differences will require further study.

Table 1. Hypophysectomy, dietary protein and liver composition

	Hypox + 18% casein	Normal 0% casein pair-fed	Normal 18% casein pair-fed
Liver wt g	4.7	7.1	8.1
Cell protein μμg/cell	407	308	752
DNA/nucleus μμg	10.8	10.6	16.5
Ribosomes (PSC-DPM × 10^{-6}/cell)			
Total	349	338	1371
Bound	324	286	1180
Free	25	52	191
Amino acid mμμ/cell			
Essential	7.0	9.3	22.0
Free	44.1	72.7	123.4

Endocrine Gland Function and Nutrition

Hypophysis. With the advent of radioimmunoassays PIMSTONE et al. (1966) recorded elevated serum levels of growth hormone in PCM children. Subsequent studies confirmed the elevated hGH levels in children exhibiting kwashiorkor but increased, unchanged, or even depressed levels were associated with marasmus (TURNER, 1972; GARDNER and AMACHER, 1973). Then too, the anticipated responses to arginine, lysine, glucose or insulin were frequently not observed. The elevated levels of growth hormone may be associated with a decrease in somatomedin formation in the liver as well as a deficient neural feed back, rather than an impaired clearance. PIMSTONE et al. (1975) also found that somatostatin caused an acute inhibition of growth hormone in PCM. Malnutrition increased hGH levels in adults, with the male being the more responsive (MERIMEE et al., 1976). Refeeding of children and adults reduced growth hormone levels to normal in 3-5 weeks.

In contrast to the human response to inanition, growth-hormone levels decline in the rat. A decrease of growth hormone in both putiutary and serum followed 5 weeks of protein-free feeding or 7 days of starvation (CAMPBELL et al., 1977). Furthermore, a 6% casein diet decreased growth-hormone synthesis (SHRADER and ZEMAN, 1973). The decreased serum levels of growth hormone in starved rats were associated with a decrease in hypothalamic GH-RF (DICKERMAN et al., 1969). However the inappropriate release of growth hormone by TRH noted in PCM in children was not found in starved rats. Neuroendocrine controls in the rat may be different from man as glucose, ether, insulin and epinephrine all inhibit the release of GH in the rat in contrast with man (TAKAHASHI et al., 1971), whereas pentobarbital anesthesia caused a significant rise of GH in the rat.

Inanition in sheep and cow does not alter serum growth hormone (TRENKLE, 1971). On the other hand, inanition caused an increase in serum GH in rabbits, that was not lowered by arginine or glucose (TURNER, 1973), and the dog responded in similar fashion. Severe protein restriction in swine favored a reduction in serum GH levels (TURNER, 1972), but more recently ATINMO et al. (1976) found that protein- or energy-restricted diets fed during the postweaning period resulted in an elevation of serum GH. Obviously age at which inanition is imposed, as well as the degree, may contribute to the seeming species differences in response among animals. Refeeding favors a return to normal serum-hormone levels, but the response to refeeding is slowed when inanition is imposed on the neonate (TRENKLE, 1974).

Pancreas. PCM in children is generally associated with a subnormal plasma insulin, and the individual may be unresponsive to glucose or arginine. Glucose tolerance is usually abnormal (MILNER, 1972). In addition, the return of β cell function may be months, or even years, after clinical recovery. These subnormal levels of plasma insulin may relate to reduced enteroglucagon due to atrophy of the gut mucosa, reduced release, increased insulin antagonism related to other hormonal imbalances, or to lack of potassium.

In animal experiments, low protein or low calorie feeding resulted in low plasma levels of insulin in rat, dog, sheep, pigs, and steers. In fact, a sharp reduction occurred in 24 h. The subnormal insulin levels were not due to a change in half-life, but rather to a decreasing in secretion rate (TRENKLE, 1971). Furthermore, the activity of the liver enzyme that controls insulin degradation was not modified by the feeding of a protein-free diet for 10 days (PETRI et al., 1976).

Refeeding restores plasma insulin following short-term inanition, extension of the depletion period delaying the response (YOUNG et al., 1973; KABADI et al., 1976) and reducing the capacity to respond to insulin.

In contrast to insulin, plasma glucagon is elevated in malnourished children, but secretion rate may be imparied (MILNER, 1972). KABADI et al. (1976) found no change in plasma glucagon in rats fed a low-protein diet, although insulin declined. However, a high-protein, but carbohydrate-free diet increased glucagon with no effect on insulin. Reducing food intake 50% elevated plasma glucagon in rats fed a 5% casein diet.

Thyroid. Information on thyroid function in clinical and experimental PCM is conflicting and, indeed, both the thyroid gland and the pituitary have been regarded as potential sites of involvement. In general, a thyroid hypofunction occurs in marasmus, in which serum thyroxine and TSH are reduced. Administration of TSH or hypothalamic TRF stimulates the thyroid; however, 36 h of fasting reduces the response to TRF. Fasting also reduces serum T_3 and results in the formation of reverse T_3; lesser malnutrition can reduce T_3 without increasing rT_3 (SPAULDING et al., 1976). In kwashiorkor, T_4 is reduced, but less of the hormone is bound, and TSG levels are normal.

Starvation can increase MIT, DIT, T_3, and T_4 in the rat thyroid gland while reducing TSH. In fact after 48 h of fasting, serum T_4 was elevated as peripheral deiodination and fecal loss were reduced (INGBAR and DALTON, 1975). Long-term restriction of food intake (50%) reduces binding. Not only can the degree of malnutrition influence the results, but also the age at which the food reduction is imposed. Thus SHRADER et al. (1977) fed 24% and 4% casein to rats prenatally, and recorded subnormal levels of serum T_3, T_4 and TSG in neonates. Furthermore, limited nursing time to day 12 resulted in subnormal hypothalamic TRH. The pituitary responded to TRH, suggesting a nutritionally induced hypothalamic deficit (SHAMBAUGH and WILBER, 1974).

Adrenal Cortex. Infants and children with marasmus exhibit elevated levels of plasma cortisol, whereas with kwashiorkor the corticoid levels may or may not be elevated. Furthermore, adrenal production is normal, half-life is increased, and protein binding is decreased as serum albumin and transcortin are reduced, possibly due to a change in liver metabolism. The adrenal will respond to ACTH administration, but an incomplete suppression of the hypothalamic-pituitary axis was noted with dexamethasone. Similar results were obtained with PCM adults in which plasma ACTH was maintained in spite of the elevated plasma F (SMITH et al., 1975). ACTH secretion must be maintained by another stimulus that might signal an alteration in hypothalamic amines.

Starvation or protein deprivation elevates plasma corticosterone in rats, due in part to a prolonged half-life, and also abolishes diurinal rhythms. Malnutrition reportedly increases hypothalamic CRF.

Nutritional restriction at critical times in development must be considered. In the rat, the functional maturation of the hypothalamo-pituitary-adrenal axis occurs during pregnancy and the neonatal period (DUPOUY et al., 1975). However, feeding 4% casein during pregnancy does not modify normal basal levels of B in offspring of 4 and 8 days of age (PARSONS et al., 1976). Furthermore, 200 cal/kg, 100 cal/kg and 10% casein feeding during pregnancy followed by full feeding after birth to day 15 results in normal basal corticosterone levels, but competence to respond to ether stress is subnormal in 100 cal/kg or 10% casein feeding, suggesting that a modified brain-pituitary axis as a response to ACTH is normal. On the other hand, food or protein restriction in pregnancy and lactation resulted after weaning in an elevated basal levels of corticosterone, but subnormal responses to ether stress (ADLARD and SMART, 1972; SHOEMAKER and DALLMAN, 1973). Furthermore, refeeding for 15 weeks failed to restore the stress response to normal. Subsequently TIGNER and BARNES (1975) fed 12% casein during lactation, and noted elevated levels of corticosterone on day 21, that returned to normal on refeeding. Stress response was not tested. When caloric intake was restricted during lactation only, the basal levels of serum corticosterone on day 15 were normal, but response to ether stress was exaggerated. On day 20, elevated basal levels were observed, but an over-response to stress did not occur. Adrenal content of corticosterone was greater in postnatal calorie-restricted rats, suggesting enhanced hormone synthesis.

Circadian periodicity of plasma corticosteroids in adult rats can be influenced by restricting access to food and water to 2 h in the morning for 15 days. A shift of 12 h in the time of the circadian peak can occur (KREIGER, 1974). The influence of food intake has been reemphasized recently (TAKAHASHI et al., 1977).

Hormones and "Catch-Up" Growth

During growth, all organs and tissues of the body increase in cell number and size. Moreover, early growth in most tissues is predominantly hyperplastic, whereas later growth is hypertrophic. Caloric restriction from birth to weaning reduces organ DNA in rats, and may blunt full recovery on refeeding. On the other hand, adult animals that are protein- or calorie-depleted indicate an enhanced protein metabolism on refeeding. In general, the refeeding process will correct the serum hormone levels, but in clinical PCM the additional administration of growth hormone may or may not be useful. Little effort has been given to evaluating the role of hormones during nutritional repletion; an aspect that can be studied in experimental animals by gland ablation.

Pituitary. It is well known that pituitary ablation results in an abrupt cessation of growth with a marked effect on nitrogen retained and organ protein content. Hypophysectomy reduces protein-synthetic competence of the ribosomes, cell size and RNA content. However, at least part of the physiologic changes ascribed to pituitary ablation do not occur if the protein stores are depleted prior to hypophysectomy. Thus, adult rats fed a protein-free diet for 30-40 days, then hypophysectomized, and refed 18% casein for 20 days, will gain weight and retain as much nitrogen as pair-fed normal controls. Hypophysectomy followed by protein refeeding results in an increase in liver protein and cell size, but prevents the increase in RNA noted in normal rats. In contrast to the liver, the normal capacity of the kidney to regain protein and RNA on refeeding is blocked by hypophysectomy. The gastrocnemius muscle exhibits an intermediate position with subnormal increases in protein and DNA, and no change in cell size. Thus distribution of retained nitrogen is modified by hypophysectomy. Comparable results were obtained with protein-calorie depletion prior to hypophysectomy (LEATHEM and KOISHI, 1972).

Pancreas. The fact that hypophysectomy does not negate the anabolism of protein repletion does not rule out a hormone contribution, as insulin is still present. Thus, the influence of diabetes on protein repletion was examined in adult rats initially fed a protein-free diet for two months, then given alloxan. A blood-sugar level of 400 mg % was obtained, and the animal was refed 18% casein for 20 days. Gain in body weight was restricted to 45 g compared with 122 g in pair-fed controls, and nitrogen retention was subnormal. Unlike hypophysectomy, serum albumin increased, as did kidney and heart weight. On the other hand, diabetes retarded rebuilding of muscle protein and cell size (LEATHEM and KIOSHI, 1972).

Nutrition and Hormone Action

In malnutrition, the hormone-tissue interaction is impaired, and thus the levels of circulating hormones may not reveal tissue responsivity. Low carbohydrate diets can cause a reduction in tissue sensitivity to insulin. Then too, in severe marasmus, response to treatment is better with combined dietary and growth hormone therapy. Several aspects of this problem have been investigated in our laboratory.

Insulin. Alloxan-diabetic immature rats fed 20% casein for 14 days gained 9 g whereas normal controls gained 54 g. 0.5 μ PZ insulin daily improved weight gain to 28 g in diabetic rats. Insulin improved muscle weight gain, DNA, RNA, and restored muscle protein and glycogen. Feeding a protein-free diet for 8 days prior to administration of alloxan, followed by 14 days of 20% casein refeeding, permitted a 32-g gain in body weight that did not respond to insulin. However, insulin improved muscle weight gain, protein, and nucleic acid content, as well as glycogen, but not to normal levels. Both protein depletion and diabetes reduced muscle protein-synthetic competence, but response to insulin during refeeding was not altered by prior protein depletion.

Growth Hormone. Protein-depleted rats, when hypophysectomized prior to refeeding 18% casein, revealed a subnormal gain in body weight and distribution of nitrogen retained. Growth hormone, thyroxine, insulin, androgen and corticoids have been provided during repletion with only

Table 2. Protein repletion in hypophysectomized adult male rats and response to human growth hormone (0.5 mg)

	0% casein 30 days;		18% casein 20 days
	Hypox[a]	Hypox + hGH	Normal control
Body wt gain g	30	104	103
Nitrogen balance g/kg/20 days	8.0	9.5	8.4
Liver wt g	8.3	11.2	10.4
Protein g	1.4	2.3	1.9
Kidney wt g	1.7	2.1	2.5
Protein g	0.28	0.34	0.43

[a] Hypophysectomy prior to refeeding 18% casein.

growth hormone being effective. The hormone increased gain in body weight without increasing food intake, enhanced nitrogen retention and counteracted renal loss protein (Table 2). Since amino acid levels may influence the responses to growth hormone, 18% lactalbumin was compared with 18% wheat gluten for responsiveness to bovine growth hormone during protein repletion of hypophysectomized rats. Growth hormone restored gain in body weight in rats fed lactalbumin, normalized liver composition, and markedly improved muscle and kidney protein and nucleic acids. By contrast, the feeding of 18% wheat gluten essentially failed to provide a nutritional base on which growth hormone could express an action.

Adrenal Steroids. Initial investigations with cortisone acetate revealed that removal of protein from the diet negated the life-maintaining action of this steroid in immature adrenalectomized rats. Since aldosterone is secreted by the rat adrenal, this steroid was studied in immature male rats fed 20% casein after adrenalectomy, 2 µg daily provided 100% survival for 20 days and a 46-g body weight gain. However, a 0% casein diet rendered the hormone totally ineffective even at 4 µg dosages. Feeding proteins of lesser nutritional value than casein, i. e., wheat gluten and gelatin, reduced survival to 70% and 0%, respectively. Lactalbumin permitted an improved gain in body weight and retained serum NPN and urea N at normal levels. A similar impact of quantity and quality of protein was noted when corticosterone was used as replacement treatment. The diet influenced steroid actions on serum urea N and muscle glycogen responses. Finally, a reduction in calories by 50% markedly reduced corticosterone effectiveness. Despite replacement therapy of 300 µg/day that provides 100% survival for 20 days in full-fed rats, no adrenalectomized rat survived for 20 days, despite being given steroid, when caloric intake was reduced 50%. Thus, as we proceed to deploy these hormones, we must recognize that the nutritional base on which they are acting can markedly influence their effectiveness.

References

ADLARD, B.P.F., SMART, J.L.: Adrenocortical function in rats subjected to nutritional deprivation in early life. J. Endocrinol. 54, 99-105 (1972)

ANTHONY, L.E., EDOZIEN, J.C.: Experimental protein and energy deficiencies in the rat. J. Nutr. 105, 631-648 (1975)
ATINMO, T., BALDIJAO, C., POND, W.G., BARNES, R.H.: Immunoreactive growth hormone levels in pigs fed protein or energy restricted diets during the preweaning period. J. Nutr. 106, 947-951 (1976)
CAMPBELL, G.A., KURCZ, M., MARSHALL, S., MEITES, J.: Effects of starvation in rats on serum levels of FSH, LH, TSH, STH, and LTH. Response to LH-releasing hormone and thyrotropin releasing hormone. Endocrinology 100, 580-587 (1977)
DICKERMAN, E., NEGRO-VILAR, A., MEITES, J.: Effects of starvation on plasma GH activity, pituitary GH and GH-RF levels in the rat. Endocrinology 84, 814-820 (1969)
DUPOUY, J.P., COFFIGNY, H., MAGRE, S.: Maternal and foetal corticosterone levels during late pregnancy in rats. J. Endocrinol. 65, 347-352 (1975)
GARDNER, L.I., AMACHER, P.: Endocrine Aspects of Malnutrition. Santa Ynez, Calif.: The Kroc Foundation, 1973
INGBAR, D.H., GALTON, V.A.: The effect of food deprivation on the peripheral metabolism of thyroxine in rats. Endocrinology 96, 1525-1532 (1975)
KABADI, V.M., EISENSTEIN, A.B., STRASK, I.: Decreased plasma insulin but normal glucagon in rats fed low protein diets. J. Nutr. 106, 1247-1253 (1976)
KREIGER, D.T.: Food and water restriction shifts corticosterone. Temperature, activity and brain amine periodicity. Endocrinology 95, 1195-1201 (1974)
LEATHEM, J.H., KOISHI, H.: Cellular growth in hypophysectomized or diabetic adult rats during protein repletion. Am. J. Anat. 135, 169-177 (1972)
MERIMEE, T.J., PULKKINEN, A.J., BURTON, C.E.: Diet induced alteration in hGH secretion in man. J. Clin. Endocrinol. 42, 931-937 (1976)
MILNER, R.D.G.: Insulin secretion in human protein-calorie deficiency. Proc. Nutr. Soc. 31, 219-224 (1972)
MULINOS, M.G., POMERANTZ, L.: Pseudo-hypophysectomy. A condition resembling hypophysectomy produced by malnutrition. J. Nutr. 19, 493-504 (1940)
PARSONS, P.L., SHRADER, R.E., ZEMAN, F.J.: Adrenal function in young of protein-deprived pregnant rats. J. Nutr. 106, 392-404 (1976)
PETRI, W., Jr., RODRIGUEZ, J., PITOT, H.C.: Environmental effects of glutathione-insulin transhydrogenase in rat liver. Proc. Soc. Exp. Biol. Med. 152, 610-614 (1976)
PIMSTONE, B.L., BECKER, D., KRONHEIM, S.: Disappearance of plasma growth hormone in acromegaly and protein calorie malnutrition after somatostatin. J. Clin. Endocr. 40, 168-171 (1975)
PIMSTONE, B.L., WITTMAN, W., HANSEN, J.D.L., MURRAY, P.: Growth hormone and kwashiorkor; role of growth hormone homeostasis. Lancet 2, 779-780 (1966)
SHAMBAUGH, G.E., WILBER, J.F.: The effect of caloric deprivation upon thyroid function in the neonatal rat. Endocrinology 94, 1145-1149 (1974)
SHOEMAKER, W.J., DALLMAN, M.F.: Pituitary-adrenal function in perinatally undernurished rats. Federation Proc. 32, 909 (1973)
SHRADER, R.E., FERLATTE, M.I., HASTINGS-ROBERTS, M.H., SCHOENBORNE, B.M., HOERNICKE, C.A., ZEMAN, F.J.: Thyroid function in prenatally protein deprived rats. J. Nutr. 107, 221-229 (1977)
SHRADER, R.E., ZEMAN, F.E.: In vitro synthesis of anterior pituitary growth hormone as affected by maternal protein deprivation and postnatal food supply. J. Nutr. 103, 1012-1016 (1973)
SMITH, S.R., BLEDSOE, T., CHHETRI, N.K.: Cortisol metabolism and the pituitary-adrenal axis in adults with protein-calorie malnutrition. J. Clin. Endocrinol. 40, 43-52 (1975)
SPAULDING, S.W., CHOPRA, I.J., SHERWIN, R.S., LYALL, S.S.: Effect of caloric restriction and dietary composition on serum T_3 and reverse T_3 in man. J. Clin. Endocrinol. 42, 197-200 (1976)
TAKAHASHI, K., DAUGHADAY, W.H., KIPNIS, D.M.: Regulation of immunoreactive growth hormone secretion in male rats. Endocrinology 88, 909-917 (1971)
TAKAHASHI, K., INONE, K., TAKAHASHI, Y.: Parallel shift in circadian rhythms of adrenocortical activity and food intake in blinded and intact rats exposed to continous illumination. Endocrinology 100, 1097-1107 (1977)
TIGNER, J.C., BARNES, R.H.: Effect of postnatal malnutrition of plasma corticosteroid levels in male albino rats. Proc. Soc. Exp. Biol. Med. 149, 80-82 (1975)

TRENKLE, A.: Effect of diet upon levels of plasma growth hormone in sheep. J. Anim. Sci. 32, 111-114 (1971a)
TRENKLE, A.: Postprandial changes in insulin secretion in sheep. J. Nutr. 101, 1099-1103 (1971b)
TRENKLE, A.: Hormonal and nutritional interrelationships and their affects on skeletal muscle. In: Protein Synthesis and Muscle Growth. Am. Soc. Animal Sci., 1974, pp. 1142-1149
TURNER, M.R.: Dietary effects on the secretion and actions of growth hormone. Proc. Nutr. Soc. 31, 205-213 (1972)
TURNER, M.R.: Protein deficiency, reproduction and hormonal factors in growth. Nutr. Rep. Int. 7, 289-308 (1973)
YOUNG, V.R., VILLAIRE, G., NEWBERNE, P.M., WILSON, R.B.: Plasma insulin and amino acid concentrations in rats given an adequate or low protein diet. J. Nutr. 103, 720-730 (1973)

3. Endocrine Responses to Malnutrition in Man

K. S. JAYA RAO

Protein-calorie malnutrition (PCM) continues to be one of the major nutritional and public health problems that confront the developing countries today. In view of the high nutrient demands of growth, children between 1 and 4 years of age, generally referred to as pre-school children, are most vulnerable to the ravages of malnutrition. The primary and the characteristic response to PCM is retardation of growth, the degree of which in any child depends on the extent of calorie and protein deficiency, its duration, the age of weaning, weaning practices, exposures to infections and their severity, etc. Hence PCM does not manifest itself as a single syndrome, but comprises a wide spectrum with varying degrees of retardation of growth. At the extreme end of this spectrum, the two clinically characteristic pictures of marasmus and kwashiorkor stand out as striking testimonies to a continuing human tragedy. Nearly 80%-90% of the pre-school children in India suffer from mild and moderate forms of malnutrition, whereas 2%-3% suffer from kwashiorkor and marasmus.

Apart from the clear-cut differences in their clinical picture, marasmus and kwashiorkor also exhibit striking differences in their biochemical profile. While the child with kwashiorkor exhibits gross alterations in various biochemical constituents of blood, in marasmus such alterations, if seen, are generally minimal (Table 1). These alterations, or the ability to resist them, cannot arise without preceding endocrine alterations.

Table 1. Salient biochemical differences between marasmus and kwashiorkor

	Marasmus	Kwashiorkor
Serum albumin	Almost normal	Low
Serum ligand-binding proteins	Normal	Low
Serum enzymes	Normal	Low
Serum urea	Normal	Low
Serum creatinine	Normal	Low
Serum amino acids	Normal	Low
Serum triglyceride	Normal	Low
Serum cholesterol	Normal	Low
Serum FFA	Raised	Raised
Blood glucose	Normal	Normal or Low
Glucose tolerance	Normal	Impaired

The question that remains unanswered is that of the manifestation of two clinically distinguishable syndromes in response to the same form of stress, namely calorie and protein deficiency. Various theories emphasizing differences in dietary pattern (BEHAR et al., 1958), weaning practices (MCLAREN, 1966) etc., have been proposed. GOPALAN (1968) speculated that the degree of adaptation to the stress of malnutrition may determine the clinical picture.

Hormones play an important role in adaptation processes, and SELYE (1952) assigned a central role to the adrenal cortex. Our hypothesis is that in response to the stress of restricted food intake, the adrenal cortex may secrete more cortisol. This catabolic hormone is known to stimulate breakdown of muscle protein, and amino acids so released will be taken up by organs with high protein turnover like the liver, pancreas and the intestinal tract (Fig. 1). Thus visceral integrity

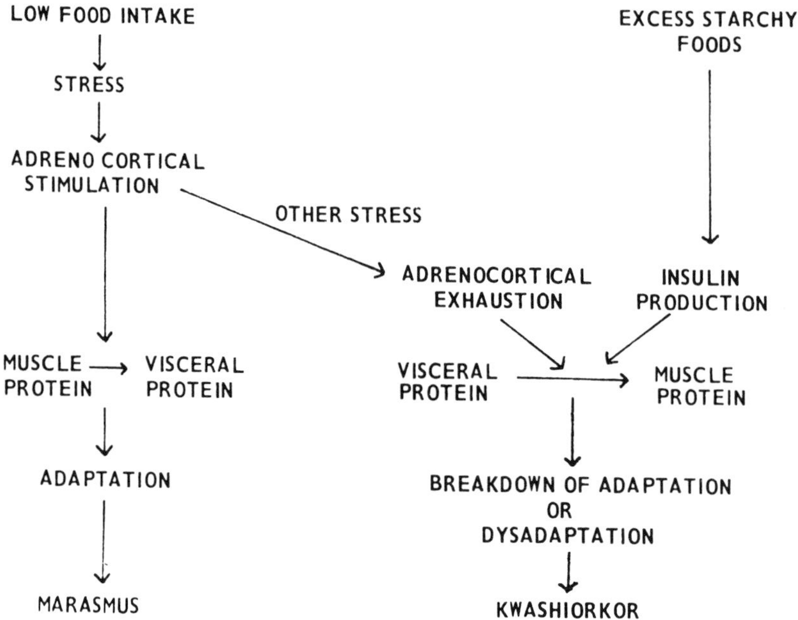

Fig. 1. Theory of adaptation to protein-calorie malnutrition and its breakdown

would be maintained at the expense of muscle, a picture characteristic of marasmus. The observations of WATERLOW (1968) that protein turnover rate is not altered in the liver, but is reduced in muscle, fits in well with this scheme. Should such a response of the adrenal cortex fail, inadequate diversion of amino acids to the liver could ultimately lead to development of kwashiorkor, reflecting the breakdown of the adaptation process. A nondiversion of amino acids from muscle to the viscera could also occur under the influence of insulin (MUNRO, 1964). In the following pages, I review salient data regarding alterations in certain endocrine secretions, and discuss how the adrenal cortex may play a crucial role in the response of the organism to PCM.

Plasma Cortisol

Plasma cortisol levels are elevated in children suffering both from kwashiorkor and marasmus (Table 2) but higher in the latter (JAYA RAO et al, 1968). The persistent high levels would indicate a breakdown of the normal adreno-hypophysial feedback relationship.

Table 2. Mean plasma cortisol levels in kwashiorkor (μg per 100 ml)

Reference	Normal	Kwashiorkor
ALLEYNE and YOUNG (1966)	13.1	29.1
ABBASSY et al. (1967)	11.7	24.1
JAYA RAO et al. (1968)	19.2	24.9
BEITINS et al. (1975)	13.5	18.3

The rise in plasma cortisol following corticotropin administration has also been found to be exaggerated in marasmus, but normal or sub-normal in kwashiorkor (JAYA RAO et al., 1968). This may be interpreted to indicate that adrenocortical activity is in fact high in marasmus, but may not be so in kwashiorkor. Similar differences in response to stimuli have also been observed with regard to blood glucose (JAYA RAO, 1965). The high basal levels of cortisol in kwashiorkor have been attributed to an impaired rate of catabolism of the hormone (ALLEYNE and YOUNG, 1967). These findings may then be interpreted to indicate that adrenocortical activity is high in marasmus, and that in kwashiorkor it is not increased to the same extent.

Thyroid Hormones

Circulating levels of thyroid hormones are low in kwashiorkor, but generally normal in marasmus (Table 3). Some workers have reported low

Table 3. Mean serum thyroxine levels in protein-calorie malnutrition (μg per 100 ml)

Reference	Normal	Kwashiorkor	Marasmus
BEAS et al.[a] (1966)	5.4	-	3.4
JAYA RAO and KHAN[a] (1974)	6.3	3.8	6.2
GRAHAM et al. (1973)	12.3	4.6	9.5

[a] Hormone measured as BEI or PBI.

levels even in marasmus, but it is pertinent to note that these reports are from countries known to be endemic areas of iodide deficiency. The low levels in kwashiorkor are not due to an impaired biosynthesis of the hormone, but due to decreased availability of binding proteins in plasma (GRAHAM et al., 1973; INGENBLEEK et al., 1974). This again is a reflection of the well-recognized fact that various proteins derived from the liver are reduced in kwashiorkor (GOPALAN, 1968).

Plasma Insulin

Reports on plasma insulin levels during fasting in kwashiorkor are conflicting. Some workers, including ourselves (JAYA RAO and RAGHURAMULU, 1972) have reported normal values, and others, low values (Table 4). Unlike in South-East Asia where the staple food is a cereal, in areas where low insulin levels have been recorded, the diet consists of mostly starchy tubers. The high carbohydrate content of such diets may lead to an initial, excess stimulation of the beta bells, followed by an exhaustion.

Table 4. Mean plasma insulin levels in kwashiorkor (μU/ml)

Reference	Normal	Kwashiorkor
MILNER (1971a)	16	9
JAYA RAO and RAGHURAMULU (1972)	4.2	2.8
PARRA et al. (1973)	5-7	5-10
ROBINSON et al. (1973)	4.5	2.7

The response of the hormone to stimuli such as glucose, given orally (JAYA RAO and RAGHURAMULU, 1972) or parenterally (ROBINSON et al., 1973), and to amino acids and glucagon (MILNER, 1971a) is impaired. Earlier in the discussion, a possible role of insulin in preventing mobilization of muscle amino acids to the viscera was suggested. The available data may be interpreted to indicate that the role of insulin in the adaptation process, if any, may be limited.

Plasma Growth Hormone

Earlier, it was believed that secretion of growth hormone may be impaired in PCM. This view arose from the reports of MONCKEBERG et al. (1964) that malnourished children respond well to nutritional therapy, when supplemented with injections of growth hormone. In fact, chronic undernutrition has been described as a state of pseudohypophysectomy (MULINOS and POMERANTZ, 1940). Later studies measuring the hormone in blood have shown unequivocally raised levels in kwashiorkor (Table 5). In contrast to the consensus on kwashiorkor, the opinions on marasmus

Table 5. Mean plasma growth hormone levels in protein-calorie malnutrition (ng per ml)

Reference	Normal	Kwashiorkor	Marasmus
PIMSTONE et al. (1968)	7.0	23.8	26.0
BEAS et al. (1971)	7.8	25.6	4.1
MILNER (1971b)	8.7	24.5	-
PARRA et al. (1973)	-	50-70	6-7
RAGHURAMULU and JAYA RAO (1974)	3.5	30.5	5.5

are conflicting. Many workers have reported normal or low levels (Table 5), but PIMSTONE et al. (1968) have reported increased levels.

The controversy regarding growth-hormone levels in marasmus can be resolved when the values are considered in relation to serum albumin levels of the children. The marasmic children studied by us had serum albumin levels of more than 2.0 g% and their plasma growth-hormone levels were not elevated (Fig. 2). Similar observations have been made by

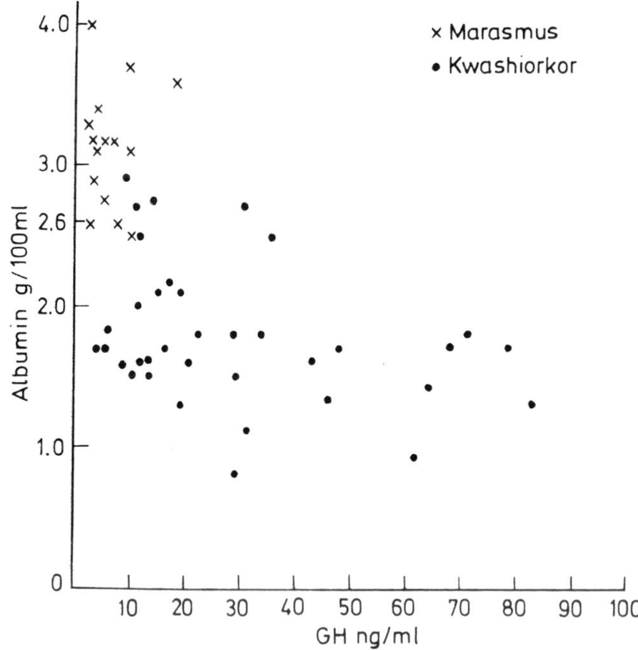

Fig. 2. Relationship between serum albumin and growth hormone levels in PCM

other workers (SAMUEL and DESHPANDE, 1972; LUNN et al., 1973), and a scrutiny of the data of PIMSTONE et al. (1968) also shows a similar trend. In kwashiorkor, serum albumin levels were generally less than 2.0 g%, and all the children had elevated levels of growth hormone (RAGHURAMULU and JAYA RAO, 1974).

The response of plasma growth hormone to various stimuli has been found to be adequate in kwashiorkor, but not in marasmus (BEAS et al., 1971; RAGHURAMULU and JAYA RAO, 1974). These findings may be interpreted that growth hormone secretion is increased in kwashiorkor, but not in marasmus.

The elevated growth hormone levels in kwashiorkor have been interpreted by WATERLOW and ALLEYNE (1971) as a part of an adaptive response to protein deficiency. On the other hand, PERLOFF et al. (1954) considered a decreased activity as an adaptive mechanism. In marasmus, despite the severe stunting of growth, the biochemical profile is essentially normal. The absence of elevation in growth hormone levels, and the failure to respond to a stimulus, seem more likely to be adaptive phenomena, leading to a preservation of metabolic integrity through mechanisms restricting growth.

Based on the above findings, an attempt has been made to integrate and interpret the gamut of changes observed in PCM (JAYA RAO, 1974) and to substantiate the postulate put forward by GOPALAN (1968) that marasmus is the end-result of adaptation to the stress of PCM, and kwashiorkor reflects a breakdown of such an adaptation process.

The Hypothesis

The elevated levels of plasma cortisol, and their exaggerated response to corticotropin in marasmus may be interpreted as an optimal response of the adrenal cortex to the stress of restricted food intake. Due to the catabolic activity of cortisol, muscle protein will be broken down, and plasma amino acids maintained in the normal range. The liver thus maintains adequate protein synthesis. The higher cortisol levels are probably instrumental in the failure of the pituitary to respond to stimuli (BLODGETT et al., 1956; PECILE and MÜLLER, 1966). Thus, physical growth is restricted, but metabolic integrity is maintained, and this may be construed as a state of extreme adaptation (Fig. 3).

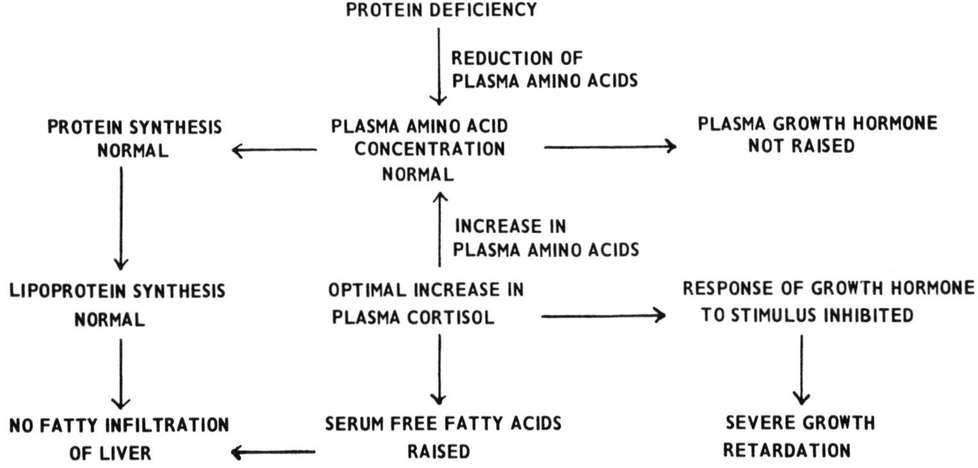

Fig. 3. Probable course of development of marasmus

The increase in plasma cortisol being inadequate in kwashiorkor, breakdown of muscle protein will be low, and this will explain the low plasma amino acids in this condition (EDOZIEN et al., 1960; JAYA RAO and RAGHURAMULU, 1972). This may operate as a feedback, stimulating the secretion of excess growth hormone. The evidence for this is the observation that oral infusion of amino acids can immediately lower growth hormone levels (MILNER, 1971b). Serum-free fatty acids are also high in kwashiorkor (LEWIS et al., 1964; JAYA RAO and PRASAD, 1966). The liver, however, fails to synthesize enough apolipoproteins, and consequently triglycerides are not released, leading to the characteristic fatty liver of kwashiorkor. Inadequate hepatic synthesis of proteins is also reflected in the low levels of serum albumin and other proteins. This may then lead to the host of other metabolic changes seen in these children (Fig. 4).

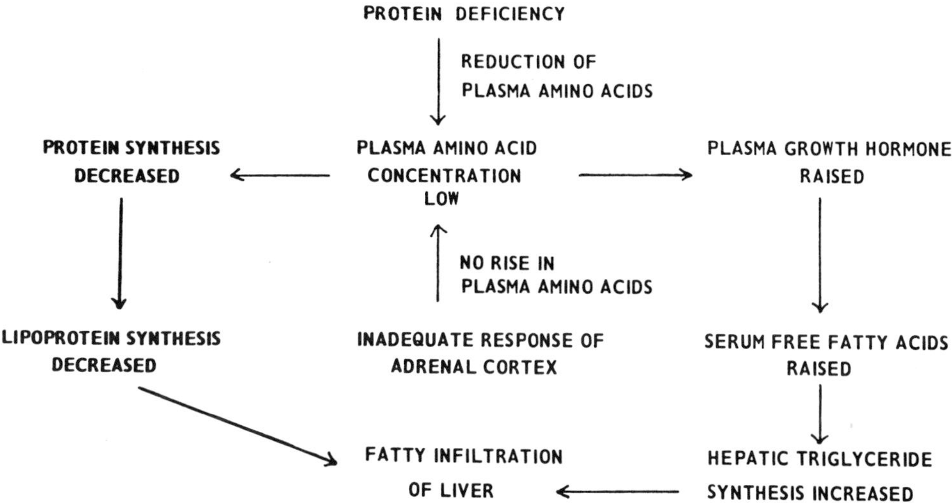

Fig. 4. Probable course of development of kwashiorkor

Conclusions

These studies thus show that the response of the adrenal cortex may be the crucial endocrine response to malnutrition, and is probably the primary event in the necessary adaptation of the growing organism to the stress of PCM. Such adaptation taken to an extreme end may result in marasmus. When the response fails to be maintained at a level necessary to meet the demands of the situation, metabolic homeostasis breaks down, leading to the development of kwashiorkor. These arguments have now received support from the studies of LUNN et al. (1976) that show that injections of cortisone into protein-deficient rats increase the serum albumin and hepatic-protein concentration and lower muscle-protein content.

A question that may legitimately be raised is whether the state of adaptation as represented by marasmus is necessarily of benefit to the organism. Adaptation, according to DU NOUY (1947), is not progressive, but protective and defensive. When perfect adaptation is attained, the organism makes no further attempt at transformation till the stress is removed. Adaptation is never a goal but a means, a means to survival. The immediate need of the organism is to develop resistance against the stress, and whether the ultimate result is of benefit to the species becomes inconsequential.

References

ABBASSY, A.S., MIKHAIL, M., ZEITOUN, M.M., RAGAB, M.: The suprarenal cortical function as measured by the plasma 17-hydroxysteroid level in malnourished children. J. Trop. Pediat. 13, 87-95 and 154-162 (1967)

ALLEYNE, G.A.O., YOUNG, V.H.: Adrenal function in malnutrition. Lancet 1, 911-912 (1966)

ALLEYNE, G.A.O., YOUNG, V.H.: Adrenocortical function in children with severe protein-calorie malnutrition. Clin. Sci. 33, 189-200 (1967)
BEAS, F., CONTRERAS, I., MACCIONI, A., ARENAS, S.: Growth hormone in infant malnutrition: the arginine test in marasmus and kwashiorkor. Brit. J. Nutr. 26, 169-175 (1971)
BEAS, F., MONCKEBERG, F., HORWITZ, I.: The response of the thyroid gland to thyroid-stimulating hormone (TSH) in infants with malnutrition. Pediatrics 38, 1003-1008 (1966)
BEHAR, M., VITERI, F., BRESSANI, R., ARROYAVE, G., SQUIBB, R.L., SCRIMSHAW, N.S.: Principles of treatment and prevention of severe protein malnutrition in children. Ann. N.Y. Acad. Sci. 69, 954-968 (1958)
BEITINS, I.Z., KOWARSKI, A., MIGEON, C.L., GRAHAM, G.G.: Adrenal function in normal infants and in marasmus and kwashiorkor. J. Pediat. 86, 302-308 (1975)
BLODGETT, F.M., BURGIN, L., IEZZONI, D., GRIBETZ, D., TALBOT, N.B.: Effects of prolonged cortisone therapy on the statural growth, skeletal maturation and metabolic status of children. New Engl. J. Med. 254, 636-641 (1956)
EDOZIEN, J.C., PHILLIPS, E.J., COLLIS, W.R.F.: The free amino acids of plasma and urine in Kwashiorkor. Lancet 1, 615-618 (1960)
GOPALAN, C.: Kwashiorkor and marasmus. Evolution and distinguishing features. In: Calorie Deficiencies and Protein Deficiencies. McCance, R.A., Widdowson, E.M. (eds.). London: J. & A. Churchill, 1968, pp. 49-58
GRAHAM, G.G., BAERTL, J.M., CLAEYSSEN, G., SUSKIND, R., GREENBERG, A.H., THOMPSON, R.G., BLIZZARD, R.M.: Thyroid hormonal studies in normal and severely malnourished infants and small children. J. Pediat. 83, 321-331 (1973)
INGENBLEEK, Y., DE NAYER, PH., DE VISSCHER, M.: Thyroxine binding globulin in infant protein-calorie malnutrition. J. Clin. Endocrinol. Metab. 39, 178-180 (1974)
JAYA RAO, K.S.: Kwashiorkor and marasmus. Blood sugar levels and response to epinephrine. Am. J. Dis. Chil. 519-522 (1965)
JAYA RAO, K.S.: Evolution of kwashiorkor and marasmus. Lancet 1, 709-711 (1974)
JAYA RAO, K.S., KHAN, L.: Basal energy metabolism in protein calorie malnutrition. Am. J. Clin. Nutr. 27, 892-896 (1974)
JAYA RAO, K.S., PRASAD, P.S.K.: Serum triglycerides and nonesterified fatty acids in kwashiorkor. Am. J. Clin. Nutr. 19, 205-209 (1966)
JAYA RAO, K.S., RAGHURAMULU, N.: Insulin secretion in kwashiorkor. J. Clin. Endocrinol. Metab. 35, 63-66 (1972)
JAYA RAO, K.S., SRIKANTIA, S.G., GOPALAN, C.: Plasma cortisol levels in protein-calorie malnutrition. Arch. Dis. Childh. 43, 365-367 (1968)
LEWIS, B., HANSEN, J.D.L., WITTMAN, W., KRUT, L.H., STEWART, F.: Plasma free fatty acids in kwashiorkor and the pathogenesis of the fatty liver. Am. J. Clin. Nutr. 15, 161-168 (1964)
LUNN, P.G., WHITEHEAD, R.G., BAKER, B.A., AUSTIN, S.: The effect of cortisone acetate on the course of development of experimental protein-energy malnutrition in rats. Brit. J. Nutr. 36, 537-550 (1976)
LUNN, P.G., WHITEHEAD, R.G., HAY, R.W., BAKER, B.A.: Progressive changes in serum cortisol, insulin and growth hormone concentrations and their relationship to the distorted amino acid pattern during the development of kwashiorkor. Brit. J. Nutr. 29, 399-422 (1973)
MCLAREN, D.S.: A fresh look at protein-calorie malnutrition. Lancet 1, 485-488 (1966)
MILNER, R.D.G.: Metabolic and hormonal responses to glucose and glucagon in patients with infantile malnutrition. Peadiat. Res. 5, 33-39 (1971a)
MILNER, R.D.G.: Metabolic and hormonal responses to oral amino acids in infantile malnutrition. Arch. Dis. Childh. 46, 301-305 (1971b)
MONCKEBERG, F., BEAS, F., HORWITH, I., DABANCENS, A., GONZALEZ, M.: Oxygen consumption in infant malnutrition. Pediatrics 33, 554-561 (1964)
MULINOS, M.G., POMERANTZ, L.: Pseudohypophysectomy. J. Nutr. 19, 493-504 (1940)
MUNRO, H.N.: General aspects of the regulation of protein metabolism by diet and by hormones. In: Mammalian Protein Metabolism. Vol. I. Munro, H.N., Allison, J.B. (eds.). New York-London: Academic Press, 1964, pp. 381-481
NOUY, L. DU: Human Destiny. London: Longmans, Green & Co., 1947
PARRA, A., GARZA, C., KLISH, W., GARCIA, G., ARGOTE, R.M., CANSECO, L., CUELLAR, A., NICHOLS, B.L.: Insulin-growth hormone adaptations in marasmus and kwashiorkor as seen in Mexico. In: Endocrine Aspects of Malnutrition. Gardner, L.I., Amacher, P. (eds.). Santa Ynez (Calif.): Kroc Foundation, 1973, pp. 31-43

PECILE, A., MULLER, E.: Suppressive action of corticosteroids on the secretion of growth hormone. J. Endocrinol. 36, 401-408 (1966)

PERLOFF, W.H., LASCHE, E.M., NODINE, J.H., SCHNEEBERG, N.G., VIEILLARD, C.B.: The starvation state and functional hypopituitarism. J. Am. Med. Assn. 155, 1307-1313 (1954)

PIMSTONE, B.L., BARBEZAT, G., HANSEN, J.D.L., MURRAY, P.: Studies on growth hormone secretion in protein-calorie malnutrition. Am. J. Clin. Nutr. 21, 482-487 (1968)

RAGHURAMULU, N., JAYA RAO, K.S.: Growth hormone secretion in protein-calorie malnutrition. J. Clin. Endocrinol. Metab. 38, 176-180 (1974)

ROBINSON, H., COCKS, T., KERR, D., PICOU, D.: Fasting and postprandial levels of plasma insulin and growth hormone in malnourished Jamaican children, during catch-up growth and after clinical recovery. In: Endocrine Aspects of Malnutrition. Gardner, L.I., AMACHER, P. (eds.). Santa Ynez (Calif.): Kroc Foundation, 1973, pp. 45-72

SAMUEL, A.M., DESHPANDE, U.R.: Growth hormone levels in protein-calorie malnutrition. J. Clin. Endocrinol. Metab. 35, 863-867 (1972)

SELYE, H.: The Story of the Adaptation Syndrome. Montreal, Canada: Acta Inc. Medical Publishers, 1952

WATERLOW, J.C.: Observations on the mechanism of adaptation to low protein intakes. Lancet 2, 1091-1097 (1968)

WATERLOW, J.C., ALLEYNE, G.A.O.: Protein malnutrition in children. Advances in knowledge in the last ten years. Adv. Prot. Chem. 25, 117-241 (1971)

Subject Index

E.B. Edney

Water Balance in Land Arthropods

1977. 109 figures, 36 tables. XII, 282 pages
(Zoophysiology and Ecology, Volume 9)
ISBN 3-540-08084-8

The book reviews knowledge about the various avenues for gain and loss of water by land arthropods, the internal and external factors that determine the rate and extent of such water movements, and the means of control either by adaptations resulting from evolutionary changes, or by relatively short-term, reversible, physiological mechanisms. Regulation of body temperature is dealt with insofar as this involves water economy. Where appropriate, these subjects are related to the various environments in which the animals referred to normally live. Areas in which research is likely to be active are indicated. There is now a need to integrate all the components of water balance with reference to whole animals operating in real environments. To achieve this, cooperation between physiologists and ecologists is necessary.

Contents: Introduction. – Water content. – Water loss – cuticular. – Water loss – respiratory. – Water loss by evaporative cooling. – Excretion and osmoregulation. – Uptake of liquid water. – Metabolic water. – Absorption of water vapour. – Water balance in eggs. – Conclusions. – Subject Index.

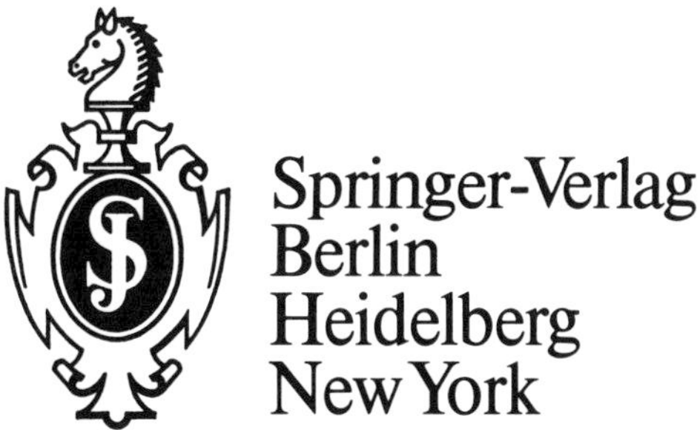

H.-U. Thiele

Carabid Beetles in Their Environments

A Study on Habitat Selection by Adaptations in Physiology and Behaviour
Translated from the German by J. Wieser

1977. 152 figures, 58 tables. XVII, 369 pages
(Zoophysiology and Ecology, Volume 10)
ISBN 3-540-08306-5

Why do organisms live where they live? In many cases there is no morphological explanation of the different ecological distribution of related species. Perhaps it is to be sought in individual physiological requirements or in behavioral differences. There seems to be justification for the use of ground beetles (Carabidae) in investigating these questions: only a few insect families can equal or exceed in numbers the 40.000 species of carabids (more than 4% of all insect species). Comprising a single family, they exhibit a relatively high degree of uniformity in morphological structure, and are thus especially suitable for studying the ecophysiological adaptations by which they cope with the demands of the environment to which they are exposed, and which are responsible for their having become so successful as a group, penetrating, despite a simple structure, environments all over the world.

Contents: Variations in the Body Structure of Carabids in Adaptation to Environment and Mode of Life. – Quantitative Investigations on the Distribution of Carabids. – The Connections Between Carabids and Biotic Factors in the Ecosystem. – Man and the Ground Beetles. – The Differences in Distribution of Carabids in the Environment: Reactions to Abiotic Factors and Their Significance in Habitat Affinity. – Ecological Aspects of Activity Patterns in Carabids. – Choice of Habitat. – The Influence of Connections Between Demands upon Environmental Factors and Activity Rhythms. – Dispersal and Dispersal Power of Carabid Beetles. – Ecological Aspects of the Evolution of Carabids. – Concerning the Reasons Underlying Species Profusion Manifest by the Carabids.

P. Dustin

Microtubules

1978. 177 figures. XIV, 451 pages
ISBN 3-540-08622-6

This book surveys the field of microtubule research and provides a detailed analysis of the large amount of literature on the subject. The fact that the author has followed this work closely over several decades puts this study in its proper perspective. None of the several recent conferences on aspects of microtubule activity have attempted to embrace all aspects of the problem: the 1975 Conference of the New York Academy of Sciences did not study ciliary motion, the more recent conference held at Cold Spring Harbor in 1976 was mainly devoted to cell motility rather than the static functions of microtubules.

The literature covered is vast, and although about 2000 references are mentioned in the text, this is only a small fraction of the total number of papers on microtubules, published mainly since 1964. It is hoped that, by covering in one monograph, the functions of microtubules in fields as different as secretion, neuroplasmic transport, cell shape, cell movement, and mitosis, and the many recent data on the biochemistry and physiology of the tubulins and their assembly into microtubules, the general properties of microtubules and their functions will be clarified, and may be used as a reference source for future work.

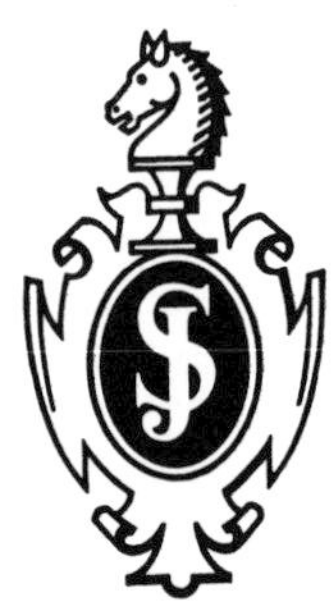

Contents: Historical Background. – Structure and Chemistry of Microtubules. – General Physiology of Tubulins and Microtubules. – Microtubule Structures: Centrioles, Basal Bodies, Cilia, Axonemes. – Microtubule Poisons. – Cell Shape. – Cell Movement. – Secretion, Exo- and Endocytosis. – Neurotubules: Neuroplasmic Transport, Neurosecretion, Sensory Cells. – The Role of MT in Mitosis. – Pathology and Medicine. – Outlook.

Springer-Verlag
Berlin
Heidelberg
New York